PHARMACOLOGY - RESEARCH, SAFETY TESTING AND REGULATION

ACE INHIBITORS

MEDICAL USES, MECHANISMS OF ACTION, POTENTIAL ADVERSE EFFECTS AND RELATED TOPICS

VOLUME 2

PHARMACOLOGY - RESEARCH, SAFETY TESTING AND REGULATION

Additional books in this series can be found on Nova's website
under the Series tab.

Additional e-books in this series can be found on Nova's website
under the e-book tab.

PHARMACOLOGY - RESEARCH, SAFETY TESTING AND REGULATION

ACE INHIBITORS

MEDICAL USES, MECHANISMS OF ACTION, POTENTIAL ADVERSE EFFECTS AND RELATED TOPICS

VOLUME 2

MACAULAY AMECHI ONUIGBO
EDITOR

NOVA BIOMEDICAL

New York

Library of Congress Cataloging-in-Publication Data

Library of Congress Control Number: 2013954142

ISBN: 978-1-62948-422-8

Published by Nova Science Publishers, Inc. † New York

CONTENTS

SPECIAL PREVIEW

Zbylut J. Twardowski* MD PhD FACP
Division of Nephrology, Department of Medicine, University of Missouri,
Columbia, MO, US

The book you have in your hands has been conceived and created by Macaulay A. Onuigbo, MD MSc FWACP FASN MBA, Associate Professor of Medicine, College of Medicine, Mayo Clinic, Rochester, MN; Former Regional Director, North Eastern Region, Mayo Health System Practice-Based Research Network (MHS PBRN); Nephrologist/Hypertension Specialist/Transplant Physician, Department of Nephrology, Mayo Clinic Health System Eau Claire, 1221 Whipple Street, Eau Claire, WI 54702, USA, and MBA Executive, Eau Claire, WI, USA.

Dr. Onuigbo received his medical degree from the University of Nigeria in 1981. His post-graduate studies took him to Enugu, Nigeria, Birmingham, United Kingdom, Houston, Texas, and Baltimore, Maryland. He is Double Board Certified in the United States of America in Internal Medicine and Nephrology, with the American Board of Internal Medicine. He had earlier served as an Associate Professor of Medicine/Senior Lecturer, Department of Medicine, College of Medicine, University of Nigeria, Enugu Campus, Nigeria, March 1990 – June 1994. He is a Nephrologist/Transplant Physician/Hypertension Specialist, Mayo Clinic Health System, Eau Claire, WI, USA, September 2002 - 2013. He is an Associate Professor of Medicine, College of Medicine, Mayo Clinic, Rochester, MN, USA since 2010 and has served as Vice Chairman, Department of Nephrology, Mayo Clinic Health System, Eau Claire, WI, USA. He is a Fellow of the West African College of Physicians (FWACP – Nephrology), a Fellow of the American Society of Nephrology (FASN), and a former Regional Director, North-Eastern Region of the Mayo Health System Practice-Based Research Network. Dr. Onuigbo's recent professional awards include the Mayo Clinic MacMillan Scholar Award (2009-2011) and the Mayo SOAR Research Grant Award in 2011. He has over 100 publications including several book chapters and books. In 2013, he co-edited a major textbook on hemodialysis titled "Hemodialysis, When, How, Why" with Claudio Ronco MD, Biagio Raffaele Di Iorio MD PhD and August Heidland MD. Dr. Onuigbo described the following previously unreported syndromes - late onset renal failure

* E-mail: twardowskiz@health.missouri.edu.

from angiotensin blockade (LORFFAB) in 2005, the syndrome of rapid onset end stage renal disease (SORO-ESRD) in 2010, and introduced the terms "Ethicomedicinomics" and "Cognitive Drift in the EMR" into current medical literature in 2012. He introduced the concept of "Quadruple Whammy" in the Spring of 2013, a publication in the British Medical Journal. He has a Master of Science (MSc) degree in Medical Biochemistry from the University of Nigeria (1988). He recently completed an MBA (Healthcare) in May 2012 from the University of Wisconsin Consortium and was named the 2012 University of Wisconsin MBA Consortium Outstanding Graduate.

Dr. Onuigbo's research interest encompasses a vast area of nephrology and hypertension that include: chronic kidney disease, acute kidney injury, end-stage renal disease, renoprotection, end-of-life care, non-dialytic therapy of end-stage renal disease, healthcare cost management, and "ethicomedicinomics". One of his major interests is the role of angiotensin converting enzyme inhibitors and angiotensin receptor blockers in renoprotection. This may be the major reason that he conceived and created this book.

Dr Onuigbo is one of the most industrious researchers and practitioners in the field of nephrology. He submitted eleven abstracts for the 33rd Annual Dialysis Conference held in Seattle, WA, USA, in March 2013. The abstracts were reviewed blindly and all were accepted for presentations. The Organizing Committee of the 33rd Annual Dialysis Conference was amazed when it was found that all these abstracts were submitted by one person, Dr. Onuigbo. His sedulousness was the major reason that he was able to accomplish publication of this book. He selected topics, authors from all over the world, solicited authors and helped them to finish their tasks, and contributed 9 chapters to this book. The book consists of 36 chapters in 8 sections, most on angiotensin and it role in nephrology and hypertension. Dr. Onuigbo is also interested in appropriate approach to the treatment of patients which is dependent on individualization of medical care. During the 33rd Annual Dialysis Conference in Seattle, where he presented his eleven abstracts, he was able to participate in discussions in several other sessions. He also participated in a discussion after the debate on the value of randomized controlled trials in dialysis research. He liked our emphasis on the individualization of medical care and asked us to contribute a chapter to his book. Several other chapters, including 4, and 22, address also this problem.

FOREWORD

Richard J. Glassock, MD MACP
Emeritus Professor of Medicine
Geffen School of Medicine at UCLA
Los Angeles, CA

The elaboration of the renin-angiotensin system (RAS), beginning more than a half-century ago, is one of the most compelling stories of all human biology. This system is now regarded as playing pivotal roles in such phenomena as blood pressure regulation, body fluid homeostasis, aldosterone syntheisis, glomerular filtration and permeability, fibrosis, inflammation, cardiac hypertrophy, neural activity and aging, to name a few. Soon after discovery of the RAS, pharmacologic agents capable of inhibiting the crucial enzyme for conversion of Angiotensin I to Angiotensin II were developed; first, S*aralasin*, an intravenous preparation in 1974, and a few years later, *Captopril*, an oral preparation, in 1978. Inhibitors of the receptor for Angiotensin II were developed later. These agents quickly came into wide use for management of hypertension and cardiac failure. Experimental studies clearly demonstrated their efficacy in altering progression of chronic kidney disease, perhaps by modifying intra-glomerular hypertension and proteinuria. In a seminal observation two decades ago, *Captopril* was demonstrated to modify the course of nephropathy in Type 1 diabetes mellitus; this setting the stage for numerous intervention trials in chronic kidney disease, both of diabetic and non-diabetic origin. Today, use of agents antagonizing the RAS is widespread and investigation into the details of the mechanisms of action of RAS inhibition in chronic kidney and cardiovascular disease continue unabated.

Thus, a volume bringing together authors with a variety of interests related to the RAS, most specifically angiotensin converting enzyme (ACE) inhibitors, is both timely and valuable. This collection of essays, original papers, reviews and editorial opinions, skillfully chosen and edited by Dr. Macaulay Onuigbo, provides a glimpse of this very dynamic and constantly evolving field. Considerable emphasis has been given to the utility of these agents for interruption of the relentless progression of chronic kidney disease ("reno-protection"), but aspects concerning clinical use of RAS inhibition in general and cardiovascular medicine, during renal replacement therapy, in renal arterial stenosis, intensive care, sickle cell disease, HIV nephropathy and other diseases has not been ignored. A unique aspect of the volume is the description of use of RAS inhibition in defined populations, such as in Western Africa, the Caribbean, Spain, United Kingdom and South America. Appropriately, basic studies of pathophysiology have received attention. Unlike many contemporary reviews, this volume spends significant effort in describing and explaining the adverse event profile of RAS inhibition, particularly in the elderly and in subjects with chronic kidney disease. Throughout this comprehensive collection of well-written papers, a theme of critical analysis of conventional wisdom pervades; providing new insights into highly clinically relevant issues and some speculation as to the future of these agents, in combination with other active drugs, to safely and effectively ameliorate the consequences of chronic kidney disease. The reader of this volume will not be disappointed - there is much enlightenment provided and much to ponder concerning the future of inhibition of the RAS in human disease.

PREFACE

This is the most authoritative reference collection of expert-contributed related articles ever put together on ACE inhibition. Top experts in the various fields of nephrology, hypertension, cardiovascular medicine, pharmacotherapeutics and related fields from around the world, drawn from all five continents, have contributed essays, original papers, reviews and editorial opinions in this book which appears in two volumes, Volume 1 and Volume 2, respectively.

This volume represents the most comprehensive and up-to-date collection of current literature on angiotensin inhibition and related topics, in medicine, nephrology and cardiovascular medicine ever put together. This book has turned out to become the most authoritative reference source on ACEIs, contributed to by leading experts in their various fields of medicine, from the USA, Europe including the United Kingdom, South America, Australia-New Zealand, Asia including Japan, and Africa.

Some of the chapters have reference sources cited from the current relevant literature in excess of over 100 references. This volume should indeed serve as a major literature resource for physicians in general, internists, researchers, cardiologists and hypertension specialists and more especially practitioners of the art of nephrology in all the countries of the world. Medical students and the various physicians' training programs should reach for a copy of this volume as a research and teaching tool for so many years to come. There is also a place here for research scientists in the pharmaceutical industry to review current and new emerging indications for angiotensin inhibition and the future of reno-protection.

Critically vital clinical topics covered in this book by top world-renowned experts in the different subspecialties include classic topics such as the efficacy of ACE inhibition as antihypertensives among the various ethnicities and races, as written from an American, an African, a Caribbean and a European perspectives, the use of ACE inhibition in the renal transplant recipient, ACE inhibition in heart failure, ACE inhibition in the pediatrics population, and ACE inhibition in the patient with renal artery stenosis. New emerging topics covered include the role of ACE inhibition in the ICU, ACE inhibition in cardiorenal syndrome, ACE inhibition in the hemodialysis patient and in the peritoneal dialysis patient, ACE inhibition in sickle cell disease, and ACE inhibition as it relates to chronotherapy in hypertension management. New developments covered here on angiotensin inhibition include angiotensin receptor blockade in HIV nephropathy, and angiotensin inhibition directed at arterial stiffness and endothelial dysfunction. Basic research topics on ACE inhibition covered in this book include an analysis of the antioxidant and cardioprotective activity of

Zofenopril, the pharmacotherapeutic mimicry between ACE inhibition and MMP-9 inhibition, ACE inhibitory peptides derived from Cowpea (Vigna unguiculata), and a histochemical examination of ACE inhibition in rat cardiac microvessels. Related and very exciting new topics covered in this book include the new concept of hypertension-misattributed kidney disease and ACE inhibition, the various presentations of AKI on CKD complicating concurrent angiotensin inhibition as it is related to the newly described syndrome of late onset renal failure from angiotensin blockade (LORFFAB) and the other newly described syndrome of rapid onset end stage renal disease (SORO-ESRD), the yet newly described syndrome of "quadruple whammy" as it relates to post-operative AKI in CKD patients on "triple whammy" medications, and a critical review of the pitfalls of randomized controlled trials in the current nephrology literature with a chapter dealing with the vexed question of the overuse and abuse of composite renal surrogates as measures of renal outcomes in the current (nephrology) literature as critically re-examined in the ALTITUDE, RENAAL, IDNT, EVOLVE and TEMPO trials.

VOLUME 1

In the first introductory chapter of this book, Onuigbo and Achebe, writing from Mayo Clinic College of Medicine, Rochester, MN, USA, and Mayo Clinic Health System, Eau Claire, WI, USA, have narrated a historical review of the introduction of angiotensin inhibition as typified by ACE inhibitors and ARBs in clinical medicine. This chapter includes a brief review of the physiology and biochemistry of the angiotensins and the various clinical uses and indications of these drug classes since their full introduction into clinical medicine in the early 1990s as a result of the pioneering work of Squibb Laboratory scientists started as far back as 1971.

Emeritus Professor Twardowski and Misra, writing from the University of Missouri, Columbia, MO, USA, did an excellent job of reviewing the drawbacks of randomized controlled trials (RCTs) especially as applied to nephrology in general, and renal replacement therapy, in particular. They very astutely, brilliantly and dispassionately, have called for caution in the interpretation of results of RCTs, bearing in mind several potential areas for errors, be it type I, II, III and IV errors, etc [Twardowski & Misra, 2013]. They also addressed the very critical but often neglected paradigm of the need to at least attempt to distinguish between statistical significance and clinical significance. The misuse of renal surrogate end-points in RCTs was referred to, a topic that is more fully addressed in another chapter of this book. Finally, these two eminent professors of the art of nephrology called for the need for nephrologists in particular, and physicians in general, to never forget the need to individualize medical care, one patient at a time – this is a mantra that we have continuously called for in many of our CKD publications. This very elaborately put together and expansive chapter on the foibles of the RCTs with special emphasis on the nephrology literature by Twadowski and Misra is a one that you start to read and you don't want to put down.

Onuigbo, from Mayo Clinic College of Medicine, Rochester, MN, USA, and Mayo Clinic Health System, Eau Claire, WI, USA, in the third chapter of this book has expanded on a recent letter to the Editor, New England Journal of Medicine, published in the Spring of 2013, to draw attention to the potential albeit unintended consequences and negative implications and connotations of the overuse and abuse of the use of renal surrogate endpoints in the nephrology literature. The NEJM letter was addressed specifically to the recently reported findings from the Aliskiren Trial in Type 2 Diabetes Using Cardiorenal Endpoints (ALTITUDE) Trial. In this commentary, similar concerns were raised with regards to several other published trials in recent nephrology literature. This chapter details the problems inherent with the use of combination renal surrogate endpoints in statistical analysis as if these represented independent endpoints. Such approaches threaten the internal validity of such statistical analysis and create the phenomena of ecologic fallacy and Simpson's Paradox. The resulting likelihood of false and potentially overrated reported trial outcomes remains major concerns among critical thinkers in this field of medicine and nephrology. We submit that such approaches are dangerous, possibly academically immoral and indefensible, and may arguably be tantamount to albeit unintended deception. We recommend that the reading physician audience must interpret the reported outcomes in such trials with a lot more caution and watchfulness.

Onuigbo et al, from Mayo Clinic College of Medicine, Rochester, MN, USA, and Mayo Clinic Health System, Eau Claire, WI, USA, brought together various concepts in medicine, nephrology, the management sciences and engineering in a novel chapter that attempts to address the CKD enigma as it relates to our limited knowledge of the natural history of CKD, the vagaries of the so-called 'CKD-ESRD-Death trilogy', the existence and interplay of asymmetric information in medical practice in general and in nephrology in particular, and the role of 'Ethicomedicinomics' in present day healthcare interactions. We then introduced the new IT Software program, "The CKD Express©", which we developed in 2010, and that is currently in US Patent application. It is our strong belief that when patented, the new "The CKD Express©" IT Software Program will help attenuate these current disparities in CKD care both here in the USA and around the world, with the enhanced ability to improve easier and convenient CKD care access, improve CKD outcomes, advance our current knowledge of the natural history of CKD, while reducing healthcare costs and eliminating waste, at the same time as achieving all these deliverables Finally, it remains our hope that meritoriously, and from a pragmatic point of view, that Medicare should become very interested in the deployment of this new "The CKD Express©" IT Software Program.

Fournier, writing from Laboratoire de Pharmacologie Médicale et Clinique, Toulouse, France. France produced the piece on "triple whammy". This review could not have come from a more apt source. Fournier has produced a concise masterpiece of results of several years of hard detective and epidemiological work on pharmacovigilance and the potential for iatrogenic renal injury from administered medications in clinical practice, with special reference to NSAIDs, diuretics and angiotensin inhibition, or "triple whammy". In this chapter, Fournier first described how the concept of Triple Whammy was coined and evaluated in observational studies in the early 2000s by Thomas, Boyd and Loboz. Then he examined the historical evolution of the epidemiology of this phenomenon in medical practices and ends with a description of how pharmacovigilance and pharmocoepidemiology have recently identified the "triple hhammy" phenomenon both in France and in the United Kingdom. Lastly, Fournier demonstrated how laboratory monitoring of serum creatinine was insufficiently performed to prevent the "triple whammy" effect. As a spin off from "triple whammy", the next chapter describes a new related syndrome of "quadruple whammy", first described in the British Medical Journal in the Spring of 2013 by Onuigbo [Onuigbo 2013].

Onuigbo et al, from Mayo Clinic College of Medicine, Rochester, MN, USA, and Mayo Clinic Health System, Eau Claire, WI, USA, reported on the newly described syndrome of 'Quadruple Whammy'. This new syndrome describes preventable AKI on CKD in CKD patients on triple whammy medications (diuretics, angiotensin inhibition, and NSAIDs) in the post-operative setting. This new syndrome was first described by Onuigbo & Onuigbo in the British Medical Journal in the Spring of 2013. We had therefore coined the new term 'Quadruple Whammy' to describe this new syndrome of preventable AKI on CKD in patients on 'triple whammy' resulting from the superimposition of peri-operative stressors especially hypotension in a patient with a priori stable CKD on triple whammy medications following a surgical intervention. We presented these two cases here, in much greater detail and profile, and once again have revisited the need for enhanced pharmacovigilance to reduce iatrogenic renal failure from prescription and over-the-counter medications. This chapter dovetailed from the preceding chapter by Fournier on 'triple whammy'. Knowledge regarding this new syndrome is expected to evolve over the coming years and will soon prove the validity of it occupying its merited place in the annals of a great nephrology reference text such as this one. Besides, we have demonstrated that the preemptive discontinuation of potential nephrotoxic agents such as ACEIs before major surgical procedures together with aggressive measures to prevent or rapidly correct peri-operative hypotension, a protocolized paradigm that we dubbed renoprevention, leads to less AKI, better renal salvage, reduced inpatient morbidity, reduced length of stays and huge dollar savings.

Onuigbo and Achebe, in yet another chapter, writing from Mayo Clinic, Rochester, MN, USA, and Mayo Clinic Health System, Eau Claire, WI, USA, have given an extended and elaborate account of the historical discovery and development of the concept of late onset renal failure from angiotensin blockade (LORFFAB), first reported in 2005 by Onuigbo & Onuigbo. This is the accelerated but potentially reversible iatrogenic renal failure from angiotensin blockade, that occurs in usually older CKD patients, despite normal renal arteries, absent traditionally acknowledged precipitating risk factors, and while remaining on the same dose of angiotenisn blockade for >3 months. In this chapter, we described the various criteria for the definition of this syndrome, and presented data from our 68-month prospective cohort analysis that was completed in May of 2008. We end the chapter by once again calling attention to the need for providers to show more awareness for preventative nephrology as applied in the principles of reno-prevention, a concept that we first reported in 2009. The need to practice reno-prevention, the pre-emptive withholding of potentially nephrotoxic agents including ACEIs and ARBs, in those clinical settings that predispose to AKI aggravation such as during critical illness, in the peri-operative period, and with iodinated contrast exposure, cannot be overemphasized.

Onuigbo, from Mayo Clinic College of Medicine, Rochester, MN, USA, and Mayo Clinic Health System, Eau Claire, WI, USA, described the potential variable renal outcomes in AKI-on-CKD, ranging from complete recovery, partial recovery and immediate, acute yet irreversible renal failure, synonymous with the syndrome of rapid onset renal failure from angiotensin blockade, first described by Onuigbo in 2010, in the journal *Renal Failure*. Undeniably, the variable renal outcomes that could follow AKI on CKD events could indeed best be described as the several colors of the rainbow. Finally, we must all recognize that except for the institution of RRT, so far modern medicine is yet to device a cure for AKI. Unquestionably, at least for now, no specific pharmacologic therapy is effective in patients with established AKI, and the care of such patients is limited to supportive care, and renal-replacement therapy when otherwise indicated. Prevention, and we dare say, reno-prevention, indisputably, is therefore better than cure. We must acknowledge that the impact of AKI on CKD-ESRD progression and pathogenesis remains fertile grounds for ground-breaking research in the 21st century.

Onuigbo et al, writing from Mayo Clinic College of Medicine, Rochester, MN, USA, and Mayo Clinic Health System, Eau Claire, WI, USA, describe in detail, the experience at four Mayo Clinic Dialysis Units of the newly described syndrome of rapid onset end stage renal disease or SORO-ESRD, which was first described by Onuigbo in 2010. The incidence of SORO-ESRD in the last 100 consecutive incident Northwestern Wisconsin Mayo Clinic chronic hemodialysis patients, 2010-2011, was detailed out as retrospective analysis. The description of SORO-ESRD as contrasted with the so-called classic ESRD, and the analogy with cold frozen Chicago in March versus warm green and sunny Seattle, WA, in March, a scenario of a tale of two different cities, made for a superlative read. In another vein, the analogy drawn between classic ESRD as all know it versus the newly described syndrome of SORO-ESRD with the smooth cadence of a modern airliner making a planned and calibrated descent and landing from 30,000 feet over 15-30 minutes versus an emergency landing by the same modern airliner, again from 30,000 feet to the ground literally over a few minutes, could not have been more apt. Furthermore, the incrimination of older age or renal senescence and concurrent exposure to potentially nephrotoxic agents including ACEIs and ARBs, with the pathogenesis of SORO-ESRD demands serious circumspection and further study. This may imply the mandate for a more heightened awareness among providers of the propensity of older CKD patients to have poorer renal outcomes with certain nephrotoxic exposures including angiotensin inhibition. Finally, we most emphatically will submit that it is ethically unconscionable, in 2012, for any practicing nephrologist or physician for that matter, to refuse to acknowledge the implications of SORO-ESRD in contemporary nephrology and dialysis practice, after all. Doing so, in our opinion, is tantamount to potentially doing harm to our patients.

In a related chapter, Onuigbo, writing from Mayo Clinic College of Medicine, Rochester, MN, USA, and Mayo Clinic Health System, Eau Claire, WI, USA, has further narrated a simulated debate titled "Geriatric Nephrology Debate: Angiotensin Inhibition Should be Withdrawn In Older Adults with Later Stage CKD – A 2013 Mayo Clinic Health System Nephrologist's Perspective and The Unmet Need For Newer Kidney-Friendly Renoprotective Agents For the 21st Century". This represented a formal extension of a similar debate stance in which the author participated in, under the auspices of the Geriatric Nephrology Advisory Group of the American Society of Nephrology (ASN), under the chairmanship of Emeritus Professor Richard Glassock at the 2012 ASN Renal Week activities held in San Diego, CA, USA in October-November 2012. Professor Robert Toto, of the University of Texas Southwestern Medical Center debated a 'pro' position to continue angiotensin inhibition in the older adult with stage IV CKD, whereas Onuigbo debated the 'con' position, recommending the withdrawal of angiotensin inhibition. In this chapter, several case presentations from the Clinic were described that demonstrate clearly, a cause-effect association between concurrent angiotensin inhibition and sometimes reversible AKI-on-CKD, more so in the older adult (>65 years old) with later stage (>III) CKD. Recent reports in the literature showing such reversal of AKI following withdrawal of angiotensin inhibition were also highlighted.

Evangelista, writing from Menarini Ricerche spa, Via Sette Santi 1, 50131 Firenze, Italy describes the peculiar characteristics of zofenopril, an inhibitor of angiotensin converting enzyme (ACE), characterized by a thiolic function which acts as the zinc ligand for the enzyme catalytic site, with high lipophilicity as one of its main characteristics. This enhanced lipophilicity determines various biological properties, such as oral absorption, an appreciable degree of biliary excretion and, probably more importantly, an enhanced tissue penetration. Moreover, zofenopril, like captopril, but unlike other ACE inhibitors, contains a sulfhydryl moiety, which is capable of scavenging oxygen free radicals. This property is likely to determine some pharmacological properties of zofenopril that are not shared with many other ACEIs. These properties include an increase in coronary blood flow, reversal of nitrates tolerance, in vitro and in vivo anti-ischemic effects, and enhanced left ventricular relaxation. Thus, zofenopril demonstrates a marked cardio-protective activity on both functional and biochemical parameters. There is also experimental evidence of important protective effects on the endothelium (e.g. reduction of endothelin-1 release, reduction of LDL oxidating capacity, reduction of intracellular formation of reactive oxygen species and superoxide anions). The conclusion is that zofenopril may thus be considered as the ACEI with one of the most potent activities of tissue inhibition at the cardiac and vascular levels of the renin-angiotensin system, and of local generation of reactive oxygen species and consequently excellent capacities for controlling hypertension and exerting cardio- and endothelium-protection.

Yamamoto et al, from Biomedical Computation Center, Osaka Medical College, 2-7 Daigakuchou, Takatuski, Osaka 569-8686, Japan, discuss the molecular mechanism and pharmacological implications of MMP-9 inhibition by ACE inhibitors, including an overview of the biochemical implications of MMP-9 molecular structure. MMP-9 levels are known to increase after myocardial infarction in humans and animal models, and cardiac dysfunction and mortality after myocardial infarction are suppressed by MMP-9 inhibitors and in MMP-9 null mice. In addition, recent reports that ACE inhibitors inhibit MMP-9 in an in vitro assay system and in infarcted left ventricles have led the authors to postulate direct interactions between ACE inhibitors and MMP-9.

Koyama of Hokkaido University, Sapporo, Japan, reviewed the experimental evidence supporting the class-specific effects of ACEIs and ARBs on the cardiac myocyte microvessels. The administration of ACEIs and ARBs reduced the cross sectional area of cardiomyocytes and capillary domain areas, and ACE inhibition resulted in a decrease in the blood pressure with a concomitant reduction in the cardiac myocyte capillary domain area. These results suggest the advantageous effects of ACE inhibition and angiotensin receptor blockade to help recover the biological balance between oxygen supply and consumption in the cardiac myocyte. The available data from the above experimental data on the cardiac myocyte microvessels support the view that ACEIs and ARBs possess an additional advantage over other drug classes in the management of hypertension, as they appear to offer additional class-specific cardioprotective effects, independent of blood pressure lowering.

Betancur-Ancona, writing from Campus de Ingenierías y Ciencias Exactas, Universidad Autónoma de Yucatán, 97203 Mérida, Yucatán, México, described ACE inhibitory peptides that were released by enzymatic proteolysis of the cowpea, Vigna unguiculata. The resulting peptides, purified by HPLC, showed strong affinity toward ACE, inhibited the enzyme in a competitive manner, and the presence of hydrophobic residues seemed to play an important role in its inhibitory activity. Although less potent than synthetic ones, they did not exhibit known side effects of ACE inhibitors. Efforts to develop safer, effective and economical ACE inhibitors are necessary for the prevention and remedy of hypertension and the present study as reported in this chapter represents the beginning of the development of nutraceuticals with physiological functions against ailments such as hypertension.

Shahin from Hull York Medical School and University of Hull, Hull, UK, examined the effect of Angiotensin Converting Enzyme Inhibitors on Arterial Stiffness and Endothelial Dysfunction. This chapter examined carotid-femoral pulse wave velocity index as the gold standard for the measurement of arterial stiffness. The other vascular index assessed in this chapter as a measure of arterial stiffness was the augmentation index, a ratio calculated from the blood pressure waveform as augmentation pressure divided by pulse pressure. The conclusion from an extensive review of the relevant literature was that in terms of arterial stiffness, ACE Inhibitors reduce PWV and augmentation index which are markers of arterial stiffness in patients with different pathological conditions. However, due to the lack of high quality and properly powered randomized controlled trials, it is not clear whether ACE Inhibitors are superior to other antihypertensive agents in their effect on arterial stiffness. Regarding endothelial dysfunction, ACE Inhibitors improve brachial FMD which is a marker of endothelial function and are superior to calcium channel blockers (CCBs) and β-blockers.

VOLUME 2

Hermida et al, writing from Bioengineering & Chronobiology Laboratories, University of Vigo, Campus Universitario, Vigo, Spain, observed that correlation between BP level and target organ damage, cardiovascular disease (CVD) risk, and long-term prognosis is greater for ambulatory blood pressure monitoring (ABPM) than clinic measurements. Furthermore, the renin-angiotensin-aldosterone system (RAAS), which is highly circadian rhythmic, activates during the second half of nighttime sleep. Accordingly, bedtime versus morning ingestion of the full daily dose of ACEIs better reduces asleep BP, with the additional benefit, independent of drug terminal half-life, of converting the 24h BP profile into a more normal dipper pattern. Such a therapeutic restoration of normal physiologic BP reduction during nighttime sleep, a novel therapeutic target best achieved by the ingestion of the entire daily dose of $\geq$1 hypertension medications at bedtime, has been identified in a recent outcome trial as the most significant independent predictor of decreased CVD risk, both in patients with and without CKD. Such a bedtime therapeutic strategy, preferably including a medication that blocks the renin-angiotensin-aldosterone system represents a good and strong case for a novel concept - chronotherapy of hypertension with ACEIs and CKD, albeit a new solution to an old problem. This review, most extensively referenced, is a pearl of information on the new concept of chronotherapy in hypertension management.

Norris et al, writing from the David Geffen School of Medicine, University of California, Los Angeles, CA, USA observed that African Americans exhibit a disproportionate burden of hypertension, as well as an earlier onset and a more rapid progression of CKD. In the USA, blacks are known to develop hypertension earlier in life than whites, and have a much higher average blood pressure, and greater rates of premature hypertensive complications such as CKD, stroke and heart disease. In the USA, the prevalence of early-stage CKD is similar across ethnic groups in the US, but the incidence of end-stage renal disease is 1.5–4 fold higher among minority populations (and highest for African Americans) than among whites indicating a marked racial/ethnic difference in the rate of CKD progression. While the prevalence of hypertensive ESRD is about five fold greater among African Americans than among whites, African American men between the ages of 24 and 44 are nearly 20 times more likely to have hypertension-related ESRD than their white counterparts. Therefore, our understanding of the complex factors that predispose African Americans to hypertension and hypertension-related complications is evolving and this chapter exhaustively reviewed the current relevant literature in this area. Furthermore, the authors acknowledged that even though several studies have suggested that the blood pressure lowering efficacy of ACE inhibition is attenuated in African Americans, nevertheless, the ability of inhibition of the renin–angiotensin system (RAS) to protect against the progression of CKD in African Americans is preserved. Typically, hypertension in African Americans is characterized by disproportionately high rates of blood pressure sensitivity to sodium and low circulating plasma renin levels. High renin levels have been implicated in contributing to poor vascular and cardio-renal outcomes. However African Americans still experience severe hypertension-related end-organ complications such as proteinuria and cardio-renal disease despite low circulating renin levels. This could be explained by a dissociation of circulating renin/angiotensin from intrarenal and tissue renin/angiotensin in this patient subgroup. Despite lower circulating renin levels and a less significant fall in blood pressure in response to renin angiotensin system (RAS) blockade in African Americans, RAS inhibition still remains a mainstay of therapy for treating hypertension especially in the presence of CKD in this population. In this chapter, the authors extensively reviewed the relevant literature on hypertension and CKD in the African American, and have discussed the rationale and use of RAS inhibition in African Americans in the context of emerging pathophysiologic and clinical trial data. A greater understanding of the pathophysiology of hypertension in African Americans can enhance the appreciation of risk factor reduction strategies, as well as the rationale for pharmacologic interventions.

Achebe, writing from Capital Medical Center, Olympia, WA, USA, described the utility of ACEIs in General Medical Practice, as seen from an internist's perspective. This well written chapter reminded one of the excellent literary works in fiction-faction by this very gifted physician-author in her debut novel "Onaedo – The Blacksmith's Daughter". This chapter traced the history of the introduction of ACEIs into clinical practice and then narrated the various indications for ACE inhibition as seen from an internist's perspective. Indeed, the author had made reference to an editorialist comment about a "pril for every ill" when reflecting on the multifarious and increasing indications for ACEIs as antihypertensives, renoprotection in diabetic and non-diabetic nephropathies, cardioprotection in heart failure and so on. The rhetorical question had been posed in this chapter - Do ACEIs represent the magic bullet in cardiovascular pharmacology? This chapter ended with a discussion of the potential for nephrotoxicity with angiotensin inhibition especially as it related to the older adult with later stage CKD. The author made references to the current nephrology literature as it related to "triple whammy" and "quadruple whammy", topics discussed in greater detail in two other chapters of this book. The chapter in conclusion had called for caution, and had recommended to 'start low and go slow' with dose titration of angiotensin inhibition, and more pharmacovigilance with very close and indefinite monitoring of serum creatinine, potassium and GFR, in the older adult with later stage CKD on angiotensin inhibition [Onuigbo, QJM 2009].

Madu et al, writing from the Heart Institute of the Carribbean, Kingston, Jamaica, narrate a Caribbean perspective of the utility of ACE inhibition with special reference to heart failure management. The Caribbean region has experienced an epidemiological transition over the past sixty years, evident in the shift from communicable disease predominance to a rising prevalence of non-communicable diseases, particularly cardiovascular diseases (CVD). To address the rising prevalence of cardiovascular diseases in the Caribbean, a systematic evaluation of the drivers of CVDs and treatment modalities must be part of a unified strategy to combat the epidemic. The authors critically examined the strong evidence in the literature to support the universal acceptance of ACEIs in the treatment of cardiovascular disease, worldwide. ACEIs, the authors noted, decreased mortality in congestive heart failure and in left ventricular dysfunction after myocardial infarction, delayed the progression of diabetic nephropathy in some patients and have proved effective in the treatment of hypertension. The authors also examined the pleiotropic effects of ACEIs as it related to fighting cardiovascular disease, different from just blood pressure lowering. The authors contend that although ACEIs are generally effective in reducing blood pressure but appear to be less potent in hypertensive blacks than whites, therefore this observation underscored the need to use higher doses of ACE inhibitors in black patients whether in the Caribbean or elsewhere. The authors concluded that ACEIs are viable therapeutic options for the Caribbean population with high cardiovascular risk or established cardiovascular conditions like hypertensive, diabetic, or ischemic heart disease and heart failure from different causes, because, when appropriately prescribed, (as monotherapy or combination therapy), they are cost effective and the results are clinically beneficial. Finally, ACEIs remain unique in the range of their proven benefits, justifying their central role in the armamentarium of the Cardiovascular Specialist and occupy an important place in the therapeutic management of cardiovascular disorders in the Caribbean.

Ulasi et al, writing from the University of Nigeria Teaching Hospital, Enugu, Nigeria, my alma mater medical school, carried out a thorough and extensive historical review of the epidemiology of increasing CKD prevalence in the developing countries, the physiology of ACE inhibition, the indications for ACE inhibition, together with a global review of current guidelines in the management of hypertension and CKD. This chapter then detailed the experience of the use of ACEI at the center. The authors concluded that ACEIs are important agents in management of CKD patients with considerable improvement in mortality. One of the most important side effects of ACEIs is a dry cough which occurs in about 5-20% of patients. A less common but significant side effect of ACEIs is angioedema which occurs in 1 to 2 per 1000 patients in Caucasians and about double this rate in blacks.

Musso and Alfie, writing from Hospital Italiano de Buenos Aires, Buenos Aires, Argentina, on the use of ACEis in the older adult, observed that ACEIs were the commonest antihypertensive agents prescribed in Argentina. They are effective in the elderly with potentially for additional benefits independent of blood-pressure lowering. However at the same time, the elderly are more prone to adverse drug effects such as hypotension, hyponatremia, hyperkalemia, acutely worsening renal failure and the newly described syndrome of rapid onset end stage renal disease (SORO-ESRD).

De Santo and Cirillo, writing from Second University of Naples, Naples, Italy, completed an exhaustive review of the transitions of man's dietary tastes over the past millennia and went on to review the relevant past trials on the impact of salt restriction on cardiovascular risks, both clinical and experimental. The general consensus is sodium intake restriction in childhood is considered as an effective and powerful maneuver to prevent the increase of blood pressure with age. Also, animal studies, studies in low salt populations, migration studies, cohort studies, randomized controlled trials, limited controlled intervention studies, studies on surrogate markers of outcomes and WHO recommendations unanimously support the benefits of a lower sodium intake. Furthermore, past studies had demonstrated that patients with hypertension uncontrolled by ACE-inhibitor and HCTZ will benefit of sodium restriction. Similar effects have been reported for ARBs, Aliskiren, and beta blockers with diuretics, but not with some calcium channel blockers. Furthermore, studies also suggest that the renoprotective effect of angiotensin receptor blockade is lost with excess dietary sodium intake. Finally, the data point out that sodium restriction in combination with antihypertensive drugs significantly increase the anti-hypertensive effect in hypertensive patients and in CKD patients, with the possible exception of calcium channel blockers, likely due to the mild sodiuretic effects of these drugs.

Di Iorio et al, writing from the Division of Nefrologia, Ospedale A. Landolfi, Solofra, Italy, reviewed the experimental and clinical evidence in support of the efficacy of RAAS blockade, including ACEIs and ARBs in the management of HIVAN, in addition to the use of HAART. The conclusion was that the current use of ACEIs or ARBs in HIVAN relied upon experimental and observational data. Although there was a strong rationale and encouraging preliminary data, the role of RAAS blockage in HIVAN remains to be elucidated. The authors called for RCTs to help resolve these cogent questions.

Molony, writing from the Division of Renal Diseases and Hypertension AND Center for Clinical Research and Evidence-based Medicine, University of Texas Houston Medical School, Houston, TX, USA, has critically examined the evidence-base for the benefits and potential harm of the continued use of ACEIs and ARBs in ESRD patients on maintenance hemodialysis or peritoneal dialysis. He observed that AECIs and ARBS are widely prescribed to individuals receiving dialysis for the treatment of ESRD. These medications are used to treat hypertension especially if the patient has other comorbid conditions such as congestive heart failure (CHF), left ventricular hypertrophy, proteinuria, or diabetes mellitus. Based largely on evidence from non-ESRD patient populations, thought leaders in nephrology have advocated the use of ACEIs/ARBs for the treatment of hypertension and CHF in ESRD undergoing dialysis. Potential benefits include ACEI/ARB therapy-related regression of left ventricular hypertrophy and preservation of residual renal function. Each of these outcomes is supported by some RCT evidence. The authors also reviewed the potential role of ACEI/ARB in preserving dialysis modality in patients treated with peritoneal dialysis. The more fundamental question of whether improvements in these intermediate outcomes translate into real improvements in morbidity or mortality is less well supported by the epidemiologic and experimental evidence. There is limited RCT evidence comparing ACEI/ARB treatment to standard of care, and moreover, systematic reviews with meta-analysis of this evidence fail to support a survival advantage with the use of ACEI/ARB compared to other antihypertensive medications. Furthermore, the RCT evidence might provide a distorted or biased reflection of the truth and this chapter, in a most elaborately researched and referenced manner, has successfully and most expertly reviewed some of the potential sources of this bias. If indeed there is a survival advantage for ESRD patients, it is likely that this benefit is either subpopulation/comorbid disease state-specific or that the overall advantage is smaller than predicted form the experience in non-ESRD populations and may require more rigorous, larger, long-term clinical trials to prove and characterize.

Weir and Mavanur, writing from the University of Maryland School of Medicine Medical Center, Baltimore, MD, USA has very astutely observed that overall, the benefit to risk balance for using RAAS inhibitors and in particular ACE inhibitors, post-transplantation, is in favor of using these drugs. The authors discussed the pathogenesis of hypertension in the renal transplant recipient. There does not appear to be any data to suggest that patients need to be placed on these drugs immediately post-transplantation. The authors suggested that once graft function and immunosuppression had been stabilized, that these medications be employed at about 2-3 months post-transplantation. At that point, serum creatinine and potassium can be monitored more capably and appropriate adjustments in dose and other medications can be considered. In the renal transplant recipient, renin angiotensin system blockers are well tolerated and are as effective as other commonly used drugs in lowering blood pressure. The likelihood that they would precipitate acute kidney injury in a patient with occult renin artery stenosis is remote, but was addressed. What is not known is whether these drugs may prove to be an important contributor to better long-term graft function, either through reducing proteinuria or reducing interstitial fibrosis and tubular atrophy or simply, through their effects on lowering blood pressure, and perhaps glomerular capillary hypertension. Despite the controversial literature on the lack of confirmatory prospective randomized controlled trials, the authors concluded that these drugs should be considered for use in the majority of transplant recipients as there is substantial convincing data in the general population that those individuals with established heart disease and kidney disease do derive a 20% relative risk reduction benefit for cardiovascular and renal events.

Singh et al, writing from Chicago Medical School, North Chicago, IL, USA, reviewed the current literature on the use of ACEIs and ARBs in patients with renal artery stenosis. The conclusion is that optimal medical therapy is the backbone of treatment for atherosclerotic renal artery stenosis (ARAS) whether intervention is required or not. The goals of therapy are to control blood pressure, stabilize renal function, and reduce cardiovascular complications. ACEIs are of particular benefit for patients with ARAS, and their use is supported by societal guidelines. ARBs can be used as an alternative. Although angiotensin blockade may induce acute renal failure in some patients with ARAS, it is generally seen with bilateral severe stenosis, high-grade stenosis in one kidney, or advanced chronic kidney disease and the probability of this complication appears to be low, and in most cases, it is reversible with the discontinuation of treatment.

Robles, writing from Universidad de Salamanca, Spain, completed a most balanced and comprehensive review of the experimental and clinical basis of renoprotection with ACEIs and ARBs. He also reviewed the increasing new literature on renal failure associated with angiotensin blockade. Taken all data altogether, Nicolas Robles conclude that the evidence in the literature suggested a higher renoprotective effect of ACEIs in renal disease, either diabetic or non-diabetic, compared with other antihypertensive drugs. He however cautioned that although ACEIs seems to be reno-protective, patient selection with reference to age, baseline kidney function, presence of co-morbidities and exposure to other nephrotoxins should be taken into account. In elderly CKD patients, the recommendation with reference to dosing of ACEIs (and obviously ARBs) would be to 'start low and go slow' with dose titration, with very close monitoring of serum creatinine, potassium and GFR [Onuigbo, QJM 2009].

Guha and Sharma, writing from the National Heart and Lung Institute, Imperial College London, Dovehouse Street, London, United Kingdom, described the evolution of the pharmacological management of left ventricular systolic dysfunction over the last few decades. Whereas once the treatment options were limited to digitalis extract and mercurial diuretics, there has been introduced the incorporation of multiple neuro-hormonal agents. Furthermore, the discovery of the role of the renin-angiotensin-aldosterone system in the pathobiology of heart failure initiated the impetus to investigate the actions of novel neuro-hormonal inhibitors. The realization, and importantly, the adept clinical testing in small and large clinical trials of the inhibitors of the renin-angiotensin-aldosterone system has rapidly established ACEIs as a cornerstone of modern heart failure pharmacotherapy. This short report provided a brief synopsis of this fascinating area of cardiovascular medicine.

Byrne and Yaqoob, writing from Queen Mary College, University of London, United Kingdom, noted that the risk of developing CKD and cardiovascular complications of hypertension and DM is significantly greater amongst black, Asian and minority ethnic (BAME) communities. However, there are no specific randomized controlled trials focusing on these high-risk groups and comparing the effects of RAS blockade against either placebo or an alternative agent. Instead BAME groups are treated with RAS blockers based on evidence derived predominantly from white patients. This review examines the evidence for cardio- and reno-protection with ACEIs and ARBs, when compared to other antihypertensive classes. The authors have raised doubts in this review about claims of superior cardio-renal protection with ACEIs and ARBs, independent of blood pressure lowering. They also allude to growing new concerns about potential for nephrotoxicity with these agents, especially as it realted to the older later stage CKD patients. The authors submit that guidelines should be viewed as desirables and should not replace a common sense clinical approach to patient care by an autonomously practicing competent clinician. Moreover, the role of RAS blockade in the prevention of cardiovascular and renal disease should be re-examined in general and more importantly in high risk ethnic populations.

Okechukwu and Tasem, writing from Temple University, Philadelphia, PA, explored the effect and role of the RAAS in the cardio-renal syndrome and evaluate the utility of manipulating the RAAS as part of the overall therapeutic strategy for the management of the cardio-renal syndrome. This comprehensive review details the history of the recognition and modern classification of cardio-renal syndrome. The pathophysiology of the syndrome was extensively reviewed. The different therapeutic paradigms available as options to manage cardiorenal syndrome were evaluated, more so the utility of RAAS blockade. In conclusion, although the pathophysiology of the cardiorenal syndromes involved the complex interplay of various systems including maladaptive neurohormonal pathways, the authors acknowledged that the renin-angiotensin-aldosterone system plays a central role in the pathogenesis and pathophysiology of the cardiorenal syndromes. The authors concluded that ACE inhibitors and angiotensin receptor blockers use should be continued in many patients despite a small initial rise in creatinine, as long as renal dysfunction does not progressively worsen and/or significant hyperkalemia does not develop. They cautioned that renal function and serum potassium should be assessed within 1 week of initiation of therapy and periodically thereafter.

Ugochukwu, writing from the Nnamdi Azikiwe University Teaching Hospital, Nnewi, Nigeria, reported on the utilization of ACEIs in pediatric practice in Southeastern Nigeria. The commonest indications for ACEI therapy were heart failure (48.3%), renoprotective effect (37.8%), and hypertension (13.9%). Although the use of ACEIs in pediatric patients has not been quite robust, they have proved reasonably efficacious in the various clinical entities they have been used to treat cardiac failure, proteinuria and hypertension and they have also been well tolerated with minimal side effects.

Kashani and Khairallah, writing from Mayo Clinic College of Medicine, Rochester, MN, USA, examined the role of ACEIs in the Intensive Care Unit. Notably, the authors observed that one instance where the use of ACEIs is justified in AKI is in systemic sclerosis renal crisis. Although ACEIs have become one of the main treatments for chronic heart failure, blocking the RAAS could be deleterious in these patients and create a more severe state of hypoperfusion. On the other hand, due to the significant importance of ACEIs in the treatment of heart failure, discontinuation of this medications are not recommended unless they are associated with progressive kidney dysfunction, hypotension or hyperkalemia. Patients having suffered an ST segment elevation MI have been shown to benefit from ACEI. As an important precaution, when starting this class of medication, is to start from a low dose, and up-titrate to reach a maximum tolerable dose. Thus, in non-hypotensive post MI patients, it is recommended to start ACEI. This is arguable in individuals above 75, whose risk from ACEI induced hypotension outweighs the benefits. Considerations of ACE inhibition in cardiogenic shock and septic shock were also examined. In many clinical scenarios in ICU the role of ACEIs is not very well defined. This class of medications potentially can cause hypotension, hyperkalemia and acute kidney injury, if they are used in high risk patients. Therefore, the authors suggested prescribing these medications based on the individual cases after balancing the risks and benefits associated with them.

Adebirigbe et al, writing, from the University of Illorin Teaching Hospital, Ilorin, Nigeria, described the increasing role of ACEIs in the management of sickle cell disease, a genetic disorder that affects 3% of the Nigerian population, with 25% of the population carrying the sickle cell disease trait. This chapter discussed in great detail the genetic basis for sickle cell disease, its epidemiology around the world, the increasing awareness of the potential renal burden with sickle cell disease as more adults survive to live longer with the disease. The authors traced the pathophysiology of the vaso-occlusive complications of sickle cell disease, with special focus on renal pathology and demonstrated the implications of Angiotensin II in these pathologic processed. The authors reviewed current literature as it related to evidence supporting the use of ACEIs in reducing hyperfiltration, glomerular hypertension, treating relative arterial hypertension, reducing the incidence of stroke, treatment of pain and is indicated to modulate and limit the rate of sclerosis of tissue since Angiotensin II up-regulated Fibroblast Growth Factor. Hyperkalemia may be more common in patients with sickle cell disease treated with ACEIs due to associated tubular dysfunction associated with certain sickle cell disease syndromes.

Skorecki and Wasser, writing from Technion-Israel Institute of Technology, Rambam Health Care Campus, Haifa, Israel, for the first time have weaved a most interesting plot linking the unusual presentation of hypertension and CKD in the African American with respect to ESRD outcomes and response, or non-response, to RAAS blockade, the implications of genetics including APOL1 linkages, and hypertension and CKD in African Americans and Africans, the interplay of genetic mutations with endogenous disease states and the hypertension-misattributed kidney disease (and CKD) among African Americans. The hypothesis of a "second hit" theory, linking genetic predisposition with a second viral hit to lead to observed presentations makes for a very excellent read. The question is asked whether there can be a special role for ACEIs for the treatment of hypertension in Africans not in the diaspora, based on some of these summations.

Tan et al, from the Centre for the Study and Treatment of Vascular Birthmarks, Wellington Regional Plastic, Maxillofacial & Burns Unit, Hutt Hospital, Wellington, New Zealand, report a novel and fascinating paradigm shift in the utilization of ACE inhibition to treat infantile hemangiomas. The novel finding of the expression of the ACE on a phenotypic haemogenic endothelium has recently been reported on the endothelium of the microvessels of proliferating infantile haemangioma, the most common tumour of infancy. The expression of the ACE and the role of the angiotensin II peptide in regulating cellular proliferation via the angiotensin II receptor 2, has been proposed to account for the programmed biologic behaviour of infantile haemangioma. A recent clinical trial that demonstrated the efficacy of an ACE inhibitor on infantile haemangioma confirms the crucial role of the renin-angiotensin system in the regulation of the haemogenic endothelium. The authors conclude that this concept underscores novel understanding and implications of ACE inhibition in human development, infantile haemangioma and other tumours, in general. Drug manufacturers and cancer research must take note of this new major paradigm shift.

Finally, Onuigbo, writing again from Mayo Clinic College of Medicine, Rochester, MN, USA, and Mayo Clinic Health System, Eau Claire, WI, USA, in the last chapter, an epilogue, as it were, has reviewed the place and role of angiotensin inhibition in reno-protection, summarized its drawbacks, and has made some bold predictions regarding the future of reno-protection – a most interesting read.

References

Onuigbo MA. Reno-prevention vs. reno-protection: a critical re-appraisal of the evidence-base from the large RAAS blockade trials after ONTARGET--a call for more circumspection. QJM. 2009 Mar;102(3):155-67. doi: 10.1093/qjmed/hcn142. Epub 2008 Dec 19.

Onuigbo MA, Onuigbo NTC. "Quadruple Whammy", a new syndrome of potentially preventable yet iatrogenic acute kidney injury in the ICU. BMJ 2013: Rapid Response, Published online February 25, 2013. http://www.bmj.com/content/346/bmj.f678/rr/632570.

Twardowski ZJ, Misra M, Singh AK. Con: Randomized controlled trials (RCT) have failed in the study of dialysis methods. Nephrol Dial Transplant. 2013 Apr;28(4):826-32; discussion 832. doi: 10.1093/ndt/gfs307.

Macaulay Amechi Chukwukadibia Onuigbo
MD MSc FWACP FASN MBA
August 2013.

ACKNOWLEDGEMENTS

First, I would like to thank the Good Lord for granting me this exceptional opportunity to edit this major text on angiotensin inhibition. Thanks to all the contributors for their superlative effort, meticulous detailed hard work and perseverance as they all struggled through various professional and personal tribulations to meet the various deadline submissions. Such tribulations include political turmoil in some countries, as well as personal and professional setbacks, which details, I am not allowed to get into here.

Furthermore, this work is dedicated to the majority of Nigerians who continue to suffer in poverty, destitution, deprivation amidst plenty, to Nigerians who remain continuously exposed daily to indefensible insecurity in the face of paralyzed, corrupt and weak governments and derelict governance, and we pray for better days for that country. I acknowledge the support of my mother, Mrs. Gladys Onuigbo, in Enugu, Nigeria, my children, Arinze, Odera and ChiChi, their mother, Nonye Onuigbo, who all also, by the way, had contributed in various ways in assembling a chapter in this volume. I owe and must express my very special thanks and gratitude to Ngozi Achebe MD, internist in Seattle, WA, for her total moral and professional support, most especially at the very initial and most crucial developmental stages of this book project. Finally, the book is dedicated to all my patients in three different continents - Africa, Europe and North America - without whose experiences in the last thirty-some years of medical practice, I would not have been able to have gotten this far.

Special thanks to Emeritus Professor Zbylut Twardowski for doing the special preview, and to Emeritus Professor Richard Glassock for doing the foreword.

Finally, this book is dedicated to the memory of late Professor Dimitrios Oreopoulos; he was indeed a great teacher and mentor to me.

It remains my hope that this volume will serve to meet the needs of physicians of all specialties around the world, the academics, researchers and scientists and the pharmaceutical industry as we all continue to seek ways and means to improve patient care and patient outcomes around the world.

Finally, in the words of the Psalmist:

"Let the words of my mouth, and the meditation of my heart, be acceptable in thy sight, O Lord, my strength, and my redeemer."

Macaulay Amechi Chukwukadibia Onuigbo
MD MSc FWACP FASN MBA
August 2013.

Cognitive Drift Poem

The EMR and Cognitive Drift – Click, Click, Click. And Only More Clicks.

Clicks
Clicks
Wasted Clicks
Clicks
Clicks
Wasted Clicks.

The iPhone Clicks
Minimum Clicks
The iPhone Clicks
Like Two Spacebar Clicks
Quicker For A Period Click
The iPhone Clicks
Minimum Number Of Clicks.

The EMR Clicks
Way Too Many Clicks
The EMR Clicks
Way Too Many Clicks.

Cognitive Drift
Cognitive Drift
The Swirling Hour Glass
The Never-Filling Swirling Hour Glass
At Least While Waiting For The Swirling Hour Glass
No More Clicks
No More Clicks.

Cognitive Drift
Cognitive Drift

Time To Drift
Drift To Sleep
No More Clicks
No More Clicks
While Staring At The Swirling Hour Glass
Maybe Time To Go Take A Leak
A Brief Leak
At The Restroom.

Macaulay Onuigbo MD FASN MBA, January 3 2013, Eau Claire, WI

Reference

Onuigbo MA. Physician 'cognitive drift' and medication errors--unintended consequences of the modern EMR. WMJ. 2012 Oct;111(5):198.

Section 1. ACE Inhibitors and Angiotensin Receptor Blockers in Hypertension

In: ACE Inhibitors. Volume 2
Editor: Macaulay Amechi Onuigbo
ISBN: 978-1-62948-422-8

Chapter 1

CHRONOTHERAPY OF HYPERTENSION WITH ACEIS AND CKD: A NEW SOLUTION TO AN OLD PROBLEM

Ramón C. Hermida, Ph.D.[1,*], Diana E. Ayala, MD, MPH, Ph.D.[1], Michael H. Smolensky, Ph.D.[2], Artemio Mojón, Ph.D[1], José R. Fernández, Ph.D[1] and Francesco Portaluppi, MD, Ph.D[3]

[1]Bioengineering and Chronobiology Laboratories, University of Vigo, Campus Universitario, Vigo, Spain
[2]Cockrell School of Engineering, Department of Biomedical Engineering, The University of Texas at Austin, Austin, Texas, US
[3]Hypertension Center, University Hospital S. Anna and Department of Medical Sciences, University of Ferrara, Ferrara, Italy

ABSTRACT

The prevalence of hypertension in patients with chronic kidney disease (CKD) is extremely high, escalating with diminishing renal function. Typically, the diagnosis of hypertension and the clinical decisions regarding treatment are based solely on daytime clinic blood pressure (BP) measurements. Yet, correlation between BP level and target organ damage, cardiovascular disease (CVD) risk, and long-term prognosis is greater for ambulatory (ABPM) than clinic measurements. Consistent result of numerous studies show the elevated risk and incidence of end-organ injury and fatal and non-fatal CVD events are significantly associated with blunted nighttime BP decline (non-dipper pattern), and also that CVD events are better predicted by the asleep BP mean than either the awake or 24h BP means. The prevalence of abnormally high asleep BP and non-dipping is extensive in patients with CKD, significantly increasing with advancing stage of severity. Indeed, elevated asleep BP is the major criterion for diagnosing hypertension and/or inadequate therapeutic ambulatory BP control in CKD. Endogenous circadian rhythms are known to explain statistically and clinically significant ingestion-time differences in the efficacy, duration of action, safety, and/or effects on the 24h BP pattern of at least six different classes of hypertension medications and their combinations.

---

* Corresponding author: Ramón C. Hermida Ph.D.; E-mail: rhermida@uvigo.es.

The renin-angiotensin-aldosterone system, which is highly circadian rhythmic, activates during the second half of nighttime sleep. Accordingly, bedtime versus morning ingestion of the full daily dose of the angiotensin-converting enzyme inhibitors benazepril, captopril, enalapril, lisinopril, perindopril, quinapril, ramipril, spirapril, trandolapril, and zofenopril better reduces asleep BP, with the additional benefit, independent of drug terminal half-life, of converting the 24h BP profile into a more normal dipper pattern. Therapeutic restoration of normal physiologic BP reduction during nighttime sleep, a novel therapeutic target best achieved by the ingestion of the entire daily dose of ≥1 hypertension medications at bedtime, has been identified in a recent outcome trial as the most significant independent predictor of decreased CVD risk, both in patients with and without CKD. Collectively, recent findings indicate around-the-clock ambulatory BP monitoring must be conducted on patients with CKD to accurately diagnose hypertension and assess CVD risk, and that the associated hypertension ought to be managed by a bedtime therapeutic strategy, preferably including a medication that blocks the renin-angiotensin-aldosterone system.

Keywords: Chronic kidney disease; Angiotensin-converting enzyme inhibitors; Chronotherapy; Hypertension; Cardiovascular risk; Ambulatory blood pressure monitoring; Asleep blood pressure

INTRODUCTION

The biology of human beings is not constant but predictably rhythmic over the 24h and other time scales [1, 2]. This concept is far too often disregarded in the practice of medicine, which is based on the concept of homeostasis, i.e., biological constancy, resulting in missed opportunities, not only for improved insight into the mechanisms of disease, but also for proper patient diagnosis and treatment. Blood pressure (BP) exhibits 24h variation as a consequence of cyclic day-night, or rather rest-activity, alterations in behavior (e.g., activity routine and level, diet, mental stress, and posture), environmental phenomena (e.g., ambient temperature, noise, etc.), and endogenous circadian (~24h) rhythms in neural, endocrine, endothelial, and hemodynamic variables (e.g., plasma noradrenaline and adrenaline [autonomic nervous system, ANS] and renin, angiotensin, and aldosterone [renin-angiotensin-aldosterone system, RAAS]) [3-8].

In ordinarily diurnally active hypertensive patients at elevated risk of cardiovascular disease (CVD) events, the staging, with reference to the 24h scale, of the peak and trough of several critical circadian rhythms results in increased vulnerability to thrombotic, ischemic, hemorrhagic, and arrhythmic accidents in the morning, when their environmental triggers tend to be most intense [7, 9-15].

Interestingly, the 24h patterning of ischemic [16] and hemorrhagic [17] stroke, acute aortic dissection, and other CVD events is the same in normotensive and hypertensive persons [18-21] indicating the important role played in their triggering by the 24h innate rhythms and cyclic environmental phenomena.

The medical literature indicates the prevalence of hypertension is very high in patients with chronic kidney disease (CKD), and that it increases with diminishing estimated glomerular filtration rate (eGFR), up to a reported 86% in patients with end-stage renal disease [22].

However, in our opinion, the majority of the published research involving hypertension, CKD, and CVD risk is inaccurate because of deficiencies in the design of investigative protocols, including limited patient assessment -- either occasional daytime cuff BP measurements or a single poorly-reproducible 24h ambulatory BP monitoring (ABPM) [22-26] -- and entailing only the traditional *morning*-time medication strategy. To begin to remedy these deficiencies, we intensely assess our patients with hypertension and CKD by 48h ABPM to accurately detect and quantify abnormalities of key features of the 24h BP pattern and their effect on CVD risk, and we explore the importance of bedtime versus morning treatment-time strategies. In this chapter, we communicate the recent findings of our outcomes trials, with particular focus on the effect of treatment-time, especially for those medications that modulate the RAAS, and the potential of hypertension chronotherapy -- timing of medications to circadian rhythm phenomena -- to normalize aberrant BP level and pattern and reduce CVD risk [27-33].

24H VARIATION IN BP

In many, but not all, persons with normotension or uncomplicated essential hypertension, both systolic (SBP) and diastolic BP (DBP) decline to lowest levels during nighttime sleep, rise with morning awakening, and elevate to highest values during daytime activity. The typical 24h BP pattern exhibits two daytime peaks, the first one approximately 3h after awakening and the second one around 12h after awakening, with a small nadir in between, in the afternoon [4, 8, 34, 35]. The asleep BP decrease has been mainly quantified through the so-called "sleep-time relative BP decline", percent decrease in mean BP during nighttime sleep relative to the mean BP during daytime activity (100 x [awake BP mean – asleep BP mean]/awake BP mean). Accordingly, subjects have been arbitrarily classified as dippers or non-dippers -- sleep-time relative BP decline $\geq$ or <10%, respectively [36]. This classification system has been recently extended to four categories based upon the sleep-time relative SBP decline: extreme-dippers (decline $\geq$20%), dippers (decline $\geq$10%), non-dippers (decline <10%), and risers (decline <0%, indicating asleep BP mean > awake BP mean) [29].

The usually higher daytime BP of most diurnally active normotensive and uncomplicated essential hypertensive patients derives mainly from dominance at this time of sympathetic tone [37, 38, 39, 40], shown by the attainment of highest concentrations of plasma norepinephrine and epinephrine, plus urinary catecholamines, after awakening [41-43]. The high-amplitude circadian rhythmicity in the constituents of the RAAS [44-51] -- prorenin, plasma renin activity, angiotensin-converting enzyme (ACE), angiotensin I and II, and aldosterone -- also plays a prominent role in 24h BP regulation and patterning in healthy and hypertensive individuals, independent of the alternation of body position with daytime activity versus nighttime sleep [50]. Thus, the lower BP during sleep of most normotensive individuals and some primary hypertensive patients represents the combined consequence of several predicable-in-time phenomena: decline of sympathetic and rise of vagal tone, depression of the RAAS in the first half of nighttime sleep (followed by progressive activation during the second part of sleep, reaching a peak in the early morning hours), and elevation of certain (calcitonin and atrial natriuretic gene-related) peptide vasodilators [6, 52-56].

Various circadian rhythms may also significantly affect the pharmacokinetics and pharmacodynamics, both beneficial and adverse effects, of hypertension medications [57-64]. Administration-time differences in pharmacokinetics can result from circadian rhythms in gastric pH, gastric transport systems, gastric emptying, gastrointestinal motility, biliary function, glomerular filtration, liver enzyme activity, and organ blood flow, e.g., to duodenum, liver, and kidney [65-72]. Administration-time differences in pharmacodynamics can result from the time-dependency in pharmacokinetics and/or circadian rhythms in drug-free fraction, metabolic/clearance processes, and drug-targeted sites, including receptor number/conformation, second messengers, and signaling pathways [60, 63, 64, 73-75]. Chronotherapeutics, a relatively new concept in clinical medicine, is defined as the purposeful timing of medications, whether or not they utilize special drug-release technology, to proportion their serum and tissue concentrations in synchrony with known circadian rhythms in biomarkers of disease processes and/or symptom intensity as a means of enhancing beneficial outcomes and/or attenuating or averting adverse effects [63, 74]. The chronotherapy of hypertension medications takes into account the administration-time (circadian-rhythm) determinants of their pharmacokinetics and pharmacodynamics plus the chronobiology and (chrono)epidemiology of the 24h patterns of CVD events in terms of the differential risk associated with the various circadian BP patterns. Specifically, it entails significant attenuation of the accelerated morning rise of SBP and DBP; normalization of elevated daytime, nighttime, and 24h SBP and DBP means; and conversion of the abnormal non-dipper 24h BP pattern that is associated with elevated risk to the normal dipper one that is associated with reduced risk.

24h BP Characteristics As Predictors of CVD Risk

Specific features of the 24h BP pattern of hypertensive patients might be mediators or biomarkers of injury to target tissues and triggers and/or risk factors for cardiovascular events (such as angina pectoris, myocardial infarction, cardiac arrest, sudden cardiac death, and pulmonary embolism) and cerebrovascular events (such as ischemic and hemorrhagic stroke) [7]. Numerous ABPM studies have consistently shown the blunted sleep-time relative BP decline (namely, a non-dipper or riser 24h BP pattern) is associated with heightened risk of end-organ injury and incidence of fatal and non-fatal CVD events in patients without [29, 33, 76-90] and with CKD [22-26, 31]. In addition, independent prospective studies report the asleep BP mean is a better predictor of CVD events than either the awake or 24h BP means [28-30, 32, 33, 78, 82, 84, 85, 88-96], also in patients with CKD [22, 25, 26, 31, 97].

Nonetheless, the findings of most previous studies may be imprecise because of inherent limitations of the investigative protocols, for example: (i) frequent use of fixed clock hours to define morning awakening and bedtime at night, such that the daytime and nighttime BP means were calculated without assessing and taking into account the actual rest and activity spans of the individual participants; and (ii) analysis of the prognostic value of dipping status and nighttime BP mean without proper adjustment for the daytime BP mean.

Furthermore, in our opinion, the majority of previous reported studies utilizing ABPM to predict CVD risk, except the MAPEC (Monitorización Ambulatoria para Predicción de Eventos Cardiovasculares, i.e., Ambulatory Blood Pressure Monitoring for Prediction of

Cardiovascular Events) one described below [27-33, 89, 90, 98, 99], are of limited value because of their reliance upon only a *single* baseline profile from each participant at the time of inclusion. The design of these studies is unsound because it presumes all features of the baseline-determined 24h BP pattern are maintained without change during the many subsequent years of follow-up in spite of BP-lowering therapy, aging, and/or development of target organ damage and concomitant diseases. The incorporation of periodic (at least annual) ABPM evaluations during follow-up, as done in the MAPEC Study, clearly reveals the alteration of features of the 24h BP pattern over time, and that the reduction of the asleep BP mean and increase of the sleep-time relative BP decline towards the more normal dipping pattern lessens CVD risk [29, 31, 32, 89].

AMBULATORY BP PATTERN IN PATIENTS WITH AND WITHOUT CKD

A blunted sleep-time BP decline, i.e., non-dipping BP pattern, is common in CKD [100-105]; nonetheless, its reported prevalence across different studies is highly inconsistent. This might be due to disparities in the studied populations (treated vs. untreated subjects, patients of different CKD severity, diverse criteria of CKD assessment), relatively small sample sizes, definition of daytime and nighttime periods by arbitrary fixed clock times, frequent reliance upon only a single, low-reproducible [106-109], 24h ABPM evaluation per subject at study inclusion, or other factors. Furthermore, most previous investigations did not compare the 24h BP pattern both of patients with and without CKD. For example, Davidson et al. [102] reported 57.5% prevalence of non-dipping in a retrospective cohort study of 322 patients but without specification of the exact prevalence of non-dipping among those with CKD. Moreover, no information on albuminuria was provided, and the classification of patients according to presence/absence of CKD was based only on the eGFR. Pogue et al. [104] conducted a cross-sectional 24h ABPM study of 617 participants with CKD, also only defined on the basis of reduced eGFR, in the African American Study of Kidney Disease Cohort Study (AASK), finding a very high 80.7% prevalence of non-dipping. In addition, high nocturnal BP was found to be a significant contributing factor to the misdiagnosis of hypertension when based on office cuff measurements; indeed, among patients with controlled *clinic* BP, 70% evidenced masked hypertension, i.e., ABPM-determined awake and/or asleep SBP/DBP mean values greater than recommended reference thresholds. Agarwal and Andersen [101] evaluated 232 elderly patients with CKD, reporting the prevalence of non-dipping increased from 60.0% in patients with stage 2 CKD, to 80.3%, 71.9%, and 71.4% in patients with stage 3, 4, and 5 CKD, respectively (P=0.046).

The ongoing multicenter Hygia Project [105, 110-114], entailing patients of primary care centers of Galicia (Northwest Spain), prospectively evaluates the prognostic value of ABPM and hypertension treatment-time on CVD risk. ABPM evaluation of the so far recruited 10271 hypertensive participants is conducted for 48h, rather than 24h, upon recruitment and at least annually thereafter to increase the reproducibility and quality of findings [106-109]. At baseline, 3227 of these patients had CKD, defined as eGFR <60 ml/min/1.73 m^2, albuminuria (urinary albumin excretion ≥30 mg/24h urine, or albumin/creatinine ratio ≥30 mg/gCr), or both, at least twice within a 3 month span [115].

Diagnosis of hypertension was based on accepted ABPM criteria [116]: awake SBP/DBP means ≥ 135/85 mmHg and/or asleep SBP/DBP means ≥120/70 mmHg, or BP-lowering treatment.

Figure 1 presents the average 24h pattern of SBP (left) and DBP (right) for hypertensive patients with and without CKD assessed by 48h ABPM. In CKD, ambulatory SBP is significantly elevated (P<0.001), mainly during nighttime sleep; ambulatory DBP, however, is significantly lower (P<0.001), mainly during daytime activity.

Between-group differences in SBP and DBP result in significantly greater (P<0.001) ambulatory pulse pressure (PP, i.e., SBP-DBP) over the 24h in the CKD group, even after correcting for age (Figure 2). Consistent with Figure 1, the prevalence of the non-dipper BP profile in the Hygia Project was significantly greater in patients with (60.6%) than without CKD (43.2%; P<0.001 between groups), and the sleep-time relative SBP/DBP decline progressively and significantly (P<0.001) decreased towards the more abnormal non-dipper pattern with diminishing eGFR. The prevalence of the riser BP pattern (sleep-time relative SBP decline <0) constituted the greatest difference between patients with and without CKD, respectively, 17.6% vs. 7.1% (P<0.001). The proportion of patients with CKD showing the non-dipper BP pattern significantly increased across the progressive stages of disease severity (Figure 3).

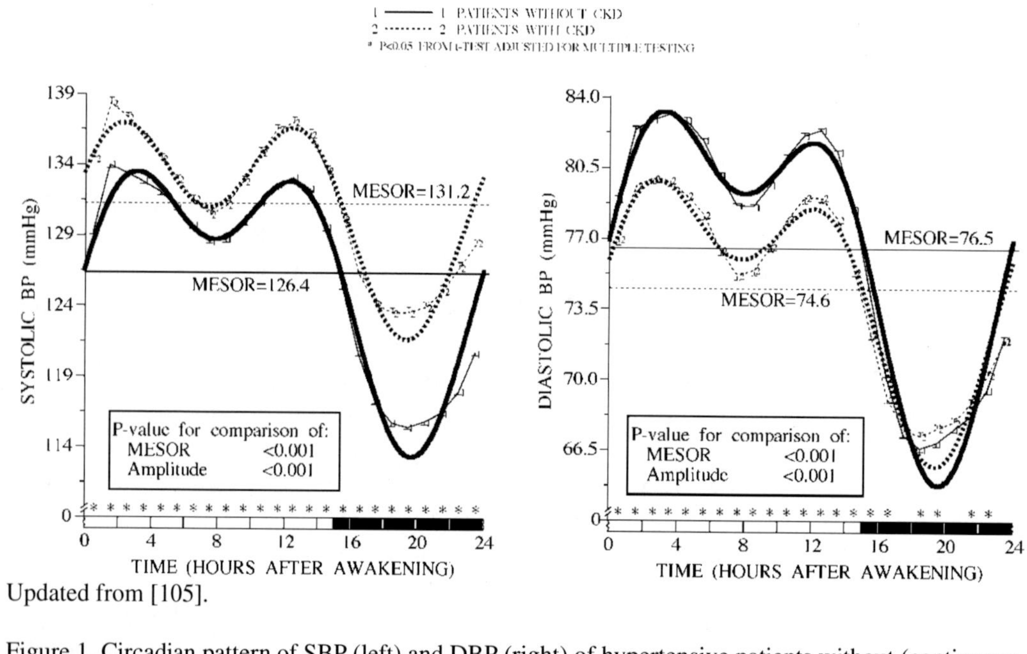

Updated from [105].

Figure 1. Circadian pattern of SBP (left) and DBP (right) of hypertensive patients without (continuous line) and with CKD (dashed line) sampled by 48h ABPM. Each graph shows hourly means and standard errors of data for each group of patients. Dark shading along lower horizontal axis of graphs denotes average hours of nighttime sleep across the patient sample. Nonsinusoidal shaped curves correspond to best-fitted waveform models derived by population-multiple-component analysis [117]. MESOR (midline estimating statistic of rhythm) is the 24-h average value of the rhythmic function fitted to the data. Amplitude is one-half the difference between maximum and minimum values of best-fitted curve. These parameters, obtained for each group of patients categorized according to presence or absence of CKD, were compared using a specially developed nonparametric test [118].

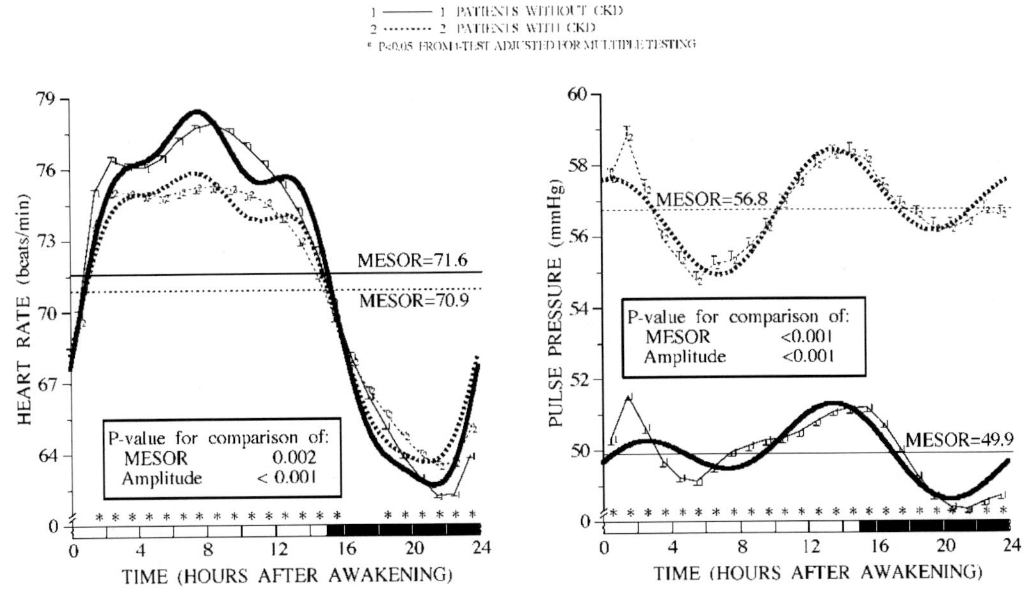

Updated from [105].

Figure 2. Circadian pattern of heart rate (left) and PP (right) of hypertensive patients without (continuous line) and with CKD (dashed line) sampled by 48h ABPM. Each graph shows hourly means and standard errors of data for each group of patients. Dark shading along lower horizontal axis of graphs denotes average hours of nighttime sleep across the patient sample. Nonsinusoidal shaped curves correspond to best-fitted waveform models derived by population-multiple-component analysis [117]. MESOR (midline estimating statistic of rhythm) is the 24-h average value of the rhythmic function fitted to the data. Amplitude is one-half the difference between maximum and minimum values of best-fitted curve. These parameters, obtained for each group of patients categorized according to presence or absence of CKD, were compared using a specially developed nonparametric test [118].

The proportion of patients with the highest CVD risk, i.e., those with the riser BP pattern, significantly and progressively increased from 8.1% for stage-1 CKD to a very high 34.9% for stage-5 CKD (Figure 3).

In actuality, the major reason for making the diagnoses of hypertension and inadequacy of therapeutic BP control in CKD was an elevated asleep SBP mean; indeed, among the uncontrolled hypertensive patients with CKD, 90.7% exhibited nocturnal hypertension [105].

Administration-Time-Differences in Effects of Hypertension Medications on Ambulatory BP

Currently, the majority of hypertensive patients, including ones prescribed combination therapy, routinely ingest the full daily dose of all their BP-lowering agents in the morning [88, 119].

However, numerous prospective trials, comprising at least six different classes of hypertension medications -- ACE inhibitors (ACEIs), angiotensin-II receptor blockers (ARBs), calcium-channel blockers (CCBs), α-blockers, ß-blockers, and diuretics -- evidence best safety, efficacy, duration of action, and effects on the 24h BP pattern when ingested at bedtime [57-64].

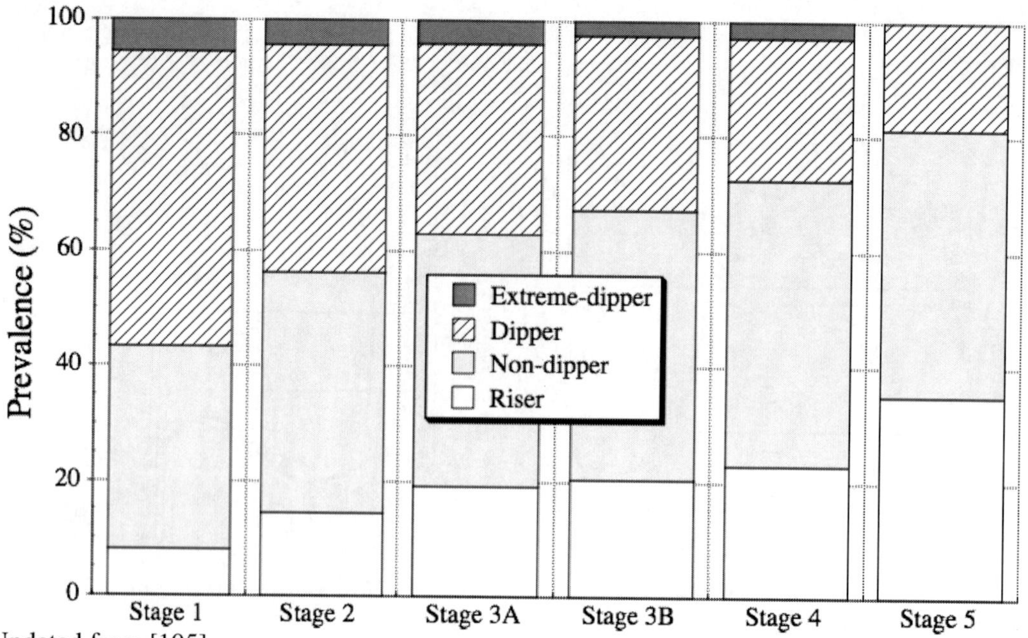

Updated from [105].

Figure 3. Prevalence of dipping classifications in terms of the sleep-time relative SBP decline -- ≥20% (extreme-dipper), 10-20% (dipper), 0-10% (non-dipper), <0% (riser) -- of hypertensive patients with CKD in relation to disease severity -- **stage 1: eGFR ≥90 ml/min/1.73 m^2**; stage 2: eGFR 60-89 ml/min/1.73 m^2; stage 3A: eGFR 45-59 ml/min/1.73 m^2; stage 3B: eGFR 30-44 ml/min/1.73 m^2; stage 4: eGFR 15-29 ml/min/1.73 m^2; stage 5: eGFR <15 ml/min/1.73 m^2.

These findings are extremely important, because they offer a convenient and cost-effective means of enhancing the BP-lowering effects and safety of conventional hypertension medications, i.e., simply by correctly timing them to the body's circadian time structure as chronotherapies. We conducted as investigators many of the studies presented in this review chapter. They entailed a prospective, randomized, open label, blinded endpoint (PROBE) design [120], and 48h ABPM before and after treatment with the specified medication(s), with BP measurements made at 20-minute intervals during daytime activity and at 30-minute intervals during sleep. Furthermore, all of our studies involved simultaneous assessment by wrist actigraphy of activity level at 1-minute intervals. This enabled us to precisely define the commencement and termination of the daytime awake and nighttime asleep spans using dedicated software [121, 122], thereby permitting for each participant accurate calculation of the awake and asleep SBP and DBP means and categorization of the 24h BP pattern (dipper versus non-dipper) before and with therapy.

Angiotensin-Converting Enzyme Inhibitors

A substantial number of clinical studies, extensively reviewed elsewhere [62, 64], demonstrate ingestion-time differences in BP effects of the ACEIs benazepril [123], captopril [124], enalapril [125-127], imidapril [128], lisinopril [129], perindopril [130], quinapril [131, 132], ramipril [133-135], spirapril [136], trandolapril [137], and zofenopril [138].

Most of these studies, which unfortunately do not detail the proportion of patients that do and do not have a diagnosis of CKD, demonstrate ACEIs, when routinely ingested in the evening or at bedtime rather than upon awakening, exert a more marked effect on the asleep than awake BP means thereby changing the 24h BP profile into the normal dipping one (Table 1).

Benazepril. Palatini et al. [123] conducted a single-blinded crossover study of 10 hypertensive patients assessed by continuous intra-arterial BP monitoring to investigate the acute effects of a single 10 mg dose of benazepril when ingested at 09:00 or at 21:00h. Morning administration achieved a more sustained BP-lowering effect than evening administration. This study, however, was too small and underpowered to assess treatment-time differences in 24h, daytime, or nighttime mean BP reductions. Moreover, the potential administration-time-dependent effects of benazepril treatment for spans longer than just a single day are still to be elucidated.

Table 1. Angiotensin-converting enzyme inhibitors: Administration-time differences in effects on the circadian BP pattern, i.e., in sleep-time relative BP decline

Medication	Dose (mg)	Treatment times	No. patients	Effect on sleep-time relative BP decline*		Reference
				Morning R_x	Evening R_x	
Benazepril	10	09:00 h vs. 21:00 h	10	=	↑	[123]
Captopril + HCTZ†	25+12.5	08:00 h vs. 20:00 h	13	↓	↑	[124]
Enalapril	10	07:00 h vs. 19:00 h	8	↓	↑	[125]
Enalapril	5	10:00 h vs. 22:00 h	12	↓	↑	[126]
Enalapril	20	Morning vs. evening	10	↓	↑	[127]
Imidapril	10	07:00 h vs. 18:00 h	20	=	=	[128]
Lisinopril	20	08:00 h vs. 16:00 h vs. 22:00 h	40	=	↑	[129]
Perindopril	4	09:00 h vs. 21:00 h	18	=	↑	[130]
Quinapril	20	08:00 h vs. 22:00 h	18	↓	↑	[132]
Ramipril	2.5	08:00 h vs. 20:00 h	33	↓	↑	[133]
Ramipril	5	08:00 h vs. 14:00 h vs. 22:00 h	30	↓	↑	[134]
Ramipril	5	Awakening vs. bedtime	115	↓	↑	[135]
Spirapril	6	Awakening vs. bedtime	165	↓	↑	[136]
Trandolapril	1	Awakening vs. bedtime	30	↓	↑	[137]
Zofenopril	30	Awakening vs. bedtime	33	↓	↑	[138]

*Sleep-time relative BP decline, an index of BP dipping, is defined as the percent decline in mean BP during nighttime sleep relative to the mean BP during daytime activity, and calculated as: ([awake BP mean – asleep BP mean]/awake BP mean) x 100.

†HCTZ: hydrochlorothiazide.

Updated from [64].

Captopril. Middeke et al. [124] reported the 25 mg/day captopril-12.5 mg/day hydrochlorothiazide combination administered to 13 hypertensive men for 3 weeks was slightly more effective in reducing nighttime BP when ingested once daily in the evening and significantly more effective (P<0.01) in reducing daytime BP when ingested once daily in the morning. In a prospective, double blind, placebo-controlled study, Qiu et al. [139] randomly assigned 121 treated non-dipper hypertensive patients to evening, at 22:00 h, 12.5 mg captopril or placebo treatment, finding the ACEI both significantly reduced nighttime BP and restored the normal dipping circadian BP rhythm in 70% of the patients. The study, however, lacked a morning-time treatment comparison group to enable proper appreciation of the findings.

Enalapril. Witte et al. [125], using a randomized crossover design, studied the cardiovascular effects plus inhibition of serum ACE by enalapril (10 mg) therapy when ingested once daily either at 07:00 or 19:00h by a small sample of eight hypertensive patients. Based on 24h ABPM, morning treatment significantly reduced BP during the day, but it was less effective at night. In contrast, evening treatment significantly further decreased sleep-time and early morning BP followed by slow increase during the day. Thus, the 24h BP profile was significantly influenced by enalapril dosing time. It is of interest that the time after ingestion to peak serum concentration of enalaprilat, the active metabolic by-product of enalapril, and time to peak BP-lowering effect occurred significantly faster, although not simultaneously, after morning than evening dosing (3.5 vs. 5.6h, and 7.4 vs. 12h, respectively, P<0.05), meaning the administration-time differences in the pharmacodynamics of enalapril cannot be attributed only to corresponding administration-time-dependent differences in pharmacokinetics [125]. A troublesome adverse effect of ACEIs, persistent dry cough, can compromise compliance to therapy. It occurs in ~12% of enalapril-treated patients [59], but it may be averted by changing the ingestion time from morning to evening [126, 140]. Fujimura et al. [140] found the dosing time of enalapril affects plasma bradykinin concentration, the chemical trigger of enalapril-induced cough; bradykinin concentration tended to increase following ingestion of the medication at 10:00h, but not after ingestion at 22:00h. Moreover, BP was still significantly reduced 24h after evening, but not morning, enalapril ingestion, indicating prolonged BP-lowering action of this ACEI is possible only with evening administration. In keeping with these combined findings, nighttime dosing has been recommended for enalapril [59,126].

Imidapril. Kohno et al. [128] found no significant morning-evening, treatment-time differences in the attenuation of the daytime or nighttime BP means by imidapril (10 mg once-daily for 4 weeks) in a crossover study involving 20 hypertensive patients.

Lisinopril. Macchiarulo et al. [129] assessed BP changes in 40 patients with grade 1-2 essential hypertension according to the treatment-time of lisinopril (20 mg once-daily for 8 weeks) either at 08:00, 16:00, or 22:00h. SBP and DBP showed significantly greater reduction between 06:00 to 11:00h with the before bedtime 22:00h treatment schedule than with either one of the two other treatment schedules. Thus, lisinopril administration close to bedtime seems to be much more effective in reducing BP during the night and also early morning when CVD risk is elevated [129].

Perindopril. Morgan et al. [130] conducted a crossover study on 20 hypertensive patients randomly assigned to perindopril (4 mg once-daily for 4 weeks) either in the morning at 09:00h or evening at 21:00h. Patients were evaluated by 26h ABPM before and after treatment. Reduction of the daytime BP mean was greater with the morning than evening treatment regimen (-8.0/-4.7 vs. -5.2/-3.9 mmHg SBP/DBP; P<0.05 for SBP), whereas reduction of the nighttime SBP mean was greater with the evening than morning treatment regimen (-11.7/-7.2 vs. -8.2/-5.2 mmHg, P<0.05 for both SBP and DBP). Although not specifically evaluated, the study showed evening compared to morning perindopril dosing resulted in increased sleep-time relative BP decline and corresponding modification of the 24h BP pattern towards a more dipping profile.

Quinapril. Palatini et al. [132] investigated 18 hypertensive patients for the BP-lowering effect of morning (at 08:00h) versus evening (at 22:00h) treatment with quinapril (20 mg once-daily for 4 weeks). The evening schedule produced more sustained BP-lowering effect, while the morning one produced smaller reduction in nighttime BP. Measurement of ACE activity showed evening quinapril administration resulted in less pronounced, yet more sustained, reduction of plasma ACE [132]. Overall, evening quinapril administration seems preferable, because it gives rise to more sustained and stable 24-h BP control, presumably through more favorable modulation of tissue ACE inhibition and/or effect on the adrenergic-induced morning BP rise [131].

Ramipril. Two different small studies [133, 134] revealed ramipril when administered once-a-day in the morning more effectively reduces daytime BP and when administered once-daily in the evening more effectively reduces nighttime BP. A larger clinical study was conducted later by Hermida and Ayala [135] on 115 previously untreated grade 1-2 essential hypertension patients randomized to an either upon-wakening or bedtime ramipril monotherapy (5 mg once-daily for 6 weeks). Evaluations by 48h ABPM before and after treatment revealed greater reduction of the 48h SBP/DBP means with the bedtime than upon-awakening schedule (-11.2/-9.5 vs. -8.5/-6.2 mmHg; P=0.059/0.004 between groups; Figure 4). Although there was no treatment-time-dependent difference in the effect upon the awake BP mean, the bedtime, compared to the upon-awakening, schedule was significantly more effective in reducing the asleep SBP/DBP means (-13.5/-11.5 vs. -4.5/-4.1 mmHg, P<0.001 between groups; [Table 2 and Figure 4]). Consequently, the sleep-time relative BP decline was attenuated toward a more non-dipping pattern when ramipril was ingested upon awakening but significantly potentiated towards a more dipping pattern when ingested at bedtime (Table 2); moreover, the proportion of patients with controlled ambulatory BP was increased from 43 to 65% (P=0.019). Overall, asleep BP regulation was significantly enhanced with the bedtime ramipril administration schedule and without any loss in efficacy during the daytime activity span. The differential administration-time-dependent effects of ramipril on BP are illustrated in Figure 5. Ramipril reached peak effect sooner when ingested at bedtime than upon awakening, giving rise to significantly greater efficacy during the first 6h following ingestion. Moreover, duration of the BP-lowering effect was shorter when ramipril was ingested upon awakening than at bedtime, resulting in BP reduction with bedtime ramipril administration being significantly greater during the last 12h of the 24h dosing interval.

Spirapril. Hermida et al. [136] explored the treatment-time-dependent efficacy of the long terminal plasma half-life (~40h) spirapril (6 mg once-daily for 12 weeks) in a study of 165 grade 1-2 essential hypertensive patients randomized to therapy either upon awakening or at bedtime. Reduction of the 48h SBP/DBP means was comparable with the morning and bedtime regimens (-8.7/-7.0 vs. -9.8/-6.6 mmHg; P>0.287 between groups [Figure 6]), and the extent of SBP reduction during daytime activity was also independent of treatment time (P=0.292 [Table 2 and Figure 6]). However, the bedtime, compared to the upon-awakening, schedule was much more effective in reducing the asleep SBP/DBP means (-12.8/-8.6 vs. -5.7/-4.6 mmHg; P<0.001 between treatment-time groups [Table 2 and Figure 6]). Accordingly, the sleep-time relative BP decline was significantly increased towards a more dipping pattern only with bedtime spirapril ingestion (P<0.001 [Table 2]), and the proportion of patients with controlled ambulatory BP was increased from 23 to 59% (P<0.001). The effects of spirapril on BP as a function of its ingestion time are illustrated in Figure 7. When dosed in the morning, spirapril starts losing its BP-lowering efficacy shortly after reaching peak effect (~3h after ingestion).

Table 2. Summary of changes from baseline (in mmHg) in awake and asleep SBP and DBP means as well as in sleep-time relative BP decline for different hypertension medications ingested as the full daily dose either always upon awakening or at bedtime by essential hypertension patients who adhered to a daytime activity and nighttime resting routine

Medication	Dose, mg	Patients	Effect on awake SBP/DBP mean		Effect on asleep SBP/DBP mean		Effect on sleep-time relative SBP/DBP decline		Reference
			Awakening R_x	Bedtime R_x	Awakening R_x	Bedtime R_x	Awakening R_x	Bedtime R_x	
Ramipril	5	115	-10.1/-6.9	-10.5/-9.0	-4.5/-4.1	-13.5/-11.5*	-3.3/-1.8	3.4/4.9*	[135]
Spirapril	6	165	-9.9/-8.0	-8.5/-5.7	-5.7/-4.6	-12.8/-8.6*	-2.5/-2.7	4.1/4.5*	[136]
Valsartan	160	90	-17.0/-11.1	-12.0/-9.8	-15.9/-10.8	-17.9/-13.3	0.2/1.3	5.4/6.3*	[141]
Valsartan	160	100[a]	-12.8/-6.6	-13.0/-8.5	-10.9/-5.5	-20.5/-11.1*	-1.0/-0.3	6.6/5.4*	[142]
Valsartan	160	200[b]	-13.1/-8.3	-12.6/-9.3	-12.9/-8.1	-21.1/-13.9*	0.4/0.9	7.2/7.1*	[143]
Olmesartan	20	133	-14.5/-12.1	-13.3/-9.6	-11.2/-8.7	-15.2/-11.5‡	-1.3/-1.4	2.9/4.6*	[144]
Olmesartan	40	72	-17.1/-10.1	-16.3/-11.5	-12.6/-8.2	-17.9/-12.5‡	-1.6/-0.2	3.0/3.8*	[145]
Telmisartan	80	215	-11.7/-8.8	-11.3/-8.2	-8.3/-6.4	-13.8/-9.7*	-1.6/-1.0	3.1/3.9*	[146]
Amlodipine	5	194	-10.2/-7.7	-11.8/-7.2	-9.6/-5.5	-11.2/-6.7	0.1/-1.6	0.2/0.7‡	[152]
Nifedipine GITS	30	238	-9.4/-6.3	-12.8/-7.7 ‡	-7.5/-5.1	-12.8/-7.8*	-0.7/-0.2	1.0/1.5‡	[158, 159]
Doxazosin GITS	4	39[c]	-2.9/-3.7	-6.0/-5.4	0.7/-1.3	-8.2/-6.5†	-2.3/-2.4	1.9/1.9‡	[163]
Doxazosin GITS	4	52[d]	-3.4/-2.9	-5.9/-4.4	0.1/-0.5	-4.9/-5.3‡	-2.3/-2.4	1.7/1.5‡	[163]
Nebivolol	5	173	-14.7/-12.4	-13.4/-10.9	-7.9/-7.4	-10.2/-8.1	-3.6/-3.0	-1.2/-1.4‡	[164]
Torasemide	5	113	-7.3/-3.7	-15.6/-9.9 *	-4.3/-2.5	-12.5/-8.0*	-1.6/-0.7	-1.3/-0.2	[165]

Sleep-time relative BP decline, an index of BP dipping, is defined as the percent decline in mean BP during nighttime sleep relative to the mean BP during daytime activity, and calculated as: ([awake BP mean – asleep BP mean]/awake BP mean) x 100. All studies followed a prospective, randomized, open label, blinded endpoint (PROBE) design. Participants (1899 in total) in all studies were grade 1 or 2 essential hypertension patients, evaluated by 48h ambulatory BP monitoring and wrist actigraphy before and after timed treatment for several (varying between studies from 6 to 12) weeks duration. Comparison of effects on BP between treatment-times: *P<0.001; †P<0.01; ‡P<0.05.

[a]Study on elderly patients (≥60 yrs of age).

[b]Study on non-dipper patients, i.e., sleep-time relative SBP decline <10%.

[c]Patients treated with doxazosin monotherapy.

[d]Patients treated with doxazosin in combination with other hypertension medications (polytherapy).

Updated from [64].

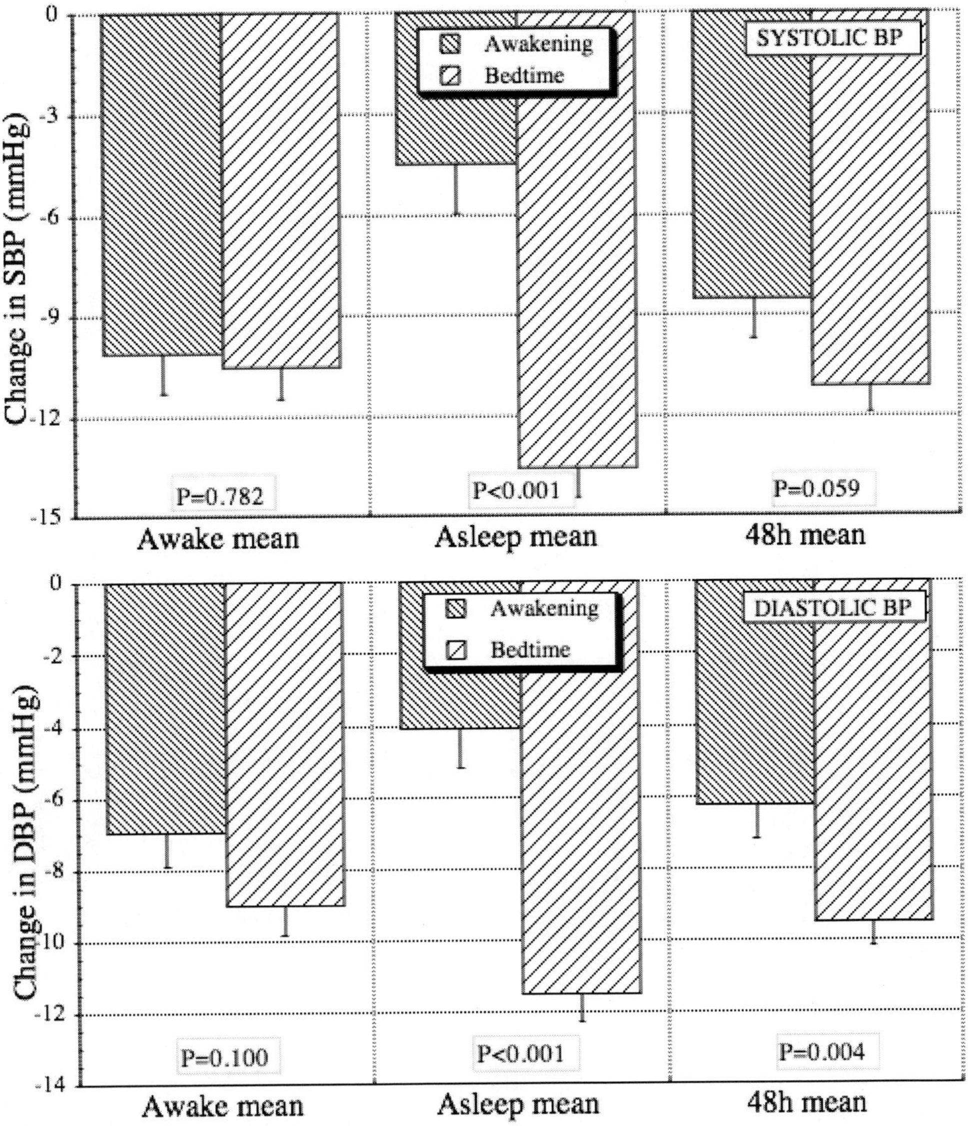

Updated from [64, 135].

Figure 4. Changes from baseline (mmHg) in awake (active span), asleep (nighttime rest span), and 48h mean of SBP (top) and DBP (bottom) with ramipril (5 mg/day) ingested upon awakening or at bedtime in patients with grade 1-2 essential hypertension studied by 48h ABPM before and after 6 weeks of timed treatment. Probability values are shown for comparison of effects between the two treatment-time groups of patients by *t* test.

In contrast, when dosed at bedtime, maximum BP-lowering effect is maintained for 8h after ingestion, thus showing greater efficacy during this time-interval relative to morning administration. With bedtime, as compared to upon awakening, spirapril administration, drug efficacy was also significantly greater during the last 4h of the dosing interval [136].

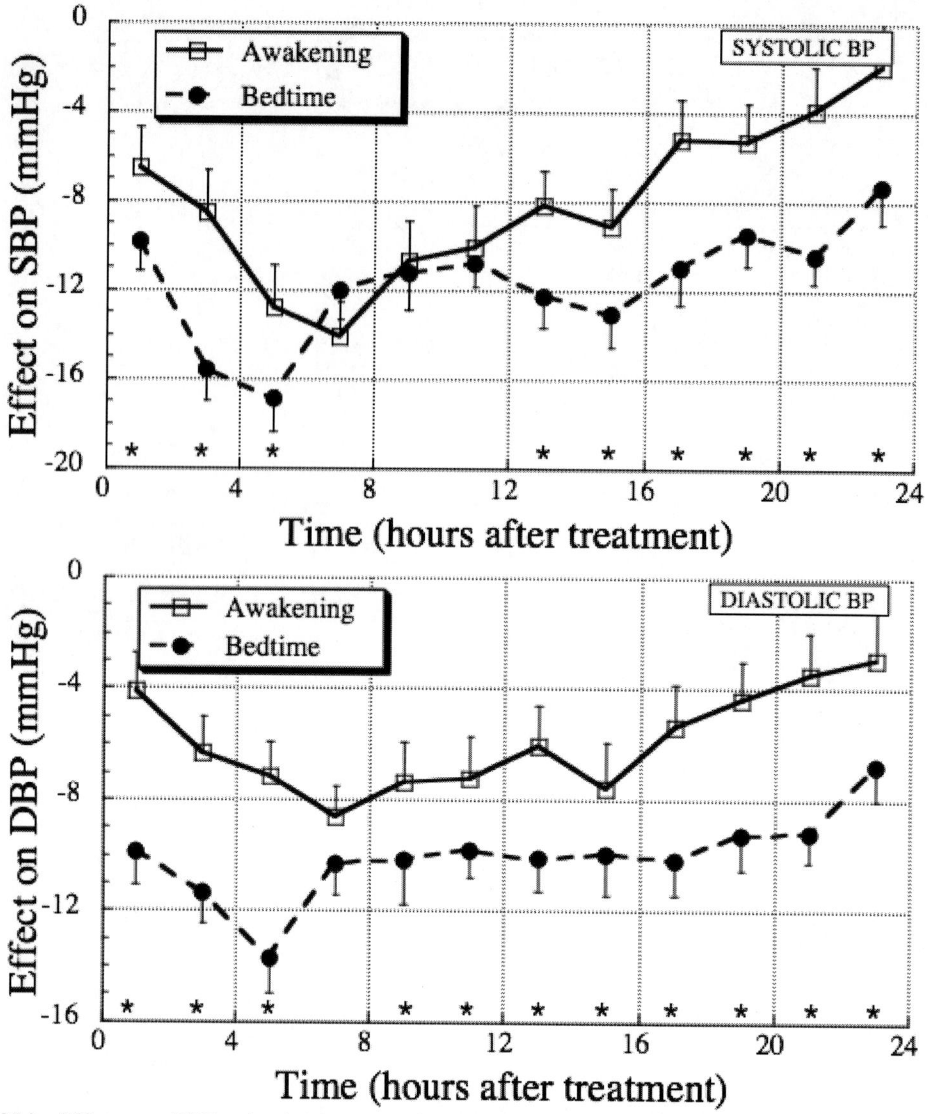

*P<0.05 in difference of BP reduction between the two treatment-time groups.
Updated from [64, 135].

Figure 5. Changes from baseline (mmHg) during the 24h in SBP (top) and DBP (bottom) after treatment with ramipril (5 mg/day) ingested either upon awakening or at bedtime in patients with grade 1-2 essential hypertension studied by 48h ABPM before and after 6 weeks of timed treatment.

Trandolapril. Kuroda et al. [137] investigated 30 hypertensive patients for the differential effects of bedtime versus morning-time therapy of the long-acting lipophilic ACEI trandolapril (1 mg once-daily for 8 weeks). With morning ingestion, the awake, but not asleep, BP was significantly reduced. In contrast, with bedtime ingestion, both the awake and asleep BP means were effectively controlled, and without induction of nighttime hypotension.

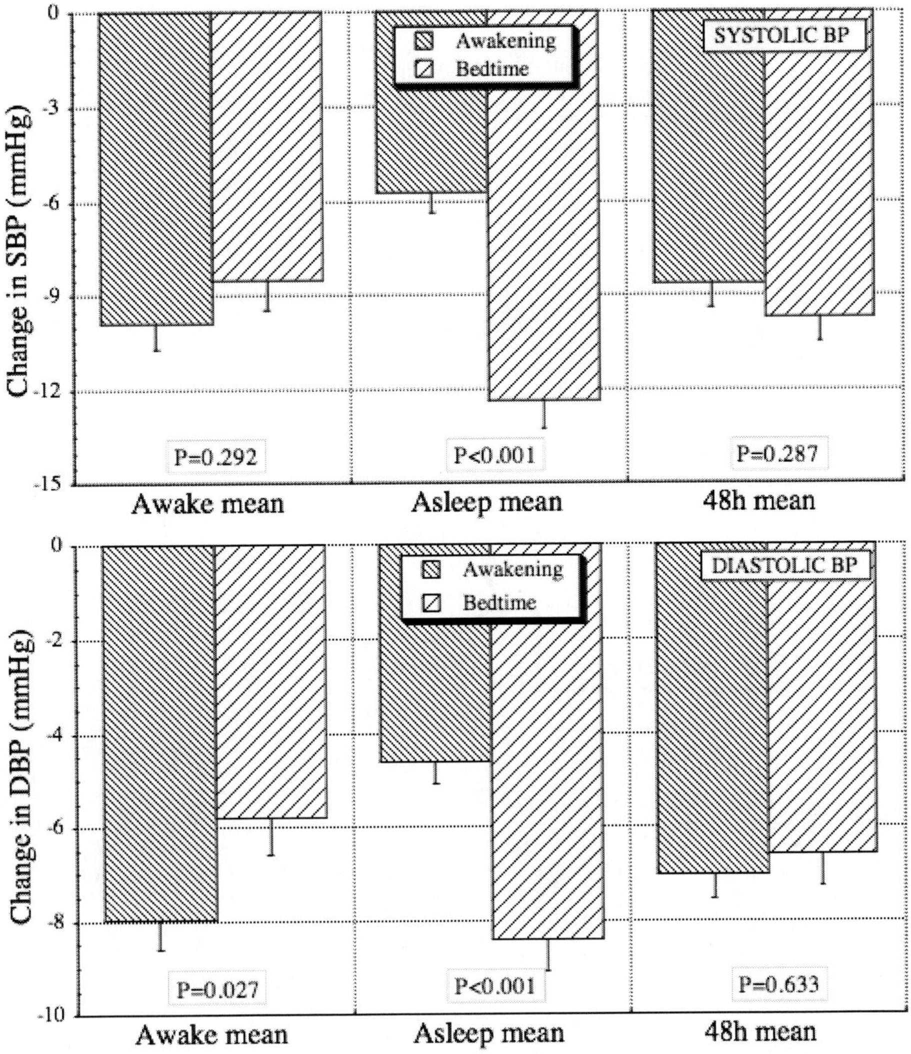

Updated from [64, 136].

Figure 6. Changes from baseline (mmHg) in awake (active span), asleep (nighttime rest span), and 48h mean of SBP (top) and DBP (bottom) with spirapril (6 mg/day) ingested upon awakening or at bedtime in patients with grade 1-2 essential hypertension studied by 48h ABPM before and after 12 weeks of timed treatment. Probability values are shown for comparison of effects between the two treatment-time groups of patients by *t* test.

Zofenopril. Balan et al. [138] investigated 33 previously untreated hypertensive patients for the differential effects of bedtime versus awakening scheduling of zofenopril (30 mg once-daily for 1 month). Both treatment-time schedules provided similar daytime BP reduction; however, bedtime dosing was more efficient than awakening dosing in attenuating the asleep BP mean. The sleep-time relative BP decline was decreased with zofenopril on awakening but significantly increased towards a more dipping pattern with zofenopril at bedtime. Finally, the proportion of patients with controlled ambulatory BP by the bedtime compared to the upon-awakening treatment schedule increased from 51.5% to 84.8% (P<0.001).

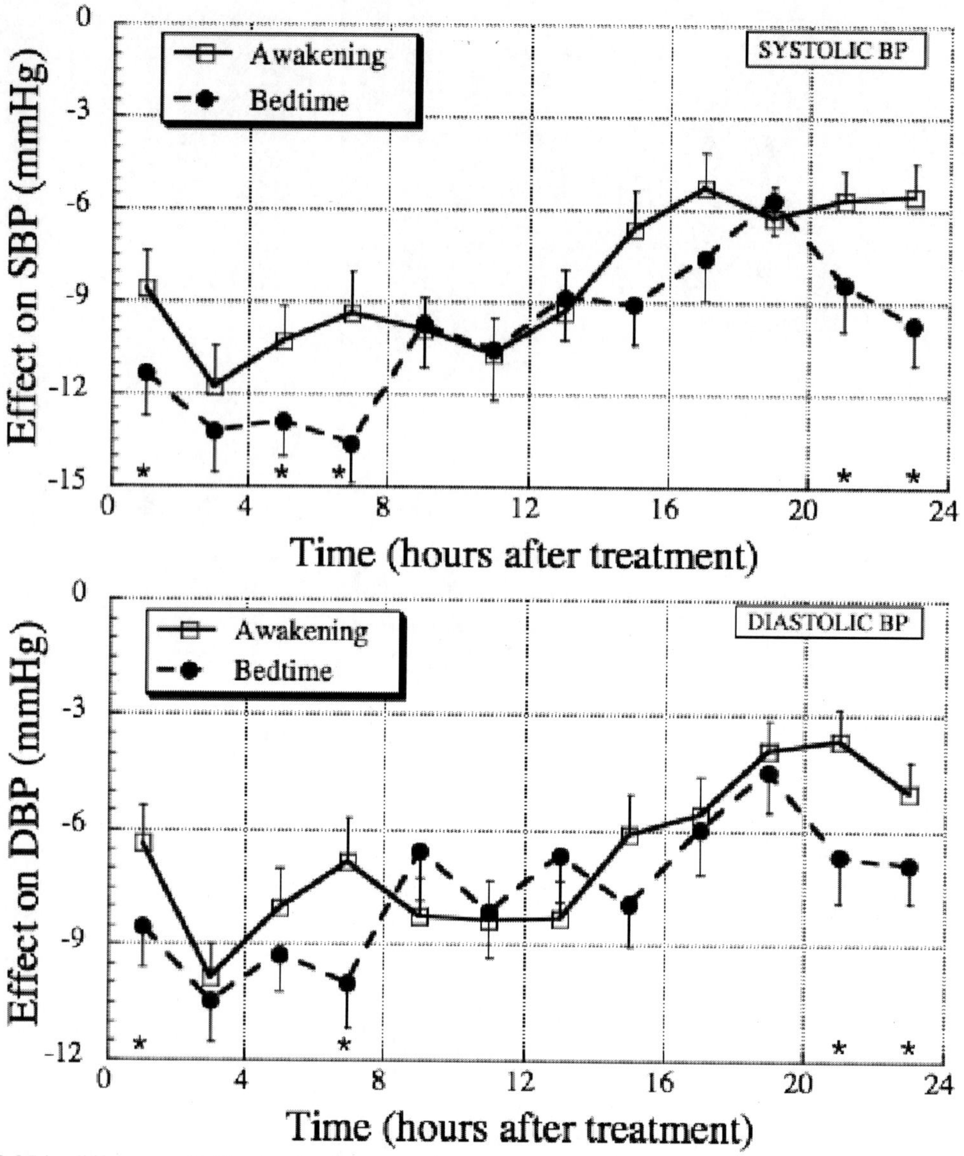

*P<0.05 in difference of BP reduction between the two treatment-time groups. Updated from [64, 136].

Figure 7. Changes from baseline (mmHg) during the 24h in SBP (top) and DBP (bottom) after treatment with spirapril (6 mg/day) ingested either upon awakening or at bedtime in patients with grade 1-2 essential hypertension studied by 48h ABPM before and after 12 weeks of timed treatment.

Other Hypertension Medications

Clinical trials also validate ingestion-time-dependent effects of the ARBs irbesartan, olmesartan, telmisartan, and valsartan [62, 64]. Independent of the considerable differences in their plasma half-life [141-146], reduction of the awake SBP/DBP means by the awakening and bedtime therapeutic regimens was similar; however, decrease of the asleep SBP/DBP means was significantly greater with the bedtime regimen.

Thus, the sleep-time relative SBP/ DBP decline was slightly attenuated when the ARBs were ingested upon awakening, while it was significantly enhanced when ingested at bedtime, thereby significantly reducing from baseline the prevalence of non-dipping. Interestingly, two different studies, one involving the bedtime ingestion of valsartan [147] and the other candesartan [148], also documented significant decline in urinary albumin excretion, which in the case of valsartan correlated with both decreased asleep BP mean and increased sleep-time relative BP decline. The circadian rhythm of the RAAS, with peak activity toward the end of the nighttime sleep span, may explain the better effect on BP regulation conveyed by the bedtime regimen of ARBs and, as reviewed above, of ACEIs [57-64].

Morning versus evening treatment-time trials of the CCBs [149-152], cilnidipine [153], diltiazem [154], isradipine [155, 156], nifedipine [157-159], nisoldipine [160], and nitrendipine [161, 162] reveal dihydropyridine derivatives, in general, reduce BP homogeneously throughout the 24h, independent of timing [64]. Nevertheless, of great clinical relevance are findings of a trial conducted on 238 previously untreated hypertensive patients randomized either to bedtime or upon awakening nifedipine GITS monotherapy (30 mg once daily for 8 weeks); bedtime, relative to upon-awakening, therapy resulted in profound and statistically significant reduction in the incidence of peripheral edema (1 vs. 13%; $P<0.001$) [158, 159].

Other hypertension medications, including the α-blocker doxazosin [163], ß-blockers carvedilol and nebivolol [164], and loop-diuretic torasemide [165], also show significantly enhanced asleep BP reduction and increased duration of BP-lowering effect with bedtime versus morning (upon awakening) therapy [64]. Combination medications -- valsartan-amlodipine [166], amlodipine-fosinopril [167], amlodipine-olmesartan [168], valsartan-hydrochlorothiazide [169], and amlodipine-hydrochlorothiazide [170] -- also evidence treatment-time differences in efficacy. Bedtime, in comparison to upon awakening, ingestion of every one of these combination therapies markedly reduces the asleep SBP/DBP means and significantly increases the proportion of patients converted from non-dipper to dipper patterning [64].

Chronotherapy and the Effect of Hypertension Medication Terminal Half-Life on Efficacy

Some proponents claim ingestion-time-dependent differences in the effects of hypertension medications on the 24h BP pattern and, in particular, asleep BP, are pertinent only for those medications that have a terminal half-life substantially shorter than 24h [171, 172]. This perspective fails to recognize that the pharmacokinetics and pharmacodynamics of a hypertension medication can vary significantly relative to treatment-time due to strong influence of the patient's circadian time structure and, in addition, that drug pharmacokinetic phenomena are not always predictive of the best and poorest pharmacodynamic effects, for example, as discussed above for enalapril [125] as well as other BP medications [57-64]). As already apparent from the presentation of findings of the various studies in previous sections and summarized in Table 2, marked ingestion-time differences in BP-lowering effects have been substantiated for long-half life (≥24 h) and controlled-release therapies, such as spirapril [136], telmisartan [146], and olmesartan [144], as well as shorter half-life ones, for instance, valsartan [141-143, 147], ramipril [135], and torasemide [165]. Ingestion-time differences in the effects of the ACEI and ARB families of medications on SBP and DBP seem to be medication-class, rather than plasma-terminal-half-life, dependent phenomena. Thus, the enhanced effects of ARB and ACEI medications when ingested at bedtime, especially the increase toward normal of the sleep-time relative BP decline and extent of 24h BP dipping, are likely the consequence of achieving the highest drug concentrations overnight when the RAAS is most activated, that is, when plasma renin activity and the plasma concentrations of ACE, angiotensin I, angiotensin II, and aldosterone are rising to highest levels [46, 49, 50, 62].

Chronotherapy in Hypertensive Patients with CKD

The impact of hypertension treatment-time regimen on 24h BP patterning and control in CKD was recently investigated by Crespo et al. [111]; among 2659 hypertensive participants with CKD enrolled in the Hygia Project, 1446 ingested all their BP-lowering medications upon awakening and 1213 patients ingested the entire daily dose of ≥1 of them at bedtime. Among the latter, 359 patients ingested all such medications at bedtime, while 854 ingested the complete daily dose of some medications upon awakening and the entire daily dose of others at bedtime. Patients ingesting ≥1 medications at bedtime, relative to those ingesting all of them upon awakening, evidenced significantly lower asleep SBP/DBP means and higher sleep-time relative SBP decline ($P<0.001$), thereby significantly reducing the prevalence of non-dipping from 68.3% in patients ingesting all hypertension medications upon awakening to 54.2% and 47.9% in ones ingesting, respectively, ≥1 or all of them at bedtime ($P<0.001$ between groups). Additionally, the prevalence of the riser BP pattern was much lower among patients who ingested the entire daily dose of some (15.7%) or all (10.6%) of their hypertension medications at bedtime rather than the complete daily dose of all of them upon awakening (21.5%; $P<0.001$ between groups). Furthermore, patients who ingested all medications at bedtime also showed a significantly higher prevalence of fully controlled ambulatory BP ($P<0.001$) that was achieved by a significantly smaller number of required hypertension medications ($P<0.001$) [111].

The prevalence of the different 24h BP patterns also varied by stage of CKD severity and treatment-time regimen [111]. In particular, stage 3 to 5 patients who ingested the complete daily dose of all their hypertension medications upon awakening (Figure 8) showed great prevalence of non-dipper pattern, with 23-26% of patients evidencing the very high CVD risk riser pattern. Prevalence of non-dipping and riser BP patterns in patients ingesting the complete daily dose of their hypertension medications at bedtime (Figure 9) was significantly lower than in those ingesting all medications upon awakening (Figure 8), with the prevalence of the riser pattern among patients of the bedtime regimen always <14%, independent of CKD stage.

Another study [173] involving 32 uncontrolled non-dipper Italian patients with CKD reported similar significant reduction of the asleep BP mean (from 114±11 to 107±12 mmHg in SBP; from 62±7 to 58±6 mmHg in DBP; $P<0.001$) and significant decrease in urinary albumin excretion (from 235 ± 259 mg/day to 167 ± 206 mg/day; $P<0.001$), after shifting one BP-lowering medication from morning to evening.

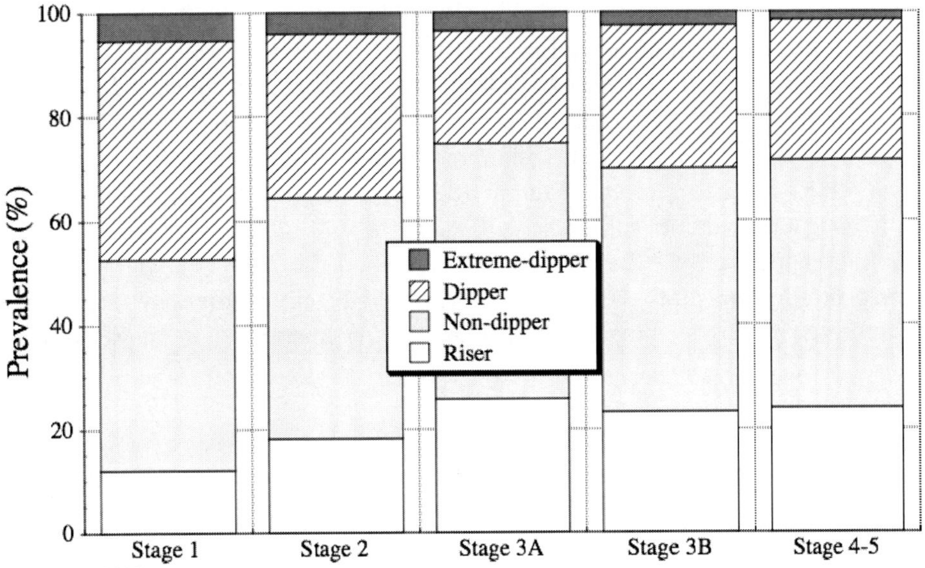

Updated from [111].

Figure 8. Prevalence of dipping classifications in terms of the sleep-time relative SBP decline -- ≥20% (extreme-dipper), 10-20% (dipper), 0-10% (non-dipper), <0% (riser) -- of hypertensive patients with CKD ingesting all BP-lowering medications upon awakening in relation to disease severity -- stage 1: eGFR ≥90 ml/min/1.73 m^2; stage 2: eGFR 60-89 ml/min/1.73 m^2; stage 3A: eGFR 45-59 ml/min/1.73 m^2; stage 3B: eGFR 30-44 ml/min/1.73 m^2; stage 4: eGFR 15-29 ml/min/1.73 m^2; stage 5: eGFR <15 ml/min/1.73 m^2.

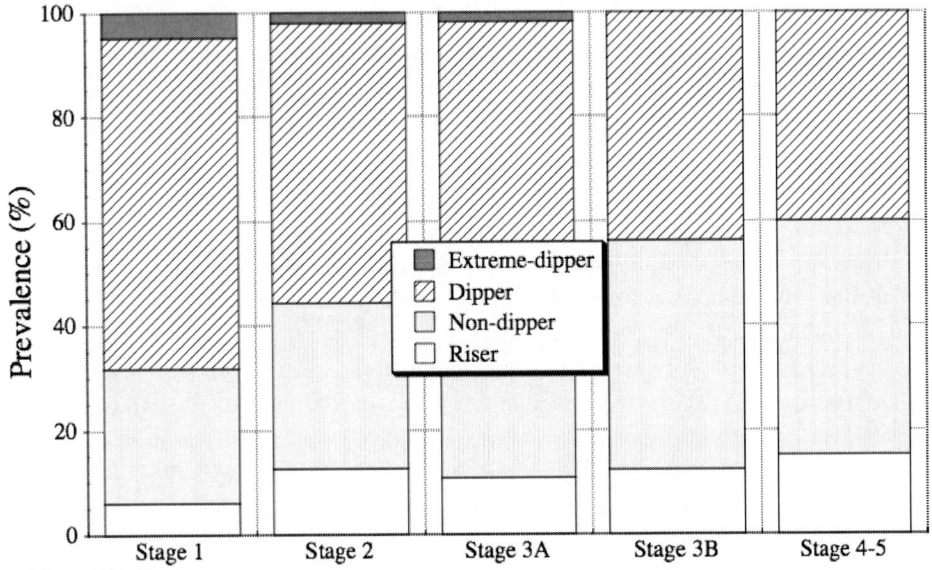

Updated from [111].

Figure 9. Prevalence of dipping classifications in terms of the sleep-time relative SBP decline -- ≥20% (extreme-dipper), 10-20% (dipper), 0-10% (non-dipper), <0% (riser) -- of hypertensive patients with CKD ingesting all BP-lowering medications at bedtime in relation to disease severity -- stage 1: eGFR ≥90 ml/min/1.73 m^2; stage 2: eGFR 60-89 ml/min/1.73 m^2; stage 3A: eGFR 45-59 ml/min/1.73 m^2; stage 3B: eGFR 30-44 ml/min/1.73 m^2; stage 4: eGFR 15-29 ml/min/1.73 m^2; stage 5: eGFR <15 ml/min/1.73 m^2.

The findings of Rahman et al. [174] entailing 151 black participants enrolled in the AASK study with controlled clinic and awake BP were somewhat different. They compared the effect on nocturnal SBP -- defined according to an assumed identical fixed clock-hour span among all participants rather than their actual sleep span -- of the shift to bedtime of an already prescribed once-a-day hypertension medication or addition of a new low-dose medication. Both strategies reduced nocturnal SBP, but not significantly (P=0.08), leading the authors to conclude bedtime chronotherapy might be of limited advantage in reducing nighttime BP in hypertensive African American patients and/or CKD.

One recent Nigerian study, however, involving 165 black hypertensives randomized to morning (10:00h) versus evening (22:00h) hypertension treatment for 12 weeks revealed significantly greater reductions in clinic DBP and left ventricular mass (P<0.001) among those treated at night [175]. Finally, a recent study by Wang et al. [176] evaluated the advantages of awakening versus bedtime scheduling of valsartan (80-320 mg once daily for one year) on 60 non-dipper Chinese patients with CKD; treatment at bedtime was significantly more effective in reducing nighttime BP, albuminuria, and left ventricular mass (P always <0.05).

Reduction of CVD Risk by Hypertension Chronotherapy

The association between prognostic ABPM parameters, CVD risk, and time-specified hypertension treatment strategy has thus far been investigated only in the MAPEC Study, specifically designed to test the hypothesis that bedtime chronotherapy with the entire dose of ≥1 hypertension medications exerts better 24h BP control and CVD risk reduction than conventional therapy, i.e., all medications ingested in the morning.

Complete details of the rationale and design of the study are described elsewhere [27, 28]. Briefly, the authors prospectively studied 3344 subjects (793 with CKD), with baseline BP ranging from normotension to sustained hypertension according to ABPM criteria [116], during a median follow-up of 5.6 years. Participants with hypertension at baseline were randomized to ingest the complete daily dose of all their prescribed hypertension medications upon awakening or the entire daily dose of ≥1 of them at bedtime.

At baseline and annually (more frequently if hypertension treatment was adjusted) thereafter, ambulatory BP was measured for 48h and physical activity was simultaneously monitored by wrist actigraphy to accurately derive the awake and asleep BP means.

The ABPM-derived asleep SBP mean was the most significant predictor of CVD outcome [29, 89]. Interestingly, large morning BP surge was significantly associated with lower, not higher, CVD risk, consistent with the highly significant relationship between increased sleep-time relative BP decline and reduced CVD risk. Exploration of the potential combined contribution of multiple BP parameters to prediction of CVD events, revealed the best jointly adjusted Cox regression model included only the asleep SBP mean (hazard ratio [HR]=1.23, 95%CI [1.16-1.32], P<0.001) and the sleep-time relative SBP decline (HR=0.98 [0.97-0.99], P=0.019). Moreover, when the asleep SBP mean was adjusted for the awake SBP mean, only the former significantly predicted CVD outcomes [29, 89]. Joint entry in the same time-dependent Cox regression model of changes in patient asleep and awake BP means during the 5.6 years of follow-up showed that only attenuation of the asleep SBP mean was significantly associated with reduced CVD risk (adjusted HR per 5 mmHg reduction in the asleep SBP mean: 0.85 [0.79-0.91], P<0.001; adjusted HR per 5 mmHg reduction in the awake SBP: 1.00 [0.94-1.05], P=0.849) [29, 89].

These results suggest the hypertension treatment-time regimen significantly impacts CVD risk. At the conclusion of the 5.6 years median follow-up span, patients who ingested the entire daily dose of ≥1 hypertension medications at bedtime showed significantly lower asleep BP mean, higher sleep-time relative BP decline, reduced prevalence of non-dipping (34 vs. 62%; P<0.001), and higher prevalence of controlled ambulatory BP (62 vs. 53%, P<0.001). Most important, routine ingestion of the full daily dose of ≥1 BP-lowering medications at bedtime, compared to routine ingestion of the complete daily dose of all such medications upon awakening, resulted in a significantly lower adjusted HR of total CVD events (HR=0.39 [0.29-0.51]; P<0.001) and major CVD events -- composite of CVD death, myocardial infarction, and ischemic and hemorrhagic stroke -- (HR=0.33 [0.19-0.55]; P<0.001) [28]. Greater benefits were observed for bedtime compared to awakening treatment with ARBs (HR=0.29 [0.17-0.51]; P<0.001) and CCBs (HR=0.46 [0.31-0.69]; P<0.001). CVD risk was higher in patients randomized to ingest the complete daily dose of all their medications upon awakening, without difference between the six different classes of BP-lowering therapy tested. Patients randomized to ingest at bedtime an ARB, in comparison to any other class of medication, with or without additional hypertension medication, however, evidenced significantly lower HR of CVD events (P<0.017) [98]. Considered together, the MAPEC Study results not only substantiate that the asleep SBP mean is the most significant prognostic marker of CVD morbidity and mortality, as previously suggested [22, 25, 26, 29, 31, 82, 84, 85, 88-92, 94-97], but they also document for the first time that decreasing the asleep SBP mean by properly timing hypertension medications significantly reduces CVD risk. These findings also have been substantiated for cohorts of participants in the MAPEC study with CKD [31], type 2 diabetes [30, 32], and resistant hypertension [33]. The beneficial effects of enhancing nighttime BP attenuation on CVD risk reduction necessitate further confirmation from prospective intervention trials, including the ongoing multicenter Hygia Project [105, 110-114].

The investigative protocols of the MAPEC Study and Hygia Project were designed to avert what we and others believe to be problems, limitations, or unanswered questions of previously conducted ABPM studies, including ones involving patients with CKD [28-33]. Specifically, the dipping/non-dipping BP pattern has been reported to have limited reproducibility when based only on a single 24h ABPM [106-109], making treatment-induced changes difficult to quantify accurately unless repeated, preferably 48h, ABPM is done during a sufficient long follow-up. Additionally, CVD risk does not seem to be significantly less in extreme-dippers than regular dippers [29, 89], even though very low asleep BP is likely to reduce vital organ perfusion. The only prospective evidence available today, derived from the results of the MAPEC Study, seems to overcome these objections and limitations, but further research is certainly required to completely resolve the concerns expressed by some.

Adherence and patient compliance might also be an influential factor in the efficacy of timed hypertension treatment. So far, there is no single randomized study yet published that compares adherence to awakening versus bedtime hypertension-treatment regimens. Although some studies have compared once versus twice-daily schedules of BP lowering medications [177, 178], they cannot be used to extrapolate adherence to awakening versus bedtime once-daily medication regimens. In the MAPEC Study, the finding that ingestion of the full daily dose of ≥1 hypertension medications at bedtime, compared with ingestion of all BP-lowering medications upon awakening, enhances medication safety, duration of action, and BP control, plus significantly reduces the risk of CVD events, is counter to an unsubstantiated assumption of compromised compliance to hypertension treatment when scheduled at bedtime.

DISCUSSION

The methods and technology for both inpatient and outpatient BP assessment are evolving rapidly. The increased application of ABPM reveals a complex picture of BP and its 24h patterning, suggesting new and clinically important targets and goals of therapy, e.g., control of morning BP rise, daytime and nighttime SBP/DBP means, plus normalization of a high-risk non-dipping 24h SBP/DBP profile [28-33, 89, 90, 96, 179]. The methods and concepts underlying the therapeutic strategies for the management of hypertension are also evolving rapidly. Herein, we presented evidence that the BP-lowering properties, and in some cases even safety, of often-prescribed medications of six different classes of hypertension therapy are significantly improved when the complete daily dose is ingested before bedtime at night rather than upon awakening in the morning. The exact mechanisms underlying these observed ingestion-time differences, although not yet completely understood, seem to involve, at least in part, circadian rhythm phenomena that affect drug pharmacokinetics and/or pharmacodynamics [57-75] relative to the staging of various other circadian rhythms, e.g., in natriuresis, nitric oxide, ANS, RAAS, etc., and day-night cycles in behavior, ambient environment, e.g., mental and physical activity and stress, posture, meal times, air temperature, noise, etc., that affect the 24h variation in blood vessel patency [4-8].

International practice guidelines recommend prescription of long-acting, once-daily hypertension medications having 24h efficacy [116] based on the assumptions they improve adherence to therapy, minimize BP variability, and provide smooth and consistent BP control. However, the typical morning-time habit of ingesting the entire daily dose of one or more hypertension medications with high 24h homogeneous and sustained efficacy is unlikely to alter the 24h BP profile. Given the high prevalence of the non-dipper BP pattern in the general population [4, 110, 119], and, particularly, in patients with CKD [100-105, 111], the routine recommendation that once-a-day therapies be taken in the morning is inappropriate, since two newly substantiated important clinical goals of hypertension pharmacotherapy -- normalization of the 24h BP pattern and control of asleep BP -- are unlikely to be achieved [60-64, 180, 181]. Findings of recently conducted long-term outcomes studies indicate asleep BP normalization can be best achieved when the full daily dose of hypertension medications are routinely ingested at bedtime rather than in the morning [28-33].

In patients with CKD, the prevalence of both non-dipper and riser BP patterns increases significantly with disease severity (Figure 3); indeed, the prevalence of the riser BP pattern, associated with highest CVD risk relative to all the other possible 24h BP patterns, is reported to be 2.5-fold greater in patients with than without CKD [105]. Thus, among patients with CKD, an elevated asleep BP mean constitutes the major criterion for the diagnoses of hypertension and inadequate therapeutic BP control, provided ABPM is routinely performed for sufficient duration (48h) and data are properly analyzed according to the actual patient's sleep and wake spans [180]. Patients with CKD who ingest the complete daily dose of ≥1 hypertension medications at bedtime, as compared to those who ingest the entire daily dose of all of them upon awakening, show significantly reduced asleep SBP/DBP means and attenuated prevalence of non-dipping, i.e., lower prevalence of these sensitive markers of CVD risk [31, 111].

Collectively, the clinical implications of the findings presented in this chapter are: (i) patients with CKD *require* around-the-clock ABPM to accurately diagnose hypertension, properly assess CVD risk, and establish and validate optimal therapeutic strategy; and (ii) bedtime hypertension chronotherapy that entails the full daily dose of ≥1 BP-lowering medications best normalizes the 24h BP profile, best decreases the sleep-time BP, and best reduces the risk of CVD morbidity and mortality of patients both with and without CKD [28-33, 182].

Consistent with the current available information, already acknowledged by the recent recommendation by the American Diabetes Association, i.e., that all hypertensive patients with diabetes ingest the complete daily dose of one or more BP-lowering medications at bedtime [183], bedtime hypertension treatment should also be recommended for hypertensive patients with CKD [180].

Nonetheless, to confirm the beneficial effects -- reduced risk of CVD events and target tissue and organ injury -- and safety of enhanced nighttime BP reduction by bedtime hypertension chronotherapy, we recognize the necessity to conduct future prospective intervention trials that incorporate 48h ABPM assessments and simultaneous diary recording of bed and wake times -- to accurately and reliably ascertain asleep BP level and dipping status -- at least annually during long-term follow-up evaluation, as done in the recently completed MAPEC Study and as now performed in the ongoing Hygia Project [105, 110-114].

ACKNOWLEDGMENTS

This chapter is dedicated to the memory of Franz Halberg, who introduced many of us into the field of Chronobiology, and Erhard Haus, our most beloved colleague and friend.

Research supported by unrestricted grants from Ministerio de Ciencia e Innovación (SAF2009-7028-FEDER); Consellería de Economía e Industria, Xunta de Galicia (INCITE-07-PXI-322003ES; INCITE08-E1R-322063ES; INCITE09-E2R-322099ES; IN845B-2010/ 114; 09CSA018322PR); European Research Development Fund and Consellería de Cultura, Educación e Ordenación Universitaria, Xunta de Galicia (CN2012/ 251 and CN2012/260); and Vicerrectorado de Investigación, University of Vigo.

Declaration of Interest: The authors report no conflicts of interest. The authors alone are responsible for the content and writing of the paper.

Reviewed by: Horia Balan, "Carol Davila" University of Medicine and Pharmacy, Bucharest, Romania.

References

[1] Duguay, D., Cermakian, N. The crosstalk between physiology and circadian clock proteins. *Chronobiol. Int.* 2009;26:1479-1513.

[2] Touitou, Y., Haus, E.,eds. *Biologic rhythms in clinical and laboratory medicine*. Berlin: Springer-Verlag, 1992;730 pp.

[3] Portaluppi, F., Vergnani, L., Manfredini, R., Fersini, C. Endocrine mechanisms of blood pressure rhythms. *Ann. N. Y. Acad. Sci.* 1996;783113-131.

[4] Hermida, R. C., Ayala, D. E., Portaluppi, F. Circadian variation of blood pressure: The basis for the chronotherapy of hypertension. *Adv. Drug Deliv. Rev.* 2007;59:904-922.

[5] Portaluppi, F., Smolensky, M. H. Circadian rhythm and environmental determinants of 24-hour blood pressure regulation in normal and hypertensive conditions. In: White, W. B., ed. *Blood Pressure Monitoring in Cardiovascular Medicine and Therapeutics.* Totowa, NJ: Humana Press, 2007;135-158.

[6] Smolensky, M. H., Hermida, R. C., Castriotta, R. J., Portaluppi, F. Role of sleep-wake cycle on blood pressure circadian rhythms and hypertension. *Sleep Med.* 2007;8:668-680.

[7] Portaluppi, F., Tiseo, R., Smolensky, M. H., Hermida, R. C., Ayala, D. E., Fabbian, F. Circadian rhythms and cardiovascular health. *Sleep Med. Rev.* 2012;16:151-166.

[8] Fabbian, F., Smolensky, M. H., Tiseo, R., Pala, M., Manfredini, R., Portaluppi, F. Dipper and non-dipper blood pressure 24-hour patterns: circadian rhythm-dependent physiologic and pathophysiologic mechanisms. *Chronobiol. Int.* 2013;30:17-30.

[9] Deedwania, P. C., Nelson, J. Pathophysiology of silent ischemia during daily life. *Circulation.* 1990;82;1296-1304.

[10] Cohen, M. C., Rohtla, K. M., Lavery, C. E., Muller, J. E., Middleman, M. A. Meta analysis of the morning excess of acute myocardial infarction and sudden cardiac death. *Am. J. Cardiol.* 1997;79:1512-1516.

[11] Chasen, C., Muller, J. E. Cardiovascular triggers and morning events. *Blood Press. Monit.* 1998;3:35-42.

[12] Elliot, W. J. Circadian variation in the timing of stroke onset. A meta-analysis. *Stroke.* 1998;29:992-996.

[13] Portaluppi, F., Manfredini, R., Fersini, C. From a static to a dynamic concept of risk: the circadian epidemiology of cardiovascular events. *Chronobiol. Int.* 1999;16:33-49.

[14] Pinotti, M., Bertolucci, C., Portaluppi, F., Colognesi, I., Frigato, E., Foa, A., Bernardi, F. Daily and circadian rhythms of tissue factor pathway inhibitor and factor VII activity. *Arterioscler. Thromb. Vasc. Biol.* 2005;25:646-649.

[15] Manfredini, R., Boari, B., Salmi, R., Fabbian, F., Pala, M., Tiseo, R., Portaluppi, F. Twenty-four-hour patterns in occurrence and pathophysiology of acute cardiovascular events and ischemic heart disease. *Chronobiol. Int.* 2013;30:6-16.

[16] Manfredini, R., Gallerani, M., Portaluppi, F., Salmi, R., Fersini, C. Chronobiological patterns of onset of acute cerebrovascular diseases. *Thromb. Res.* 1997;88:451-463.

[17] Casetta, I., Granieri, E., Portaluppi, F., Manfredini, R. Circadian variability in hemorrhagic stroke. *JAMA.* 2002;287:1266-1267.

[18] Manfredini, R., Portaluppi, F., Grandi, E., Fersini, C., Gallerani, M. Out-of-hospital sudden death referring to an emergency department. *J. Clin. Epidemiol.* 1996;49:865-868.

[19] Gallerani, M., Portaluppi, F., Grandi, E., Manfredini, R. Circadian rhythmicity in the occurrence of spontaneous acute dissection and rupture of thoracic aorta. *J. Thorac. Cardiovasc. Surg.* 1997;113:603-604.

[20] Mehta, H. R., Manfredini, R., Hassan, F., Sechtem, U., Bossone, E., Oh, J. K., Cooper, J. V., Smith, D. E., Portaluppi, F., Penn, M., Hutchison, S., Nienaber, C. A., Isselbacher, E. M., Eagle, K. A. Chronobiological patterns of acute aortic dissection. *Circulation.* 2002;106:1110-1115.

[21] Manfredini, R., Boari, B., Bressan, S., Gallerani, M., Salmi, R., Portaluppi, F., Mehta, R. H. Influence of circadian rhythm on mortality after myocardial infarction: data from a prospective cohort of emergency calls. *Am. J. Emerg. Med.* 2004;22:555-559.

[22] Agarwal, R., Andersen, M. J. Prognostic importance of ambulatory blood pressure recordings in patients with chronic kidney disease. *Kidney Int.* 2006;69:1175-1180.

[23] Liu, M., Takahashi, H., Morita, Y. Non-dipping is a potent predictor of cardiovascular mortality and is associated with autonomic dysfunction in haemodialysis patients. *Nephrol. Dial. Transplant.* 2003;18:563-569.

[24] Tripepi, G., Fagugli, R. M., Dattolo, P., Parlongo, G., Mallamaci, F., Buoncristiani, U., Zoccali, C. Prognostic value of 24-hour ambulatory blood pressure monitoring and of night/day ratio in nondiabetic, cardiovascular events-free hemodialysis patients. *Kidney Int.* 2005;68:1294-1302.

[25] Agarwal, R., Andersen, M. J. Blood pressure recordings within and outside the clinic and cardiovascular events in chronic kidney disease. *Am. J. Nephrol.* 2006;26:503-510.

[26] Minutolo, R., Agarwal, R., Borrelli, S., Chiodini, P., Bellizzi, V., Nappi, F., Cianciaruso, B., Zamboni, P., Conte, G., Gabbai, F. B., De Nicola, L. Prognostic role of ambulatory blood pressure measurement in patients with nondialysis chronic kidney disease. *Arch. Intern. Med.* 2011;171:1090-1098.

[27] Hermida, R. C. Ambulatory blood pressure monitoring in the prediction of cardiovascular events and effects of chronotherapy: Rationale and design of the MAPEC study. *Chronobiol. Int.* 2007;24:749-775.

[28] Hermida, R. C., Ayala, D. E., Mojón, A., Fernández, J. R. Influence of circadian time of hypertension treatment on cardiovascular risk: Results of the MAPEC study. *Chronobiol. Int.* 2010;27:1629-1651.

[29] Hermida, R. C., Ayala, D. E., Mojón, A., Fernández, J. R. Decreasing sleep-time blood pressure determined by ambulatory monitoring reduces cardiovascular risk. *J. Am. Coll. Cardiol.* 2011;58:1165-1173.

[30] Hermida, R. C., Ayala, D. E., Mojón, A., Fernández, J. R. Influence of time of day of blood pressure-lowering treatment on cardiovascular risk in hypertensive patients with type 2 diabetes. *Diabetes Care.* 2011;34:1270-1276.

[31] Hermida, R. C., Ayala, D. E., Mojón, A., Fernández, J. R. Bedtime dosing of antihypertensive medications reduces cardiovascular risk in CKD. *J. Am. Soc. Nephrol.* 2011;22:2313-2321.

[32] Hermida, R. C., Ayala, D. E., Mojón, A., Fernández, J. R. Sleep-time blood pressure as a therapeutic target for cardiovascular risk reduction in type 2 diabetes. *Am. J. Hypertens.* 2012;25:325-334.

[33] Ayala, D. E., Hermida, R. C., Mojón, A., Fernández, J. R. Cardiovascular risk of resistant hypertension: Dependence on treatment-time regimen of blood pressure-lowering medications. *Chronobiol. Int.* 2013;30:340-352.

[34] Hermida, R. C., Fernández, J. R., Ayala, D. E., Mojón, A., Alonso, I., Smolensky, M. Circadian rhythm of double (rate-pressure) product in healthy normotensive young subjects. *Chronobiol. Int.* 2001;18:475-489.

[35] Hermida, R. C., Ayala, D. E., Fernández, J. R., Mojón, A., Alonso, I., Calvo, C. Modeling the circadian variability of ambulatorily monitored blood pressure by multiple-component analysis. *Chronobiol. Int.* 2002;19:461-481.

[36] O'Brien, E., Sheridan, J., O'Malley, K. Dippers and non-dippers. *Lancet* (letter). 1998; 13:397.

[37] Sowers, J. R., Vlachakis, N. Circadian variation in plasma dopamine levels in man. *J. Endocrinol. Invest.* 1984;7:341-345.

[38] Furlan, R., Guzzetti, S., Crivellaro, W., Dassi, S., Tinelli, M., Baselli, G., Cerutti, S., Lombardi, F., Pagani, M., Malliani, A. Continuous 24-hour assessment of the neural regulation of systemic arterial pressure and RR variabilities in ambulant subjects. *Circulation.* 1990;81:537-547.

[39] Somers, V. K., Dyken, M. E., Mark, A. L., Abboud, F. M. Sympathetic-nerve activity during sleep in normal subjects. *N. Engl. J. Med.* 1993;328:303-307.

[40] Van de Borne, P., Nguyen, H., Biston, P., Linkowski, P., Degaute, J. P. Effects of wake and sleep stages on the 24-h autonomic control of blood pressure and heart rate in recumbent men. *Am. J. Physiol.* 1994;266 (2 Pt 2):H548-H554.

[41] Linsell, C. R., Lightman, S. L., Mullen, P. E., Brown, M. J., Causon, R. C. Circadian rhythms of epinephrine and norepinephrine in man. *J. Clin. Endocrinol. Metab.* 1985; 60:1210-1215.

[42] Lakatua, D. J., Haus, E., Halberg, F., Halberg, E., Wendt, H. W., Sackett-Lundeen, L. L., Berg, H. G., Kawasaki, T., Ueno, M., Uezono, K., Matsuoka, M., Omae, T. Circadian characteristics of urinary epinephrine and norepinephrine from healthy young women in Japan and US. *Chronobiol. Int.* 1986;3:189-195.

[43] Kawano, Y., Tochikubo, O., Minamisawa, K., Miyajima, E., Ishii, M. Circadian variation of hemodynamics in patients with essential hypertension: comparison between early morning and evening. *J. Hypertens.* 1994;12:1405-1412.

[44] Gordon, R. D., Wolfe, L. K., Island, D. P., Liddle, G. W. A diurnal rhythm in plasma renin activity in man. *J. Clin. Invest.* 1966;45:1587-1592.

[45] Katz, F., Romfh, P., Smith, J. A. Diurnal variation of plasma aldosterone, cortisol and renin activity in supine man. *J. Clin. Endocrinol. Metab.* 1975;40:125-134.

[46] Bartter, F. C., Chan, J. C. M., Simpson, H. W. Chronobiological aspect of plasma renin activity, plasma aldosterone and urinary electrolytes. In: Krieger, D. T., ed. *Endocrine Rhythms.* New York: Raven, 1979:49-132.

[47] Cugini, P., Manconi, E., Serdoz, N., Mancini, A., Meucci, R., Scavo, D. Rhythm characteristics of plasma renin, aldosterone and cortisol in five types of mesor-hypertension. *J. Endocrinol. Invest.* 1980;3:143-149.

[48] Cugini, P., Letizia, C., Scavo, D. The circadian rhythmicity of serum angiotensin converting enzyme: its phasic relation with the circadian cycle of plasma renin and aldosterone. *Chronobiologia.* 1988;15:229-232.

[49] Angeli, A., Gatti, G., Masera, R. Chronobiology of the hypothalamic-pituitary-adrenal and renin-angiotensin-aldosterone systems. In: Touitou, Y., Haus, E., eds. *Biologic Rhythms in Clinical and Laboratory Medicine*. Berlin: Springer-Verlag, 1992:292-314.
[50] Kool, M. J., Wijnen, J. A., Derkx, F. H., Struijker Boudier, H. A., Van Bortel, L. M. Diurnal variation in prorenin in relation to other humoral factors and hemodynamics. *Am. J. Hypertens.* 1994;7:723-730.
[51] Nicholls, M. G., Espiner, E. A., Ikram, H., Maslowski, A. H., Hamilton, E. J., Bones, P. J. Hormone and blood pressure relationships in primary aldosteronism. *Clin. Exp. Hypertens. A.* 1984;6:1441-1458.
[52] Winters, C. J., Sallman, A. L., Vesely, D. L. Circadian rhythm of prohormone atrial natriuretic peptides 1-30, 31-67 and 99-126 in man. *Chronobiol. Int.* 1988;5:403-409.
[53] Portaluppi, F., Trasforini, G., Margutti, A., Vergnani, L., Ambrosio, M. R., Rossi, R., Bagni, B., Pansini, R., degli Uberti, E. C. Circadian rhythm of calcitonin gene-related peptide in uncomplicated essential hypertension. *J. Hypertens.* 1992;10:1227-1234.
[54] Sothern, R. B., Vesely, D. L., Kanabrocki, E. L., Hermida, R. C., Bremner, F. W., Third, J. L. H. C., Boles, M. A., Nemchausky, B. M., Olwin, J. H., Scheving, L. E. Temporal (circadian) and functional relationship between atrial natriuretic peptides and blood pressure. *Chronobiol. Int.* 1995;12:106-120.
[55] Kanabrocki, E. L., Third, J. L. H. C., Ryan, M. D., Nemchausky, B. A., Shirazi, P., Scheving, L. E., McCormick, J. B., Hermida, R. C., Bremmer, F. W., Hoppensteadt, D. A., Fareed, J., Olwin, J. H. Circadian relationship of serum uric acid and nitric oxide. *JAMA.* 2000;283:2240-2241.
[56] Kanabrocki, E. L., George, M., Hermida, R. C., Messmore, H. L., Ryan, M. D., Ayala, D. E., Hoppensteadt, D. A., Fareed, J., Bremmer, F. W., Third, J. L. H. C., Shirazi, P., Nemchausky, B. A. Day-night variations in blood levels of nitric oxide, T-TFPI and E-selectin. *Clin. Appl. Thrombosis/Hemostasis.* 2001;7:339-345.
[57] Hermida, R. C., Smolensky, M. H. Chronotherapy of hypertension. *Curr. Opin. Nephrol. Hypertens.* 2004;13:501-505.
[58] Hermida, R. C., Ayala, D. E., Calvo, C. Administration time-dependent effects of antihypertensive treatment on the circadian pattern of blood pressure. *Curr. Opin. Nephrol. Hypertens.* 2005;14:453-459.
[59] Ohmori, M., Fujimura, A. ACE inhibitors and chronotherapy. *Clin. Exp. Hypertens.* 2005;2:179-185.
[60] Hermida, R. C., Ayala, D. E., Calvo, C., Portaluppi, F., Smolensky, M. H. Chronotherapy of hypertension: Administration-time dependent effects of treatment on the circadian pattern of blood pressure. *Adv. Drug Deliv. Rev.* 2007;59:923-939.
[61] Smolensky, M. H., Hermida, R. C., Ayala, D. E., Tiseo, R., Portaluppi, F. Administration-time-dependent effect of blood pressure-lowering medications: Basis for the chronotherapy of hypertension. *Blood Press. Monit.* 2010;15:173-180.
[62] Hermida, R. C., Ayala, D. E., Fernández, J. R., Portaluppi, F., Fabbian, F., Smolensky, M. H. Circadian rhythms in blood pressure regulation and optimization of hypertension treatment with ACE inhibitor and ARB medications. *Am. J. Hypertens.* 2011;24:383-391.
[63] Smolensky, M. H., Siegel, R. A., Haus, E., Hermida, R. C., Portaluppi, F. Biological rhythms, drug delivery, and chronotherapeutics. In: Siepmann, J., Siegel, R. A.,

Rathbone, M. J., eds. *Fundamentals and Applications of Controlled Release Drug Delivery*. Heildelberg: Springer-Verlag, 2012:359-443.

[64] Hermida, R. C., Ayala, D. E., Fernández, J. R., Mojón, A., Smolensky, M. H., Fabbian, F., Portaluppi, F. Administration-time-differences in effects of hypertension medications on ambulatory blood pressure regulation. *Chronobiol. Int.* 2013;30:280-314.

[65] Reinberg, A., Smolensky, M. H. Circadian changes of drug disposition in man. *Clin. Pharmacokinet.* 1982;7:401-420.

[66] Koopman, M. G., Koomen, G. C., Krediet, R. T., de Moor, E. A., Hoek, F. J., Arisz, L. Circadian rhythm of glomerular filtration rate in normal individuals. *Clin. Sci. (Lond).* 1989;77:105-111.

[67] Bruguerolle, B., Lemmer, B. Recent advances in chronopharmacokinetics: methodological problems. *Life Sci.* 1993;52:1809-1824.

[68] Gupta, S. K., Yih, B. M., Atkinson, L., Longstreth, J. The effect of food, time of dosing and body composition on the pharmacokinetics and pharmacodynamics of verapamil and norverapamil. *J. Clin. Pharmacol.* 1995;35:1083-1093.

[69] Bélanger, P. M., Bruguerolle, B., Labrecque, G. Rhythms in pharmacokinetics: Absorption, distribution, metabolism. In: Redfern, P. H., Lemmer, B., eds. Physiology and Pharmacology of Biological Rhythms. *Handbook of Experimental Pharmacology series,* vol 125. New York: Springer-Verlag, 1997:177-204.

[70] Lemmer, B. Chronopharmacokinetics—implications for drug treatment. *J. Pharm. Pharmacol.* 1999;51:887-890.

[71] Labrecque, G., Beauchamp, D. Rhythms and pharmacokinetics. In: Redfern, P. H., ed. *Chronotherapeutics*. London: Pharmaceutical Press, 2003:75-110.

[72] Okyar, A., Dressler, C., Hanafy, A., Baktir, G., Lemmer, B., Spahn-L49uth H. Circadian variations in exsorptive transport: In-situ intestinal perfusion data and in-vivo relevance. *Chronobiol. Int.* 2012;29:443-453.

[73] Smolensky, M. H., Portaluppi, F. Chronopharmacology and chronotherapy of cardiovascular medications: relevance to prevention and treatment of coronary heart disease. *Am. Heart J.* 1999;137 (4 Pt 2):S14-S24.

[74] Smolensky, M. H., Haus, E. Circadian rhythms in clinical medicine with applications to hypertension. *Am. J. Hypertens.* 2001;14 (9, Part 2):280S-290S.

[75] Witte, K., Lemmer, B. Rhythms and pharmacodynamics. In: Redfern, P. H., ed. *Chronotherapeutics*. London: Pharmaceutical Press, 2003:111-126.

[76] Verdecchia, P., Porcellati, C., Schillaci, G., Borgioni, C., Ciucci, A., Battistell, M., Guerrieri, M., Gatteschi, C., Zampi, I., Santucci, A., Santucci, C., Reboldi, G. Ambulatory blood pressure: an independent predictor of prognosis in essential hypertension. *Hypertension.* 1994;24:793-801.

[77] Nakano, S., Fukuda, M., Hotta, F., Ito, T., Ishii, T., Kitazawa, M., Nishizawa, M., Kigoshi, T., Uchida, K. Reversed circadian blood pressure rhythm is associated with occurrences of both fatal and nonfatal events in NIDDM subjects. *Diabetes.* 1998; 47: 1501-1506.

[78] Staessen, J. A., Thijs, L., Fagard, R., O´Brien, E. T., Clement, D., de Leeuw, P. W., Mancia, G., Nachev, C., Palatini, P., Parati, G., Tuomilehto, J., Webster, J., for the Systolic Hypertension in Europe (Syst-Eur) trial investigators. Predicting

cardiovascular risk using conventional vs ambulatory blood pressure in older patients with systolic hypertension. *JAMA.* 1999;282:539-546.

[79] Sturrock, N. D., George, E., Pound, N., Stevenson, J., Peck, G. M., Sowter, H. Non-dipping circadian blood pressure and renal impairment are associated with increased mortality in diabetes mellitus. *Diabet. Med.* 2000;17:360-364.

[80] Kario, K., Pickering, T. G., Matsuo, T., Hoshide, S., Schwartz, J. E., Shimada, K. Stroke prognosis and abnormal nocturnal blood pressure falls in older hypertensives. *Hypertension.* 2001;38:852-857.

[81] Ohkubo, T., Hozawa, A., Yamaguchi, J., Kikuya, M., Ohmori, K., Michimata, M., Matsubara, M., Hashimoto, J., Hoshi, H., Araki, T., Tsuji, I., Satoh, H., Hisamichi, S., Imai, Y. Prognostic significance of the nocturnal decline in blood pressure in individuals with and without high 24-h blood pressure: the Ohasama study. *J. Hypertens.* 2002;20:2183-2189.

[82] Dolan, E., Stanton, A., Thijs, L., Hinedi, K., Atkins, N., McClory, S., Den Hond, E., McCormack, P., Staessen, J. A., O'Brien, E. Superiority of ambulatory over clinic blood pressure measurement in predicting mortality: the Dublin outcome study. *Hypertension.* 2005;46:156-161.

[83] Ingelsson, E., Bjorklund-Bodegard, K., Lind, L., Arnlov, J., Sundstrom, J. Diurnal blood pressure pattern and risk of congestive heart failure. *JAMA.* 2006;295:2859-2866.

[84] Astrup, A. S., Nielsen, F. S., Rossing, P., Ali, S., Kastrup, J., Smidt, U. M., Parving, H. H. Predictors of mortality in patients with type 2 diabetes with or without diabetic nephropathy: a follow-up study. *J. Hypertens.* 2007;25:2479-2485.

[85] Boggia, J., Li, Y., Thijs, L., Hansen, T. W., Kikuya, M., Björklund-Bodegård, K., Richart, T., Ohkubo, T., Kuznetsova, T., Torp-Pedersen, C. H., Lind, L., Ibsen, H., Imai, Y., Wang, J., Sandoya, E., O'Brien, E., Staessen, J. A. Prognostic accuracy of day versus night ambulatory blood pressure: a cohort study. *Lancet.* 2007;370:1219-1229.

[86] Brotman, D. J., Davidson, M. B., Boumitri, M., Vidt, D. G. Impaired diurnal blood pressure variation and all-cause mortality. *Am. J. Hypertens.* 2008;21:92-97.

[87] Eguchi, K., Pickering, T. G., Hoshide, S., Ishikawa, J., Ishikawa, S., Schwartz, J., Shimada, K., Kario, K. Ambulatory blood pressure is a better marker than clinic blood pressure in predicting cardiovascular events in patients with/without type 2 diabetes. *Am. J. Hypertens.* 2008;21:443-450.

[88] Salles, G. F., Cardoso, C. R., Muxfeldt, E. S. Prognostic influence of office and ambulatory blood pressures in resistant hypertension. *Arch. Intern. Med.* 2008;168: 2340-2346.

[89] Hermida, R. C., Ayala, D. E., Fernández, J. R., Mojón, A. Sleep-time blood pressure: Prognostic value and relevance as a therapeutic target for cardiovascular risk reduction. *Chronobiol. Int.* 2013;30:68-86.

[90] Hermida, R. C., Ayala, D. E., Mojón, A., Fernández, J. R. Blunted sleep-time relative blood pressure decline increases cardiovascular risk independent of blood pressure level -- The "normotensive non-dipper" paradox. *Chronobiol. Int.* 2013;30:87-98.

[91] Kikuya, M., Ohkubo, T., Asayama, K., Metoki, H., Obara, T., Saito, S., Hashimoto, J., Totsune, K., Hoshi, H., Satoh, H., Imai, Y. Ambulatory blood pressure and 10-year risk of cardiovascular and noncardiovascular mortality. The Ohasama Study. *Hypertension.* 2005;45:240-245.

[92] Ben-Dov, I. Z., Kark, J. D., Ben-Ishay, D., Mekler, J., Ben-Arie, L., Bursztyn, M. Predictors of all-cause mortality in clinical ambulatory monitoring. Unique aspects of blood pressure during sleep. *Hypertension.* 2007;49:1235-1241.

[93] Bouhanick, B., Bongard, V., Amar, J., Bousquel, S., Chamontin, B. Prognostic value of nocturnal blood pressure and reverse-dipping status on the occurrence of cardiovascular events in hypertensive diabetic patients. *Diabetes Metab.* 2008;34:560-567.

[94] Fagard, R. H., Celis, H., Thijs, L., Staessen, J. A., Clement, D. L., De Buyzere, M. L., De Bacquer, D. A. Daytime and nighttime blood pressure as predictors of death and cause-specific cardiovascular events in hypertension. *Hypertension.* 2008;51:55-61.

[95] Fan, H. Q., Li, Y., Thijs, L., Hansen, T. W., Boggia, J., Kikuya, M., Björklund-Bodegard, K., Richart, T., Ohkubo, T., Jeppesen, J., Torp-Pedersen, C., Dolan, E., Kuznetsova, T., Stolarz-Skrzypek, K., Tikhonoff, V., Malyutina, S., Casiglia, E., Nikitin, Y., Lind, L., Sandoya, E., Kawecka-Jaszcz, K., Imai, Y., Ibsen, H., O'Brien, E., Wang, J., Staessen, J. A. Prognostic value of isolated nocturnal hypertension on ambulatory measurement in 8711 individuals from 10 populations. *J. Hypertens.* 2010; 28: 2036-2045.

[96] Hermida, R. C., Ayala, D. E., Mojón, A., Fernández, J. R. Sleep-time blood pressure and the prognostic value of isolated-office and masked hypertension. *Am. J. Hypertens.* 2012; 25:297-305.

[97] Amar, J., Vernier, I., Rossignol, E., Bongard, V., Arnaud, C., Conte, J. J., Salvador, M., Chamontin, B. Nocturnal blood pressure and 24-hour pulse pressure are potent indicators of mortality in hemodialysis patients. *Kidney Int.* 2000;57:2485-2491.

[98] Hermida, R. C., Ayala, D. E., Mojón, A., Fernández, J. R. Cardiovascular risk of essential hypertension: Influence of class, number, and treatment-time regimen of hypertension medications. *Chronobiol. Int.* 2013;30:315-327.

[99] Hermida, R. C., Ayala, D. E., Mojón, A., Fernández, J. R. Role of time-of-day of hypertension treatment on the J-shaped relationship between blood pressure and cardiovascular risk. *Chronobiol. Int.* 2013;30:328-339.

[100] Portaluppi, F., Montanari, L., Ferlini, M., Gilli, P. Altered circadian rhythms of blood pressure and heart rate in non-hemodialysis chronic renal failure. *Chronobiol. Int.* 1990; 7: 321-327.

[101] Agarwal, R., Andersen, M. J. Correlates of systolic hypertension in patients with chronic kidney disease. *Hypertension.* 2005;46:514–520.

[102] Davidson, M. B., Hix, J. K., Vidt, D. G., Brotman, D. J. Association of impaired diurnal blood pressure variation with a subsequent decline in glomerular filtration rate. *Arch. Intern. Med.* 2006;166:846-852.

[103] Agarwal, R., Peixoto, A. J., Santos, S. F. F., Zoccali, C. Out-of-office blood pressure monitoring in chronic kidney disease. *Blood Press. Monit.* 2009;14:2-11.

[104] Pogue, V., Rahman, M., Lipkowitz, M., Toto, R., Miller, E., Faulkner, M., Rostand, S., Hiremath, L., Sika, M., Kendrick, C., Hu, B., Greene, T., Appel, L., Phillips, R. A.; African American Study of Kidney Disease and Hypertension Collaborative Research Group. Disparate estimates of hypertension control from ambulatory and clinic blood pressure measurements in hypertensive kidney disease. *Hypertension.* 2009;53:20-27.

[105] Mojón, A., Ayala, D. E., Piñeiro, L., Otero, A., Crespo, J. J., Moyá, A., Bóveda, J., Pérez de Lis, J., Fernández, J. R., Hermida, R. C., on behalf of the Hygia Project

Investigators. Comparison of ambulatory blood pressure parameters of hypertensive patients with and without chronic kidney disease. *Chronobiol. Int.* 2013;30:145-158.

[106] Hermida, R. C., Calvo, C., Ayala, D. E., Fernández, J. R., Ruilope, L. M., López, J. E. Evaluation of the extent and duration of the "ABPM effect" in hypertensive patients. *J. Am. Coll. Cardiol.* 2002;40:710-717.

[107] Hermida, R. C., Ayala, D. E. Sampling requirements for ambulatory blood pressure monitoring in the diagnosis of hypertension in pregnancy. *Hypertension.* 2003;42:619-624.

[108] Hermida, R. C., Ayala, D. E., Fernandez, J. R., Mojón, A., Calvo, C. Influence of measurement duration and frequency on ambulatory blood pressure monitoring. *Rev. Esp. Cardiol.* 2007;60:131-138.

[109] Hermida, R. C., Ayala, D. E., Fontao, M. J., Mojón, A., Fernández, J. R. Ambulatory blood pressure monitoring: Importance of sampling rate and duration -- 48 versus 24 hours -- on the accurate assessment of cardiovascular risk. *Chronobiol. Int.* 2013;30:55-67.

[110] Ayala, D. E., Moyá, A., Crespo, J. J., Castiñeira, C., Domínguez-Sardiña, M., Gomara, S., Sineiro, E., Mojón, A., Fontao, M. J., Hermida, R. C., on behalf of the Hygia Project Investigators. Circadian pattern of ambulatory blood pressure in hypertensive patients with and without type 2 diabetes. *Chronobiol. Int.* 2013;30:99-115.

[111] Crespo, J. J., Piñeiro, L., Otero, A., Castiñeira, C., Ríos, M. T., Regueiro, A., Mojón, A., Lorenzo, S., Ayala, D. E., Hermida, R. C., on behalf of the Hygia Project Investigators. Administration-time-dependent effects of hypertension treatment on ambulatory blood pressure in patients with chronic kidney disease. *Chronobiol. Int.* 2013; 30:159-175.

[112] Hermida, R. C., Ríos, M. T., Crespo, J. J., Moya, A., Domínguez-Sardiña, M., Otero, A., Sánchez, J. J., Mojón, A., Fernández, J. R., Ayala, D. E., on behalf on the Hygia Project Investigators. Treatment-time regimen of hypertension medications significantly affects ambulatory blood pressure and clinical characteristics of patients with resistant hypertension *Chronobiol. Int.* 2013;30:192-206.

[113] Moyá, A., Crespo, J. J., Ayala, D. E., Ríos, M. T., Pousa, L., Callejas, P. A., Salgado, J. L., Mojón, A., Fernández, J. R., Hermida, R. C., on behalf on the Hygia Project Investigators. Effects of time-of-day of hypertension treatment on ambulatory blood pressure and clinical characteristics of patients with type 2 diabetes. *Chronobiol. Int.* 2013; 30:116-131.

[114] Ríos, M. T., Domínguez-Sardiña, M., Ayala, D. E., Gomara, S., Sineiro, E., Pousa, L., Callejas, P. A., Fontao, M. J., Fernández, J. R., Hermida, R. C., on behalf of the Hygia Project Investigators. Prevalence and clinical characteristics of isolated-office and true resistant hypertension determined by ambulatory blood pressure monitoring. *Chronobiol. Int.* 2013;30:207-220.

[115] Levey, A. S., Eckardt, K. U., Tsukamoto, Y., Levin, A., Coresh, J., Rossert, J., De Zeeuw, D., Hostetter, T. H., Lameire, N., Eknoyan, G. Definition and classification of chronic kidney disease: a position statement from Kidney Disease: Improving Global Outcomes (KDIGO). *Kidney Int.* 2005;67:2089-2100.

[116] Mancia, G., Fagard, R., Narkiewicz, K., Redón, J., Zanchetti, A., Böhm, M., Christiaens, T., Cifkova, R., De Backer, G., Dominiczak, A., Galderisi, M., Grobbee, D. E., Jaarsma, T., Kirchhof, P., Kjeldsen, S. E., Laurent, S., Manolis, A. J., Nilsson, P.

M., Ruilope, L. M., Schmieder, R. E., Sirnes, P. A., Sleight, P., Viigimaa, M., Waeber, B., Zannad, F. 2013 ESH/ESC Guidelines for the management of arterial hypertension: The Task Force for the management of arterial hypertension of the European Society of Hypertension (ESH) and of the European Society of Cardiology (ESC). *J. Hypertens.* 2013; 31:1281-1357.

[117] Fernández, J. R., Hermida, R. C. Inferential statistical method for analysis of nonsinusoidal hybrid time series with unequidistant observations. *Chronobiol. Int.* 1998;15:191-204.

[118] Fernández, J. R., Mojón, A., Hermida, R. C. Comparison of parameters from rhythmometric models with multiple components on hybrid data. *Chronobiol. Int.* 2004; 21:467-482.

[119] Hermida, R. C., Calvo, C., Ayala, D. E., Mojón, A., López, J. E. Relationship between physical activity and blood pressure in dipper and nondipper hypertensive patients. *J. Hypertens.* 2002;20:1097-1104.

[120] Smith, D. H., Neutel, J. M., Lacourciere, Y., Kempthorne-Rawson, J. Prospective, randomized, open-label, blinded-endpoint (PROBE) designed trials yield the same results as double-blind, placebo-controlled trials with respect to ABPM measurements. *J. Hypertens.* 2003;21:1291-1298.

[121] Crespo, C., Aboy, M., Fernández, J. R., Mojón, A. Automatic identification of activity-rest periods based on actigraphy. *Med. Biol. Eng. Comput.* 2012;50:329-340.

[122] Crespo, C., Fernández, J. R., Aboy, M., Mojón, A. Clinical application of a novel automatic algorithm for actigraphy-based activity and rest period identification to accurately determine awake and asleep ambulatory blood pressure parameters and cardiovascular risk. *Chronobiol. Int.* 2013;30:43-54.

[123] Palatini, P., Mos, L., Motolese, M., Mormino, P., Del Torre, M., Varotto, L., Pavan, E., Pessina, A. C. Effect of evening versus morning benazepril on 24-hour blood pressure: a comparative study with continuous intraarterial monitoring. *Int. J. Clin. Pharmacol. Ther. Toxicol.* 1993;31:295-300.

[124] Middeke, M., Kluglich, M., Holzgreve, H. Chronopharmacology of captopril plus hydrochlorothiazide in hypertension: morning versus evening dosing. *Chronobiol. Int.* 1991;8:506-510.

[125] Witte, K., Weisser, K., Neubeck, M., Mutschler, E., Lehmann, K., Hopf, R., Lemmer, B. Cardiovascular effects, pharmacokinetics and converting enzyme inhibition of enalapril after morning versus evening administration. *Clin. Pharmacol. Ther.* 1993; 54:177-186.

[126] Sunaga, K., Fujimura, A., Shiga, T., Ebihara, A. Chronopharmacology of enalapril in hypertensive patients. *Eur. J. Clin. Pharmacol.* 1995;48:441-445.

[127] Pechère-Bertschi, A., Nussberger, J., Decosterd, L., Armagnac, C., Sissmann, J., Bouroudian, M., Brunner, H. R., Burnier, M. Renal response to the angiotensin II receptor subtype 1 antagonist irbesartan versus enalapril in hypertensive patients. *J. Hypertens.* 1998;16:385-393.

[128] Kohno, I., Ijiri, H., Takusagawa, M., Yin, D. F., Sano, S., Ishihara, T., Sawanobori, T., Komori, S., Tamura, K. Effect of imidapril in dipper and nondipper hypertensive patients: comparison between morning and evening administration. *Chronobiol. Int.* 2000; 17:209-219.

[129] Macchiarulo, C., Pieri, R., Mitolo, D. C., Pirrelli, A. Management of antihypertensive treatment with Lisinopril: a chronotherapeutic approach. *Eur. Rev. Med. Pharmacol. Sci.* 1999;3:269-275.

[130] Morgan, T., Anderson, A., Jones, E. The effect on 24 h blood pressure control of an angiotensin converting enzyme inhibitor (perindopril) administered in the morning or at night. *J. Hypertens.* 1997;15:205-211.

[131] Palatini, P. Can an angiotensin-converting enzyme inhibitor with a short half-life effectively lower blood pressure for 24 hours? *Am. Heart J.* 1992;123:1421-1425.

[132] Palatini, P., Racioppa, A., Raule, G., Zaninotto, M., Penzo, M., Pessina, A. C. Effect of timing of administration on the plasma ACE inhibitory activity and the antihypertensive effect of quinapril. *Clin. Pharmacol. Ther.* 1992;52:378-383.

[133] Myburgh, D. P., Verho, M., Botes, J. H., Erasmus, Th. P., Luus, H. G. 24-Hour pressure control with ramipril: comparison of once-daily morning and evening administration. *Curr. Ther. res.* 1995;56:1298-1306.

[134] Zaslavskaia, R. M., Narmanova, O. Z., Teiblium, M. M., Kalimurzina, B. S. Time-dependent effects of ramipril in patients with hypertension of 2 stage. *Klin. Mad. (Mosk.).* 1999;77:41-44.

[135] Hermida, R. C., Ayala, D. E. Chronotherapy with the angiotensin-converting enzyme inhibitor ramipril in essential hypertension: Improved blood pressure control with bedtime dosing. *Hypertension.* 2009;54:40-46.

[136] Hermida, R. C., Ayala, D. E., Fontao, M. J., Mojón, A., Alonso, I., Fernández, J. R. Administration-time-dependent effects of spirapril on ambulatory blood pressure in uncomplicated essential hypertension. *Chronobiol. Int.* 2010;27:560-574.

[137] Kuroda, T., Kario, K., Hoshide, S., Hashimoto, T., Nomura, Y., Saito, Y., Mito, H., Shimada, K. Effects of bedtime vs. morning administration of the long-acting lipophilic angiotensin-converting enzyme inhibitor trandolapril on morning blood pressure in hypertensive patients. *Hypertens. Res.* 2004;27:15-20.

[138] Balan, H., Popescu, E., Angelescu, G. Comparing different treatment schedules of Zomen (zofenopril). *Rom. J. Intern. Med.* 2011;49:75-84.

[139] Qiu, Y. G., Zhu, J. H., Tao, Q. M., Zheng, P., Chen, J. Z., Hu, S. J., Zhang, F. R., Zheng, L. R., Zhao, L. L., Yao, X. Y. (2005). Captopril administered at night restores the diurnal blood pressure rhythm in adequately controlled, nondipping hypertensives. *Cardiovasc. Drugs Ther.* 19:189-195.

[140] Fujimura, A., Ebihara, A., Shiigai, T., Shimada, K., Tagawa, H., Gomi, T., Nakamura, Y., Suzuki, M., Yokozuka, H. A. melioration of enalapril-induced dry cough by changing dosing time from morning to evening: a preliminary trial. *Jpn. J. Clin. Pharmacol. Ther.* 1999;30:741-744.

[141] Hermida, R. C., Calvo, C., Ayala, D. E., Domínguez, M. J., Covelo, M., Fernández, J. R., Mojón, A., López, J. E. Administration-time-dependent effects of valsartan on ambulatory blood pressure in hypertensive subjects. *Hypertension.* 2003;42:283-290.

[142] Hermida, R. C., Calvo, C., Ayala, D. E., Mojón, A., Rodríguez, M., Chayán, L., López, J. E., Fontao, M. J., Soler, R., Fernández, J. R. Administration time-dependent effects of valsartan on ambulatory blood pressure in elderly hypertensive subjects. *Chronobiol. Int.* 2005;22:755-776.

[143] Hermida, R. C., Calvo, C., Ayala, D. E., Fernández, J. R., Covelo, M., Mojón, A., López, J. E. Treatment of non-dipper hypertension with bedtime administration of valsartan. *J. Hypertens.* 2005;23:1913-1922.

[144] Hermida, R. C., Ayala, D. E., Chayán, L., Mojón, A., Fernández, J. R. Administration-time-dependent effects of olmesartan on the ambulatory blood pressure of essential hypertension patients. *Chronobiol. Int.* 2009;26:61-79.

[145] Hermida, R. C., Ayala, D. E., Chayán, L., Mojón, A., Fernández, J. R. Comparison of the efficacy of morning versus bedtime administration of 40 mg/day olmesartan in essential hypertension. *J. Clin. Hypertens.* 2008;10(Suppl. A):A22.

[146] Hermida, R. C., Ayala, D. E., Fernández, J. R., Calvo, C. Comparison of the efficacy of morning versus evening administration of telmisartan in essential hypertension. *Hypertension.* 2007;50:715-722.

[147] Hermida, R. C., Calvo, C., Ayala, D. E., López, J. E. Decrease in urinary albumin excretion associated to the normalization of nocturnal blood pressure in hypertensive subjects. *Hypertension.* 2005;46:960-968.

[148] Kario, K., Hoshide, S., Shimizu, M., Yano, Y., Eguchi, K., Ishikawa, J., Ishikawa, S., Shimada, K. Effects of dosing time of angiotensin II receptor blockade titrated by self-measured blood pressure recordings on cardiorenal protection in hypertensives: The Japan Morning Surge-Target Organ Protection (J-TOP) study. *J. Hypertens.* 2010; 28: 1574-1583.

[149] Mengden, T., Binswanger, B., Spühler, T., Weisser, B., Vetter, W. The use of self-measured blood pressure determinations in assessing dynamics of drug compliance in a study with amlodipine once a day, morning versus evening. *J. Hypertens.* 1993; 11: 1403-1411.

[150] Nold, G., Strobel, G., Lemmer, B. Morning vs evening amlodipine treatment: effect on circadian blood pressure profile in essential hypertensive patients. *Blood Press. Monit.* 1998; 3:17-25.

[151] Qiu, Y. G., Chen, J. Z., Zhu, J. H., Yao, X. Y. Differential effects of morning or evening dosing of amlodipine on circadian blood pressure and heart rate. *Cardiovasc. Drugs Ther.* 2003;17:335-341.

[152] Hermida, R. C., Calvo, C., Ayala, D. E., López, J. E., Rodríguez, M., Covelo, M. Administration time-dependent effects of amlodipine on ambulatory blood pressure in patients with essential hypertension. *Am. J. Hypertens.* 2005;18 (5 part 2):61A.

[153] Kitahara, Y., Saito, F., Akao, M., Fujita, H., Takahashi, A., Taguchi, H., Hino, T., Otsuka, Y., Kushiro, T., Kanmatsuse, K. Effect of morning and bedtime dosing with cilnidipine on blood pressure, heart rate, and sympathetic nervous activity in essential hypertensive patients. *J. Cardiovasc. Pharmacol.* 2004;43:68-73.

[154] Kohno, I., Iwasaki, H., Okutani, M., Mochizuki, Y., Sano, S., Satoh, Y., Ishihara, T., Ishii, H., Mukaiyama, S., Ijiri, H., Komori, S., Tamura, K. Administration-time-dependent effects of diltiazem on the 24-hour blood pressure profile of essential hypertension patients. *Chronobiol. Int.* 1997;14:71-84.

[155] Fogari, R., Malacco, E., Tettamanti, F., Gnemmi, A. E., Milani, M. Evening vs. morning isradipine sustained release in essential hypertension: a double-blind study with 24 h ambulatory monitoring. *Br. J. Clin. Pharmacol.* 1993;35:51-54.

[156] Portaluppi, F., Vergnani, L., Manfredini, R., degli Uberti, E. C., Fersini, C. Time-dependent effect of isradipine on the nocturnal hypertension in chronic renal failure. *Am. J. Hypertens.* 1995;8:719-726.

[157] Greminger, P., Suter, P. M., Holm, D., Kobelt, R., Vetter, W. Morning versus evening administration of nifedipine gastrointestinal therapeutic system in the management of essential hypertension. *Clin. Invest.* 1994;72:864-869.

[158] Hermida, R. C., Calvo, C., Ayala, D. E., Lopez, J. E., Rodriguez, M., Chayan, L., Mojon, A., Fontao, M. J., Fernandez, J. R. Dose- and administration-time-dependent effects of nifedipine GITS on ambulatory blood pressure in hypertensive subjects. *Chronobiol. Int.* 2007;24:471-493.

[159] Hermida, R. C., Ayala, D. E., Mojón, A., Fernández, J. R. Chronotherapy with nifedipine GITS in hypertensive patients: Improved efficacy and safety with bedtime dosing. *Am. J. Hypertens.* 2008;21:948-954.

[160] White, W. B., Mansoor, G. A., Pickering, T. G., Vidt, D. G, Hutchinson HG, Johnson RB, Noveck R. Differential effects of morning and evening dosing of nisoldipine ER on circadian blood pressure and heart rate. *Am. J. Hypertens.* 1999;12:806-814.

[161] Meilhac, B., Mallion, J. M., Carre, A., Chanudet, X., Poggi, L., Gosse, P., Dallocchio, M. Study of the influence of the time of administration on the antihypertensive effect and nitrendipine tolerance in mild to moderate essential hypertensive patients. Value of ambulatory recording of blood pressure on 24 hours. *Therapie.* 1992;47:205-210.

[162] Umeda, T., Naomi, S., Iwaoka, T., Inoue, J., Sasaki, M., Ideguchi, Y., Sato, T. Timing for administration of an antihypertensive drug in the treatment of essential hypertension. *Hypertension.* 1994;23(Suppl. 1):I211-I214.

[163] Hermida, R. C., Calvo, C., Ayala, D. E., Domínguez, M. J., Covelo, M., Fernández, J. R., Fontao, M. J., López, J. E. (2004). Administration-time-dependent effects of doxazosin GITS on ambulatory blood pressure of hypertensive subjects. *Chronobiol. Int.* 21:277-296.

[164] Hermida, R. C., Calvo, C., Ayala, D. E., Rodríguez, M., Chayán, L., López, J. E. (2006). Administration time-dependent effects of nebivolol on the diurnal/nocturnal blood pressure ratio in hypertensive patients. *J. Hypertens.* 24 (suppl. 4):S89.

[165] Hermida, R. C., Ayala, D. E., Mojón, A., Chayán, L., Domínguez, M. J., Fontao, M. J., Soler, R., Alonso, I., Fernández, J. R. (2008c). Comparison of the effects on ambulatory blood pressure of awakening versus bedtime administration of torasemide in essential hypertension. *Chronobiol. Int.* 25:950-970.

[166] Hermida, R. C., Ayala, D. E., Fontao, M. J., Mojón, A., Fernández, J. R. Chronotherapy with valsartan/amlodipine combination in essential hypertension: Improved blood pressure control with bedtime dosing. *Chronobiol. Int.* 2010;27:1287-1303.

[167] Meng, Y., Zhang, Z., Liang, X., Wu, C., Qi, G. Effects of combination therapy with amlodipine and fosinopril administered at different times on blood pressure and circadian blood pressure pattern in patients with essential hypertension. *Acta Cardiol.* 2010; 65:309-314.

[168] Hoshino, A., Nakamura, T., Matsubara, H. The bedtime administration ameliorates blood pressure variability and reduces urinary albumin excretion in amlodipine-olmesartan combination therapy. *Clin. Exp. Hypertens.* 2010;32:416-422.

[169] Hermida, R. C., Ayala, D. E., Mojón, A., Fontao, M. J., Fernández, J. R. Chronotherapy with valsartan/hydrochlorothiazide combination in essential hypertension: Improved

sleep-time blood pressure control with bedtime dosing. *Chronobiol. Int.* 2011;28:601-610.

[170] Zeng, J., Jia, M., Ran, H., Zhang, Y., Zhang, J., Wang, X., Wang, H., Yang, C., Zeng, C. Fixed-combination of amlodipine and diuretic chronotherapy in the treatment of essential hypertension: improved blood pressure control with bedtime dosing—a multicenter, open-label randomized study. *Hypertens. Res.* 2011;34:767-772.

[171] Morgan, T. O. Does it matter when drugs are taken? *Hypertension.* 2009;54, 23-24.

[172] Parati, G., Bilo, G. Evening administration of antihypertensive drugs: filling a knowledge gap. *J. Hypertens.* 2010;28:1390-1392.

[173] Minutolo, R., Gabbai, F. B., Borrelli, S., Scigliano, R., Trucillo, P., Baldanza, D., Laurino, S., Mascia, S., Conte, G., De Nicola, L. Changing the timing of antihypertensive therapy to reduce nocturnal blood pressure in CKD: An 8-week uncontrolled trial. *Am. J. Kidney Dis.* 2007;50:908-917.

[174] Rahman, M., Greene, T., Phillips, R. A., Agodoa, L. Y., Bakris, G. L., Charleston, J., Contreras, G., Gabbai, F., Hiremath, L., Jamerson, K., Kendrick, C., Kusek, J. W., Lash, J. P., Lea, J., Miller, E. R. 3rd, Rostand, S., Toto, R., Wang, X., Wright, J. T. Jr, Appel, L. J. A trial of 2 strategies to reduce nocturnal blood pressure in blacks with chronic kidney disease. *Hypertension.* 2013;61 82-88.

[175] Okeahialam, B., Ohihoin, E., Ajuluchukwu, J. Chronotherapy in Nigerian hypertensives. *Ther. Adv. Cardiovasc. Dis.* 2011;5:113-118.

[176] Wang, C., Zhang, J., Liu, X., Li, C. C., Ye, Z. C., Peng, H., Chen, Z., Lou, T. Effect of valsartan with bedtime dosing on chronic kidney disease patients with nondipping blood pressure pattern. *J. Clin. Hypertens. (Greenwich).* 2013;15:48-54.

[177] Iskedjian, M., Einarson, T. R., MacKeigan, L. D., Shear, N., Addis, A., Mittmann, N., Ilersich, A. L. Relationship between daily dose frequency and adherence to antihypertensive pharmacotherapy: Evidence from a meta-analysis. *Clin. Ther.* 2002; 24: 302-316.

[178] Flack, J. M., Nasser, S. A. Benefits of once-daily therapies in the treatment of hypertension. *Vasc. Health Risk. Manag.* 2011;7:777-787.

[179] Portaluppi, F., Smolensky, M. H. Perspectives on the chronotherapy of hypertension based on the results of the MAPEC study. *Chronobiol. Int.* 2010;27:1652-1667.

[180] Hermida, R. C., Smolensky, M. H., Ayala, D. E., Portaluppi, F., Crespo, J. J., Fabbian, F., Haus, E., Manfredini, R., Mojón, A., Moyá, A., Piñeiro, L., Ríos, M. T., Otero, A., Balan, H., Fernández, J. R. 2013 ambulatory blood pressure monitoring recommendations for the diagnosis of adult hypertension, assessment of cardiovascular and other hypertension-associated risk, and attainment of therapeutic goals. Joint recommendations from the International Society for Chronobiology (ISC), American Association of Medical Chronobiology and Chronotherapeutics (AAMCC), Spanish Society of Applied Chronobiology, Chronotherapy, and Vascular Risk (SECAC), Spanish Society of Atherosclerosis (SEA), and Romanian Society of Internal Medicine (RSIM). *Chronobiol. Int.* 2013;30:355-410.

[181] Mehta, R., Drawz, P. E. Is nocturnal blood pressure reduction the secret to reducing the rate of progression of hypertensive chronic kidney disease? *Curr. Hypertens. Rep.* 2011; 13:378-385.

[182] Hermida, R. C., Ayala, D. E., Smolensky, M. H., Mojón, A., Fernández, J. R., Crespo, J. J., Moyá, A., Ríos, M. T., Portaluppi, F. Chronotherapy improves blood pressure control and reduces vascular risk in CKD. *Nat. Rev. Nephrol.* 2013;9:358-368.

[183] American Diabetes Association: Standards of Medical Care in Diabetes – 2012. *Diabetes Care.* 2012;35 (Suppl. 1):S11-S63.

In: ACE Inhibitors. Volume 2
Editor: Macaulay Amechi Onuigbo
ISBN: 978-1-62948-422-8

Chapter 2

ACEIs as Antihypertensives in African Americans: A 21st Century Perspective

Sandra F. Williams, DMD, MD*[1,2]*, Nosratola D. Vaziri, MD*[3]*,
***Susanne B. Nicholas, MD, MPH, PhD*[4] *and Keith C. Norris, MD*[5,*]**
[1]Department of Endocrinology, Cleveland Clinic, Weston, Florida (Williams), US
[2]Department of Clinical Biomedical Science, Charles E. Schmidt College of Medicine, Florida Atlantic University, Boca Raton, Florida, US
[3]Division of Nephrology and Hypertension, Departments of Medicine, Physiology and Biophysics, University of California, Irvine, Irvine California, US
[4]Division of Nephrology and Division of Endocrinology, Diabetes and Hypertension, Department of Medicine, David Geffen School of Medicine, University of California, Los Angeles, California, US
[5]Division of General Internal Medicine and Division of Nephrology, Department of Medicine, David Geffen School of Medicine, University of California, Los Angeles, California US

Abstract

African Americans exhibit a disproportionate burden of hypertension, as well as an earlier onset and a more rapid progression of chronic kidney disease (CKD). Several studies have suggested that the blood pressure lowering efficacy of angiotensin converting enzyme inhibitors (ACEI) is attenuated in African Americans. By contrast, the ability of blockade of the renin–angiotensin system (RAS) to protect against the progression of CKD in African Americans is preserved. In addition to the modifiable factors that may contribute to the more rapid progression of CKD among African Americans, there appears to be a unique role for RAS modulation beyond lowering blood pressure, with established evidence for not only reducing CKD progression, but the associated mortality risk. Typically, hypertension in African Americans is characterized by disproportionately high rates of blood pressure sensitivity to sodium and low circulating plasma renin levels. High renin levels have been implicated in contributing to poor vascular and cardio-renal outcomes.

[*] Corresponding author: Keith C. Norris MD, E-mail: knorris@ucla.edu.

However African Americans still experience severe hypertension-related end-organ complications such as proteinuria and cardio-renal disease despite low circulating renin levels. This could be explained by a dissociation of circulating renin/angiotensin from intrarenal and tissue renin/angiotensin in this patient subgroup. Despite lower circulating renin levels and a less significant fall in blood pressure in response to RAS blockade in African Americans, RAS inhibition still remains a mainstay of therapy for treating hypertension especially in the presence of CKD in this population. We discuss the rationale and use of RAS inhibition in African Americans in the context of emerging pathophysiologic and clinical trial data.

Keywords: African American, blood pressure, ethnicity, hypertension, kidney disease, angiotensin converting enzyme inhibitors

ABBREVIATIONS

BP	blood pressure
SBP	systolic blood pressure
DBP	diastolic blood pressure
CKD	chronic kidney disease
WHO	World Health Organization
CRIC	Chronic Renal Insufficiency Cohort
US	United States
KDOQI	Kidney Disease Outcomes Quality Initiative
KDIGO	Kidney Disease: Improving Global Outcomes
eGFR	estimated glomerular filtration rate
ACEI	angiotensin converting enzyme inhibitors
ARB	angiotensin receptor blockers
DRIs	direct renin inhibitors
ACR	urinary albumin-to-creatinine ratio
RAAS	Renin–Angiotensin-Aldosterone System
AASK	African American Study of Kidney Disease and Hypertension
ALLHAT	Antihypertensive and Lipid-Lowering Treatment to Prevent Heart Attack Trial
ACCORD trial	Action to Control Cardiovascular Risk in Diabetes
RENAAL study	Reduction of Endpoints in NIDDM with the Angiotensin II Antagonist Losartan
ALTITUDE	The Aliskiren Trial in Type 2 Diabetes Using Cardiovascular and Renal Disease Endpoints
IRMA-2	Irbesartan Microalbuminuria Type 2 Diabetes in Hypertensive Patients
ONTARGET	Ongoing Telmisartan Alone and in Combination with Ramipril Global End Point Trial
SPRINT	Systolic Blood Pressure Intervention Trial
NHANES	National Health and Nutrition Examination Survey
USRDS	United States Renal Data System

IMPROVE	Irbesartan in the Management of PROteinuric patients at high risk for Vascular Events
REIN	Ramipril Efficiency in Nephropathy;
UKPDS	United Kingdom Prospective Diabetes study;
HOPE	Heart Outcomes Prevention Evaluation study

INTRODUCTION

Hypertension has been reported as one of the most important modifiable risk factors for coronary disease [1]. The condition of hypertension is characterized by a persistent and frequently progressive elevation in blood pressure [2]. The level of blood pressure increases with age in many, but not all populations [2]. The level of systolic blood pressure (SBP) and/ or diastolic blood pressure (DBP), which connotes a diagnosis of hypertension, may vary depending on the presence or absence of coexisting comorbidities. Hypertension is typically defined as physician diagnosed SBP ≥140mmHg and DBP ≥90mmHg; and pre-hypertension is defined as SBP ≥120 and <140mm Hg or DBP ≥80 and <90mmHg [2]. A blood pressure ≥130/80 mmHg is often considered hypertension in the setting of diabetes or chronic kidney disease (CKD) [2]. The current classification of hypertension and the level of blood pressure that defines hypertension for the major comorbid conditions are outlined in the seventh report of the Joint National Committee on Prevention, Detection, Evaluation, and Treatment of high blood pressure [2].

In the United States (US), blacks develop hypertension earlier in life than whites, and have a much higher average blood pressure, and greater rates of premature hypertensive complications such as CKD, stroke and heart disease [3]. Although blood pressure control in the US has improved over time, rates of control remain unacceptable. Data from the National Health and Nutrition Examination Survey (NHANES) revealed that the prevalence of adequate blood pressure control during the period 1999–2004 was only 35% for whites, 29% for African Americans, and 27% for Hispanics [4], whereas by 2007-2008 blood pressure control rates reached 50% for the first time and were now similar across race/ethnicity [5]. In the Multi-Ethnic Study of Atherosclerosis the percentage of treated but uncontrolled hypertension was significantly higher in African Americans (35%), Chinese (33%), and Hispanics (32%) than in whites (24%) [6]. After adjustment for socioeconomic factors, the relative higher rates of uncontrolled hypertension for Chinese and Hispanic participants largely disappeared, but persisted in the African American population, suggesting that other factors such as biologic or other confounders accounted for the higher rates [6].

The disproportionate burden of hypertension in African Americans offer a unique challenge to our standard approach to the treatment of hypertension especially given the variations in the pathogenesis of hypertension and its response to treatment in this population. Extensive investigations have delineated the effectiveness of both non-pharmacologic and pharmacologic therapies. It has been reported that in African Americans, the blood pressure lowering efficacy of angiotensin converting enzyme inhibitors (ACEI) is attenuated in comparison to other therapeutic agents [7]. This finding had led to a reduced utilization of ACEIs in African Americans with hypertension, including those afflicted with CKD, despite emerging evidence of the beneficial effect of ACEI in patients with CKD. A greater understanding of the pathophysiology of hypertension in African Americans can enhance the appreciation of risk factor reduction strategies, as well as the rationale for pharmacologic interventions.

This chapter will review recent studies assessing the role of ACEIs and angiotensin receptor blockers (ARBs) as well as a brief overview of the optimal level of blood pressure control and targets for treating African Americans with hypertension, with a special focus on hypertension and CKD.

Chronic Kidney Disease

In 2002, the National Kidney Foundation Kidney Disease Outcomes Quality Initiative (KDOQI) defined five stages of chronic kidney disease (CKD) based on a sustained reduction in eGFR and/or sustained proteinuria (Table 1) [8]. The inclusion of early markers of kidney damage such as albuminuria in the staging criteria allows for the early identification of CKD. These early stages of CKD may be characterized by estimated glomerular filtration rate (eGFR) levels well within or near the normal limits, but the presence of proteinuria is now established as a harbinger of cardiovascular (CV) risk and should herald increased attention to commonly associated co-morbidities such as elevated blood pressure for which early and aggressive intervention may be helpful.

CKD is estimated to currently afflict as many as one in nine adults in the US or over 26 million Americans [9, 10]. In fact, it is now recognized by the World Health Organization (WHO) as a major global chronic non-communicable threat to public health in this century, accounting for significant morbidity and premature mortality in high-, middle- and low-income nations alike [9, 10]. In 2011, the WHO added CKD to the list of major chronic non-communicable threats to public health because of its substantial impact on premature morbidity and mortality, as well as its overwhelmingly burdensome cost to the healthcare system [9, 11].

Along this global spectrum, African Americans suffer from one of, if not the highest, rate of advanced CKD in the world. In the US, the prevalence of early-stage CKD is similar across ethnic groups in the US, but the incidence of end-stage renal disease (ESRD) is 1.5–4 fold higher among minority populations (and highest for African Americans) than among whites indicating a marked racial/ethnic difference in the rate of CKD progression [12, 13]. Even in the United Kingdom, a similar relationship is noted among immigrants of African descent, with the incidence of ESRD being 3-4 fold higher than in the general population [14].

Further data underscores the disproportionate impact of CKD on the African American population and the importance of optimal control of hypertension as a means of impacting CKD progression in minority populations.

In the Chronic Renal Insufficiency Cohort (CRIC) study which included a diverse cohort of racial/ethnic US minority adults (n=3,612) with CKD and an average eGFR of 43.4ml/min/1.73 m^2, 87.5% of study participants had hypertension [15] - a rate three times that of the estimated national prevalence of hypertension (28.5%) in the US adult population [5]. Given the progressively increased rates of hypertension across the spectrum of the five stages of CKD, successful management of hypertension in CKD patients could have an enormous impact on clinical outcomes. While strategies to improve blood pressure control in African Americans with CKD and the optimal approaches remain controversial, a comprehensive understanding of the role of ACEI for blood pressure control in CKD is critical to controlling the associated high rates of premature morbidity and mortality.

Table 1. Stages of Chronic Kidney Disease

Stage	Description	eGFR (mL/min/1.73m^2)	Prevalence Estimates, 1999-2004 (95% CI)
1	Slight kidney damage with normal or increased filtration	≥90	1.8% (95% CI 1.4%-2.3%)
2	Mild decrease in kidney function	60-89	3.2% (95% CI 2.6%-3.9%)
3	Moderate decrease in kidney function	30-59	7.7% (95% CI 7.0%-8.4%)
4	Severe decrease in kidney function	15-29	0.35% (95% CI 0.25%-0.45%)

eGFR; estimated glomerular filtration rate.
Adapted from reference [8].

Epidemiology of CKD in African Americans

According to the United States Renal Data System (USRDS), hypertension and diabetes are the leading primary causes of ESRD, accounting for approximately 25% and 50% of cases, respectively [9]. Hypertension is frequently present in patients with diabetes and acts as an important CKD risk and progression factor. Estimates show that while CKD is present in >10% of the US adult population with normal blood pressure, it is present in 13.9% of the pre-hypertensive population, 23.8% of the undiagnosed hypertensive population and 32.0% of the diagnosed hypertensive population [16]. Further, NHANES data revealed that patients with CKD were 2.5-3 times as likely to exhibit treatment-resistant hypertension (uncontrolled blood pressure despite ≥3 medications vs. all uncontrolled hypertensive patients) compared to those without CKD [17]. Regardless of the cause, poor blood-pressure control has been associated with increased proteinuria, reduced GFR, hypertensive nephrosclerosis and a myriad of other adverse renal outcomes [8, 9]. A comparison between persons with high-normal and optimal blood pressure revealed no significant difference in the risk of microalbuminuria among whites, but showed a trend toward increased risk of microalbuminuria (odds ratio; OR 1.16; 95% CI 0.90–1.51) among Mexican Americans and a statistically significant increase in microalbuminuria risk (OR 1.30; 95% CI 1.04–1.64) among African Americans [18].

The Multiple Risk Factor Intervention Trial found that the incidence of all-cause ESRD per 100,000 person-years of hypertension after 16 years was only 3.00 for white Americans but 16.38 for African Americans [19]. Similarly, at the 15-year examination of 3,554 randomly selected participants in the Coronary Artery Risk Development in Young Adults study, the adjusted OR of an elevated serum creatinine level was significantly higher in blacks, although there was a gender difference with the odds for black men 11.4 fold higher than white men, but only 1.5 folder higher for black women (not significant) compared to white women [20]. While the prevalence of hypertensive ESRD is about 5 fold greater among

African Americans than whites, African American men between the ages of 24 and 44 years are nearly 20 times more likely to have hypertension-related ESRD than their white counterparts [9].

The reasons for the exceptionally high rates of CKD and ESRD among young African American males in particular, are not entirely clear but likely include socioeconomic status, lifestyle choices, clinical factors (e.g. increased risks of diabetes and hypertension), and others [21].

These findings suggest an important role for gender although it is not clear how much is driven by biology and how much is driven by culture. In addition, emerging data continue to identify additional environmental, sociocultural, biologic and genetic factors that may contribute broadly to racial/ethnic differences in outcomes and in response to therapeutic intervention [22-26]. Our understanding of the complex factors that predispose African Americans to hypertension and hypertension-related complications is evolving.

Salt Sensitivity

An increase in blood pressure in response to sodium or salt intake has been termed "salt sensitivity" [27-30]. In comparison to whites, salt sensitivity has been observed at much higher rates in Caribbean and American blacks of African descent in a western society where high salt intake is pervasive.

This difference has been posited as a major pathophysiologic basis for the greater severity and frequency of hypertension in persons of African descent as compared with whites and even native black Africans, especially in the western hemisphere [31]. Wilson and Grim postulated that the slave trade from Africa to the Caribbean and Americas accelerated gene selection for sodium retention when volume depletion and cardiovascular collapse due to diarrheal diseases and limited access to water favored the survival of persons who were avid sodium retainers [31]. Consistent with this premise, Maseko et al. found no relationship between hypertension and 24h urinary sodium and potassium excretion rates in 291 city-dwelling black South Africans, supporting the theory that African slave descendants have a higher rate of salt sensitivity than native black Africans [32]. However, others have refuted this hypothesis [33].

The Renin–Angiotensin System

Since the renin–angiotensin system (RAS) is an important modulator of blood pressure, vascular disease and CKD as well as related complications, it is important to understand the mechanisms through which RAS and other key pathways may contribute to the progression of CKD (Figure 1). Hypertension may lead to chronic kidney damage via multiple mechanisms including the induction of glomerular hypertension and glomerular hyperfiltration, oxidative stress, inflammation, endothelial damage due to enhanced traffic of plasma proteins and/or increased translational and shear forces [34, 35]. These changes may stimulate widespread vascular growth and hypertrophy and activate a series of signaling pathways and promote generation of cytokines [36].

In addition, proteinuria itself has been associated with endothelial dysfunction, increased glomerular capillary pressure and permeability, and inflammatory cytokine release [37]. Glomerular hypertension and glomerular hyperfiltration may initiate a series of events, common to many forms of CKD, including mesangial cell proliferation; fibroblast transformation; matrix accumulation; local release of vasoactive compounds such as angiotensin II (Ag II), and endothelin-1, as well as inflammatory cytokines, transforming growth factor (TGF)-β1, plasminogen activator inhibitor (PAI)-1, and others which may contribute to glomerular scarring and progressive kidney disease [37].

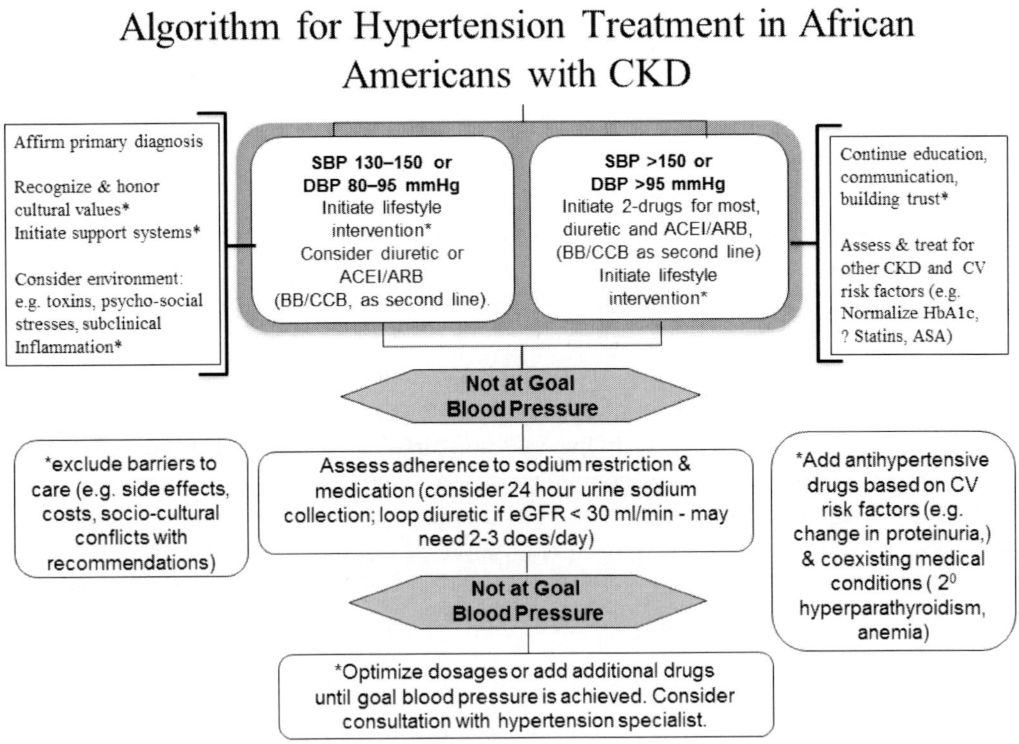

Adapted from reference [125].

Figure 1. The role of angiotensin in pathways leading to progressive renal failure.

Angiotensin II is one of the more extensively studied mediators of vascular function and has been well characterized as stimulating renal inflammation and fibrosis via upregulation of TGF-β1, tumor necrosis factor (TNF)-α, nuclear factor (NF)-κB, osteopontin (OPN), several adhesion molecules and chemoattractants, and more recently interactions with adiponectin and select microRNAs [36, 38-40]. The documented role of RAS in the progression of CKD has positioned it as a prime therapeutic target in high-risk patients. RAS blockade can reduce blood pressure, reverse endothelial dysfunction, attenuate proteinuria, and reduce renal injury independent of blood pressure changes [41]. This makes RAS blockade an important therapeutic option for treating patients with hypertension and/or CKD [42]. Of note, hypertension in older persons, African Americans and Caribbean Hispanics is associated with increased rates of both salt sensitivity and reduced plasma renin levels [43-45]. The reduced plasma renin levels suggest RAS inhibition may not be as effective in these groups. Given the documented role of RAS in the progression of CKD, an attenuated risk of hypertension-related end-organ damage might be expected in patients with low-renin hypertension. Paradoxically, however, many such individuals do experience hypertension-related end-organ complications suggesting RAS may still be important in patients with reduced plasma renin levels. This is not surprising since in nearly all forms of CKD, intra-renal RAS is up-regulated independently of the systemic RAS. The pathological upregulation of the intra-renal angiotensin system is marked by simultaneous increases in the Ag II receptor 1 (AT1) receptor expression and the number of the Ag II-producing cells in the diseased kidney. It is of interest that many of the Ag II-producing cells in the diseased kidney are macrophages, which serve as ectopic sources of this hormone [46].

In addition, the kidney contains angiotensinogen, angiotensin converting enzyme, and renin, which together make the kidney a unique organ for the production of Ag II and a recipient of its physiological and pathophysiological actions [47, 48]. Activation of the AT1 receptor by Ag II in the diseased kidney simultaneously raises superoxide production via upregulation of NAD(P)H oxidase, and causes inhibition of Nrf2 which is the master regulator of genes encoding many antioxidant and cytoprotective enzymes and related molecules. Via these actions, activation of intra-renal RAS promotes, oxidative stress, inflammation and subsequent tissue damage and dysfunction in animals and most likely humans with CKD and hypertension [49-51].

Much of our understanding of the role of the RAS in blood-pressure regulation at a tissue level derives from salt-sensitive hypertension animal models. Consumption of a high-salt diet by Dahl salt-sensitive rats results in hypertension and early onset of renal injury and dysfunction. Although it might seem counterintuitive to implicate RAS in the pathogenesis of renal and cardiovascular diseases in Dahl salt-sensitive rats because of the reductions in plasma renin activity and angiotensinogen concentration that are found in this model, these reductions in serum levels of plasma renin activity are accompanied by paradoxical elevations of renal tissue angiotensin II, tissue AT1 receptor expression and urinary angiotensinogen excretion [52].

These observations support a dissociation of the low circulating RAS from the upregulated intrarenal and tissue RAS in this model which is accompanied by renal interstitial inflammation, oxidative stress and activation of NAD(P)H oxidase in the kidney and cardiovascular tissues [53].

Despite the low circulating renin level, RAS blockade in Dahl salt-sensitive rats fed a high-salt diet attenuated proteinuria, reduced renal injury and reversed endothelial dysfunction, even though it did not normalize the blood pressure [54]. These findings suggest that the intrarenal and tissue RAS is more important in the pathogenesis of salt sensitive hypertension and hypertensive nephropathy than the circulating RAS, which may be more reflective of the regulation of sodium balance, vascular resistance and arterial blood pressure. In addition to salt sensitive hypertension, the upregulation of intra-renal RAS occurs and contributes to the development and progression of renal disease in various other forms of hypertension as seen in animals with renal mass reduction, spontaneous focal glomerulosclerosis, obese Zucker rats [55, 56], and rodents with hypertensive nephropathy induced by Ag II infusion [57].

Osteopontin (OPN), which is a secreted matrix glycoprotein that is expressed in Ag II-injured tissues, has been shown to be an important modulator of several of the Ag II-induced mechanisms of hypertensive nephropathy including inflammation and oxidative stress, which may precede the development of renal fibrosis [57]. Global deletion of OPN in hypertensive, albuminuric mice that were infused with Ag II significantly reduced tubulointerstitial macrophage infiltration, α-smooth muscle actin, fibronectin and TGF-β. At the same time, the lack of OPN promoted Ag II-induced monocyte chemoattractant protein-1, NADPH oxidase subunits (NOX2, gp47phox and NOX4) and PAI-1, compared to Ag II-infused wild-type mice [57]. Earlier studies showed that inhibition of OPN expression may account for a mechanism by which Ag II blockade attenuated renal injury following renal ablation [58], and this action may likely contribute to the beneficial effects of ACEI therapy in hypertensive nephropathy.

Genetic Factors

Genetic variations may contribute to ethnic differences in the prevalence of hypertension and CKD, and may be especially important in salt-sensitive hypertension and response to ACEI therapy. Low circulating levels of renin and sodium sensitivity and low circulating levels of renin have been linked to the 460Trp variant of alpha-adducin that was found to be twice as common among hypertensive patients in comparison to patients with normal blood pressure [59, 60].

However the 460Trp variant of alpha-adducin did not appear to contribute to plasma RAS profile in persons of African descent [61, 62], nor did a recent meta-analysis [63]. While several additional genetic factors might influence the development of salt-sensitive hypertension in ethnic minorities such as gain-in-function mutations of epithelial sodium channels (e.g. Liddle syndrome) or glucocorticoid-remediable aldosteronism [64], a systematic review by Beeks and colleagues did not find any association between polymorphisms of the angiotensin II type 1 receptor or aldosterone synthase genes and sodium-sensitive hypertension [65].

More specific to the RAS, Tiago et al. examined variants of the promoter region of the angiotensinogen gene (AGT) in over 1,000 South Africans of African ancestry and noted a marked influence of homozygosity for the –20A allele (n = 399) on the relationship between SBP and body mass index (r = 0.23; P <0.0001) [66]. However, most reports suggest AGT promoter region variants may be more influential in the response of blood pressure to select therapeutics. The AGT promoter region variants among a cohort of South Africans of African ancestry influenced the blood pressure response to an ACEI, but not to a calcium channel blocker [67]. The African-American Study of Kidney Disease and Hypertension (AASK) study showed that African Americans who were homozygous for the ACE polymorphism 12269G>A experienced a more rapid reduction in blood pressure in response to ACE inhibition than those who were heterozygous for this variant (P <0.001), but no difference to a calcium channel blocker [68].

Although a significant proportion of the early onset and accelerated progression of CKD to ESRD among minority populations derives from the higher prevalence and greater severity of diabetes and hypertension, variations in the genetic profile superimposed on nontraditional risk factors such as socio-economic status, lesser access to care, excess exposure to environmental toxins may contribute more than previously imagined [23, 69-71]. Recent genome-wide admixture mapping studies have demonstrated genetic variation in the regions of MYH9 and APOL 1 on chromosome 22 that have been estimated to explain as much as 70% of the differences in the rates of non-diabetic ESRD between white and black Americans [72-74], but to date no reports have linked those gene variants to hypertension or response to ACEI therapy.

Treatment Trials of Hypertensive CKD in African Americans

Clinical trials form the basis of guidelines and recommendations for addressing the medical care of patients with most chronic disease states.

But despite the known racial differences in the pathobiology of hypertension and CKD, there has been a paucity of clinical trial data relating to African Americans or other ethnic minority groups. As in many other areas of health care, most clinical trials of antihypertensive therapy in CKD (Table 2) included relatively few participants from ethnic minorities.

The Modification of Diet in Renal Disease study, a key study in the estimation of renal function that is widely used, only included 53 African Americans of the 548 enrollees, although a subgroup analysis did suggest that a lower mean arterial pressure might confer optimal renal protection in African Americans with hypertension or any patient with proteinuria (>1 g/day) [75]. Another landmark trial by the Collaborative Study Group, demonstrating the efficacy of ACEI in slowing the progression of CKD in 409 participants with type 1 diabetes, included only 15 African Americans [76]. Other large studies reporting beneficial effects of ACEI on the outcomes of people with CKD also enrolled low numbers of patients from ethnic minority groups [77, 78].

AASK

To date the African-American Study of Kidney Disease and Hypertension (AASK) is the largest prospective CKD study to focus on and successfully recruit African Americans [79]. The AASK trial (n=1094) was a prospective study designed to examine the effects of two levels of blood pressure control: intensive (≤120/80mmHg) and standard (~135–140/85–90mmHg), and three classes of initial antihypertensive therapy (ACEI, β-blocker or calcium channel blocker) on eGFR progression and combined clinical outcomes in a high-risk cohort with hypertension-related CKD.

Table 2. Selected trials and meta-analyses of antihypertensive therapy in patients with chronic kidney disease, with an emphasis on ACEIs and ARBs

Study	Year	Type of CKD	Patient number and ethnicity	Results
Collaborative Study Group [76]	1993	Type 1 diabetic	409 (4% African American)	ACEI reduced proteinuria, risk of doubling of serum creatinine, and combined risk of ESRD and death.
REIN [77]	1997	Nondiabetic	352 (ethnicity not reported)	ACEI plus standard therapy reduced proteinuria and rate of composite outcome[a] vs placebo plus standard therapy.
UKPDS [126]	1998	Type 2 diabetic	3867 (8% Black)	ACEI as effective as [beta]-blocker in improving clinical outcomes.
HOPE [78]	2000	Mild (serum creatinine <1.4 mg/dl or normal renal function)	980 with mild renal insufficiency and 8307 with normal renal function (ethnicity not reported)	Ramipril reduced progression of proteinuria and composite cardiovascular end point vs placebo
Jafar et al. meta-analysis [127]	2001	Nondiabetic	1860 (6% African American)	ACEI more effective than non ACEI antihypertensive (composite outcome[a])
RENAAL [90]	2001	Type 2 diabetic	1513 (~15% African American, 16.5% Asian, 18% Hispanic, 1% other ethnicity)	ARB plus standard therapy more effective than non-ARB, non-ACEI antihypertensive plus standard therapy (composite outcome[a])
IDNT [89]	2001	Type 2 diabetic	1715 (~13% African American, 5% Asian, 5% Hispanic, 4% other)	ARB more effective than calcium channel blocker or placebo (composite outcome[a])
AASK [79]	2001	Hypertensive	1094 (all African American)	ACEI more effective than β-blocker or amlodipine (composite outcome[a])
ALLHAT [128]	2006	Advanced (baseline GFR <60 ml/min)	5,662 (25% African American, 11% Hispanic, 4.5% other ethnicity)	Lisinopril as effective as chlorthalidone and amlodipine for composite outcome[a].

Table 2. (Continued)

Study	Year	Type of CKD	Patient number and ethnicity	Results
IMPROVE [129]	2007	Hypertensive (87% Type 2 diabetes)	414 (1.5% African American, 2% Asian, 3% other ethnicity).	Ramipril plus irbesartan vs. ramipril plus placebo: similar affects on microalbuminuria
Balamuthusamy et al. méta-analysis [101]	2008	Any	45,758 (ethnicity not reported)	RAS blockade more effective than placebo, and => effective than standard therapy in patients with proteinuria (cardiovascular outcomes)
ALTITUDE [99]	2013	Type 2 diabetic, 95% hypertensive	8606 (31.7 % Asian, 3.3% African American)	Aliskiren was trending to worse outcomes than placebo on top of standard therapy with ACEI or ARB.

[a]The composite outcome was a combination of renal function decline, ESRD and death.

Abbreviations: ACEI, angiotensin-converting-enzyme inhibitor; ARB, angiotensin receptor blocker; CKD, chronic kidney disease; ESRD, end-stage renal disease; GFR, glomerular filtration rate; RAS, renin–angiotensin system. REIN - Ramipril Efficiency in Nephropathy; UKPDS - United Kingdom Prospective Diabetes study; HOPE - Heart Outcomes Prevention Evaluation study RENAAL - Reduction of Endpoints in NIDDM with the Angiotensin II Antagonist Losartan; IDNT AASK - African American Study of Kidney Disease and Hypertension; ALLHAT - Antihypertensive and Lipid-Lowering Treatment to Prevent Heart Attack Trial; IMPROVE - Irbesartan in the Management of PROteinuric patients at high risk for Vascular Events; ALTITUDE - The Aliskiren Trial in Type 2 Diabetes Using Cardiovascular and Renal Disease Endpoints

Adapted from reference [42].

Individuals with substantial proteinuria (>2.5g per day) were excluded from the trial [80]. Diuretics were not among the three randomized classes of antihypertensive agents as it was assumed the majority of study participants would require diuretic therapy due to their impaired renal function and associated volume retention. This premise was validated by the finding that nearly 90% of AASK participants required concomitant diuretic therapy to achieve target blood pressure levels. While calcium channel blockers were the most commonly prescribed antihypertensive for African Americans with CKD due to their blood pressure lowering efficacy, the calcium channel blocker arm of AASK was terminated early because of increased rates of adverse events [81]. AASK demonstrated that clinical cardio-renal outcomes in African Americans: 1) did not differ between intensive (≤120/80mmHg) and standard (~135–140/85–90mmHg) blood pressure targets, and 2) were improved with ACEI in comparison to β-blocker or calcium channel blocker, with diuretics and other agents added as needed [82]. Importantly, AASK demonstrated that blood pressure can be controlled in African Americans with CKD and that combined clinical outcomes (cardiovascular and renal) can be improved by using an ACEI, beta blocker or calcium channel blocker as initial therapy to reach a usual or strict blood pressure target, with diuretics in most, and other agents added as needed [81, 82]. Also important were the findings that secondary clinical outcomes including the composite end point of development of ESRD, doubling of serum creatinine, or death were less frequent in the ACEI group than in the beta blocker or calcium channel blocker groups, suggesting that RAS inhibition should be the initial antihypertensive regimen in African Americans with hypertensive nephrosclerosis. This is contrary to previous suggestions that RAS inhibition was of limited benefit in African Americans [7].

An important finding in AASK was that the incidence of cardiovascular events was considerably lower than that observed in other major hypertension and renal outcomes trials [83]. While this low cardiovascular event rate precluded the comparison of the cardiovascular effects of the different agents studied, it did support the notion that aggressive blood pressure control by use of RAS inhibition can improve clinical outcomes in African Americans, especially since the combined clinical composite of cardiovascular outcomes, renal outcomes, and death were significantly reduced with ACEI. The rate of a first cardiovascular event (3.4% per patient-year) in AASK was <1/2 that in previous studies such as the Ramipril Efficacy in Nephropathy (REIN) study, the Reduction of Endpoints in NIDDM with the Angiotensin II Antagonist Losartan (RENAAL) study and Irbesartan in the Diabetic Nephropathy (IDNT) study (9%, 10% and 17% per patient-year, respectively) [83]. Additionally, the rate of all-cause death in AASK (2.3% per patient-year) was considerably lower than that of African American hypertensive patients with a similar mean baseline serum creatinine >2mg/dl (177μmol/l) who were enrolled in the Hypertension Detection and Follow-up Program (~5% per patient-year) [84].

RENAAL and IDNT

Unfortunately, the rate of ACEI-related serious adverse events is greater in ethnic minorities, especially Blacks and Chinese [85-88]. Thus, inclusion of ethnic minorities in studies of ARBs is of critical importance since these agents would represent the alternative to providing the benefits of RAS inhibition in those patients who cannot tolerate ACEI use.

Recent studies of irbesartan (IDNT) and losartan (RENAAL) in persons with diabetic nephropathy, most of whom had hypertension, involved slightly higher proportions of ethnic minorities than most prior renal trials: 13% African Americans and 5% Hispanics in the former and 15% African Americans and 18% Hispanics in the latter [89, 90].

Results from these two studies, although not sufficient to enable subgroup analyses according to ethnicity, strongly suggest that the positive outcomes of ARB in whites extend to ethnic minorities without evidence of increased adverse effects. A post-hoc analysis of RENAAL (1513 participants followed for 3.4 years with final SBP of 141 mmHg), found no ethnic differences in the influence of baseline albuminuria on ESRD risk, the effect of 6-month antiproteinuric response to therapy on ESRD risk, or the overall renoprotective effect of ARB therapy [91]. Further data is, however, needed for long-term treatment guidelines directed to the use of ARB therapy in the African American population.

Importantly, while the RENAAL post-hoc data support the recommendation of RAS inhibition for improving clinical outcomes in diabetic nephropathy in racial and ethnic minorities, it should also be noted that the findings of RENAAL and AASK study proved a second important point: that African Americans with hypertensive kidney disease or hypertension and diabetic kidney disease can achieve and sustain adequate blood pressure control over a long period of time.

ALLHAT

Another hypertension clinical trial which included ACEI and minority participants was the Antihypertensive and Lipid-Lowering Treatment to Prevent Heart Attack Trial (ALLHAT). ALLHAT enrolled over 33,000 high-risk hypertensive patients, of whom 32% were black and 16% were Hispanic [92].

ALLHAT analysis found that first-line therapy with chlorthalidone, amlodipine or lisinopril were equally effective in preventing fatal coronary heart disease and nonfatal myocardial infarction, and superior to alpha blocker (the alpha blocker arm was discontinued early [93]) as first line therapy [94]. Subgroup analysis by race/ethnicity revealed no significant differences from that of the overall trial results. Many authorities still favor initial therapy with RAS blockade, especially in patients with hypertension and CKD where diuretics are commonly included in treatment. In a secondary analysis of ALLHAT patients with reduced GFR, amlodipine, chlorthalidone and lisinopril were equivalent in reducing the rate of a composite end point of development of ESRD or a 50% or greater decrement in GFR [95].

ALLHAT differed from AASK in many respects. AASK focused on patients with hypertensive CKD and compared calcium channel blocker, beta blocker and ACEI, but not diuretic as the steering committee felt diuretic would be required in most if not all patients with CKD. As noted above in AASK, ACEI plus diuretic was superior to beta blocker plus diuretic, which was superior to calcium channel blocker plus diuretic in reducing composite clinical outcomes.

Recent Clinical Trials

Recent trials to investigate whether there would be enhanced efficacy with combination therapy of ACEI and ARB are important to better understand how many of the available RAS inhibitory therapies may work together. The optimism for enhanced efficacy with combination ARB/ACEI generated by the independent findings has recently dampened. The ONTARGET trial randomized 25,000 participants (11% Aboriginal/African) with vascular disease or diabetes with end-organ damage (13% with microalbuminuria), followed for 4.5 years. Baseline mean blood pressure of 142/82mmHg was reduced at 6 months by 6.4-/4.3 mmHg in the Ramipril group (ACEI), 7.4/5.0 mmHg in the Telmisartan group (ARB), and by 9.8/6.3mmHg in the combination therapy group and continued at similar levels throughout the study.

The composite primary outcome of death from cardiovascular causes, myocardial infarction, stroke, or hospitalization for heart failure did not differ between groups [96]. While combination therapy reduced proteinuria to a greater extent than monotherapy, it worsened major renal outcomes [97]. Not only did the ONTARGET trial not demonstrate any cardiovascular benefit for dual RAAS blockade (Ramipril and Telmisartan), it suggested an increased risk of major renal outcomes, although the differences were not statistically significant. There were no reports of secondary analyses for Aboriginal and/or African patients in the study. The reason for the unanticipated results were not clear, but may have been related to the paucity of patients (13%) with albuminuria [98].

The Aliskiren Trial in Type 2 Diabetes Using Cardio-Renal Endpoints (ALTITUDE) trial investigated the use of direct renin inhibitors (DRIs), another emerging potential RAS related therapy, in treating hypertension in patients with CKD. The ALTITUDE study randomized over 8600 participants with type 2 diabetes and nephropathy to either Aliskiren or placebo on top of standard therapy with ACEI or ARB [99].

The study populations included 31.7 % Asian participants, but only 3.3% African Americans. ALTITUDE was stopped early due to a low likelihood of ever demonstrating clinical benefit and a trend toward increased risk of key adverse outcomes, casting doubt on the future use of DRIs in combination with ACEI or ARB [100]. There was no subgroup analysis by race.

This notion of the overall efficacy of ACEI or ARB is supported by a recent meta-analysis of 25 randomized controlled trials (N = 45,758) by Balamuthusamy et al. who found improved or equivalent cardiovascular outcomes in patients with diabetic or non-diabetic CKD and proteinuria treated with RAS blockade (ACEI/ARB) in comparison to placebo and control (β-blocker, calcium-channel blockers and other antihypertensive-based therapy) [101]. RAS blockade reduced the combined number of cardiovascular events in many subtypes of CKD compared with placebo or control therapy (non RAS blockade antihypertensives). RAS blockade was equivalent to non-RAS blockade in hypertensive nephropathy (n >5,000) in this meta-analysis.

The ethnic composition of the meta-analysis was not provided and the results are confounded by combining studies that recruited patients with hypertension and retrospectively analyzed subgroups with reduced eGFR versus studies that specifically recruited subjects with a priori hypertensive CKD. However, the preponderance of evidence supports the important role for RAS blockade in treating patients with CKD and proteinuria.

Blood Pressure Targets

Central to the effective management of hypertension and its associated chronic complications is not only the selection of optimum agents, but the knowledge of the optimal blood pressure target to achieve maximal benefits in regards to cardio-renal outcomes. These targets are of significant importance in the African American population, which is disproportionately affected by hypertension and its related complications. One of the key studies that explored the relationship of blood pressure goal (usual goal SBP <140mmHg vs. low goal of SBP < 120mmHg) to outcomes was the Action to Control Cardiovascular Risk in Diabetes (ACCORD) trial [102]. ACCORD included 19.3% blacks and 7.2% Hispanics among the 4733 participants with type 2 diabetes mellitus followed for a mean of 4.7 years. In the study 53% of the enrollees were treated with ACEI. No benefit was found with regard to the primary composite outcome of major cardiovascular events with a SBP target of <120mmHg versus <140mmHg. There were not enough study participants to perform power analyses for black participants. Upadhyay and colleagues used MEDLINE and the Cochrane Central Register of Controlled Trials (July 2001 through January 2011) of randomized, controlled trials to compare lower versus higher blood pressure targets in adult patients with CKD. They found that a blood pressure target <130/80mmHg did not improve clinical outcomes more than a target <140/90mmHg. However their criteria led to only 3 trials being included (2272 participants) and their findings suggested that a low blood pressure target may be beneficial in subgroups with proteinuria greater than 300 to 1000mg/d [103]. After completing the trial phase, AASK patients were invited to enroll in a cohort phase in which the blood pressure target was <130/80mmHg and primary therapy was a diuretic with either ACEI or ARB. During the cohort phase, corresponding intensive and standard group mean blood pressure was 131/78mmHg and 134/78mmHg, respectively. With a combined follow-up period of 8.8 to 12.2 years across both phases, there remained no significant difference in clinical outcomes between blood pressure groups (p= 0.27). However, when stratified by baseline level of proteinuria the groups differed (p= 0.02 for interaction), with a potential benefit of original intensive blood pressure treatment in patients with a protein-to-creatinine ratio of more than 0.22 (p= 0.01) [104]. Monitoring proteinuria over time can help guide therapy as the change in the level of proteinuria is a powerful predictor of progression of hypertensive kidney disease in all patients at any given GFR [105]. The 2012 Kidney Disease: Improving Global Outcomes (KDIGO) Clinical Practice Guideline for Management of Blood Pressure in Chronic Kidney Disease indicated that the available evidence in CKD patients without albuminuria supports a target SBP of <140mmHg and DBP <90mmHg. However, in patients with an albumin excretion rate >30mg/24h the committee suggested a more aggressive SBP target of <130mmHg and DBP <80mmHg [Table 3] [106]. To achieve BP control, it is also important to recognize the value of non-pharmacologic approaches as well [Table 4]. RAS inhibition therapy is suggested in patients with an albumin excretion rate of >30mg/24h. Importantly, recommendations are essentially identical in CKD patients with and without diabetes [106, 107]. Specific recommendations were not stratified by race/ethnicity but given the KDIGO recommendations and the suggested benefit of original intensive blood pressure treatment in AASK patients when stratified by baseline level of proteinuria (protein-to-creatinine ratio of ≥0.22 compared to <0.22) a combination of ACEI and a SBP target of <130mmHg in African Americans with hypertension and proteinuria/CKD seem prudent.

Table 3. Pharmacological treatment recommendations for lowering blood pressure in chronic kidney disease patients with or without diabetes mellitus

Urine Albumin Excretion*	Target BP (evidence)	Preferred Agent (evidence)
<30 mg per 24 hours	SBP <140mmHg DBP <90mmHg (strong)	None (strong)
30-300 mg per 24 hours	SBP <130mmHg DBP <80mmHg (weak)	ARB or ACEI (modest)
>300 mg per 24 hours	SBP <130mmHg DBP <80mmHg (modest)	ARB or ACEI (strong)

*urine albumin excretion - mg per 24 hours or equivalent; ARB – angiotensin receptor blocker; ACE-I - angiotensin converting enzyme inhibitor.

Adapted from reference [112].

Special Considerations for the Use of ACEI in Treating Hypertension in African Americans

Consideration is necessary of the well-recognized common effects noted with agents that inhibit the RAS system. ACEI-related adverse events are more common in ethnic minorities. There is a 3 fold higher rate of angioedema in blacks vs. non-blacks [08, 109], and a 50% greater rate of ACEI discontinuation due to cough (9.6% vs. 2.4%) [110].

It should also be noted that chronic persistent cough is even more common among Asians, having been reported to occur in as much as 44% of Chinese patients [111]. A second important consideration is that the initiation of RAS inhibition therapy can lead to an acute reduction in GFR in patients with advanced CKD.

In most instances this reduction in GFR is a physiologic hemodynamic effect that is reversed if the therapy is reduced or discontinued. A post-hoc analysis of RENAAL trial found an initial fall in eGFR was a better predictor of long-term renoprotection [112].

Thus, the current evidence suggests modest stable reduction in eGFR in patients with later stages of CKD is usually associated with an improved long-term prognosis [113], although close care should be taken to avoid complications such as hyperkalemia or hypotension, which may occur in some patients and would warrant discontinuation.

Conclusion: A Comprehensive Approach to Blood Pressure Care in African American Patients with Chronic Kidney Disease

Many health care providers consider a patient's age, gender and ethnic background when making clinical decisions based on the evidence from clinical research findings. As in the non-African American patient, excluding secondary causes of hypertension and/or primary kidney disorders is of paramount importance in African American patients with suspected hypertensive CKD.

Table 4. Non-pharmacologic considerations to blood pressure control in African Americans

Barrier	Reason	How to manage
Overweight/obesity (body mass index >25/30 kg/m^2)	Cultural concern that a thin body means poor health	Health education. Lose weight gradually by making permanent changes in daily diet for the entire family
High dietary intake of sodium and fat	Several ethnic cultural food preferences probably started or were exacerbated during slavery, when high salt and fat content were needed to preserve food or make suboptimal food more palatable	Salt sensitivity is more common in African Americans and Caribbean Hispanics than in whites. Eat fewer processed foods, fast foods, and fried foods. If blood pressure is not controlled, check 24h urinary sodium excretion to assess dietary adherence

Table 4. (Continued)

Barrier	Reason	How to manage
Low dietary calcium intake	High prevalence of lactose intolerance, especially in African Americans	Calcium and/or vitamin D supplementation
Stressful lifestyle	Associated neuro-hormonal stimulation may lead to poor BP control and accelerated vascular disease	Develop coping skills for specific stressors in work and/or home environment by use of meditation, relaxation, yoga, biofeedback, etc.
Poor adherence to treatment plan	Some medications have adverse effects (diuretics and [beta] blockers cause impotence; angiotensin-converting-enzyme inhibitors cause angioedema in African Americans and chronic cough in Asians) High rate of poverty, low rate of health insurance	Assess biobehavioral barriers (health beliefs and practices) and family support structure Recognize distrust of the medical establishment, even if not expressed Check prescription plan and ability to pay for prescribed drugs and adjust therapy as needed
Missed office appointments	Transportation difficulties: many patients do not have a car, and many cities have poor mass-transportation systems Competing priorities, such as caring for a child, grandchild, or elder (often related to extended family home structure and geographic disconnection of child-care and elder-care facilities from health-care centers) Limited ability to leave work to keep health-care appointments in many jobs	Have office staff work proactively with all patients to assess potential barriers and facilitators, and modify scheduling to best accommodate the patient's schedule.

Adapted from reference [109].

In particular, renal artery stenosis can mimic hypertensive nephrosclerosis and may require a different treatment approach to improve blood pressure and stabilize renal function [114-116]. Both African Americans and non-African Americans with established hypertension and kidney disease will require a comprehensive approach to slow the progression of kidney disease and its complications, often necessitating aggressive care of the primary etiology, assessment and medication of select lifestyle and socio-cultural issues, and the use of two or more antihypertensive agents for control of BP and/or proteinuria (Figure 2).

The existing data highly supports the initial therapy for treating hypertension in patients with CKD to comprise RAS inhibition in combination with diuretic, because this approach seems to confer additional renal and cardiovascular protection beyond that offered by other antihypertensive agents administered with a diuretic. Despite reports that African Americans have lower blood pressure response rates than whites to ACEI therapy and other agents [7, 117], there is significant patient level variability [118]. Importantly, ACEI or ARB therapy has been shown to improve clinical outcomes in African Americans and in other ethnic minorities, especially in the presence of CKD and proteinuria [119]. Thus, until more data are available, ethnicity should not be the primary criterion for selecting a given class of antihypertensive therapy, especially in patients with hypertension and CKD [23, 42, 119]. The overall treatment decision should be guided by individual patient response, coexisting risk factors and potential sociocultural considerations such as cost of medications and insurance coverage, which affect adherence to both pharmacologic and non-pharmacologic interventions [120].

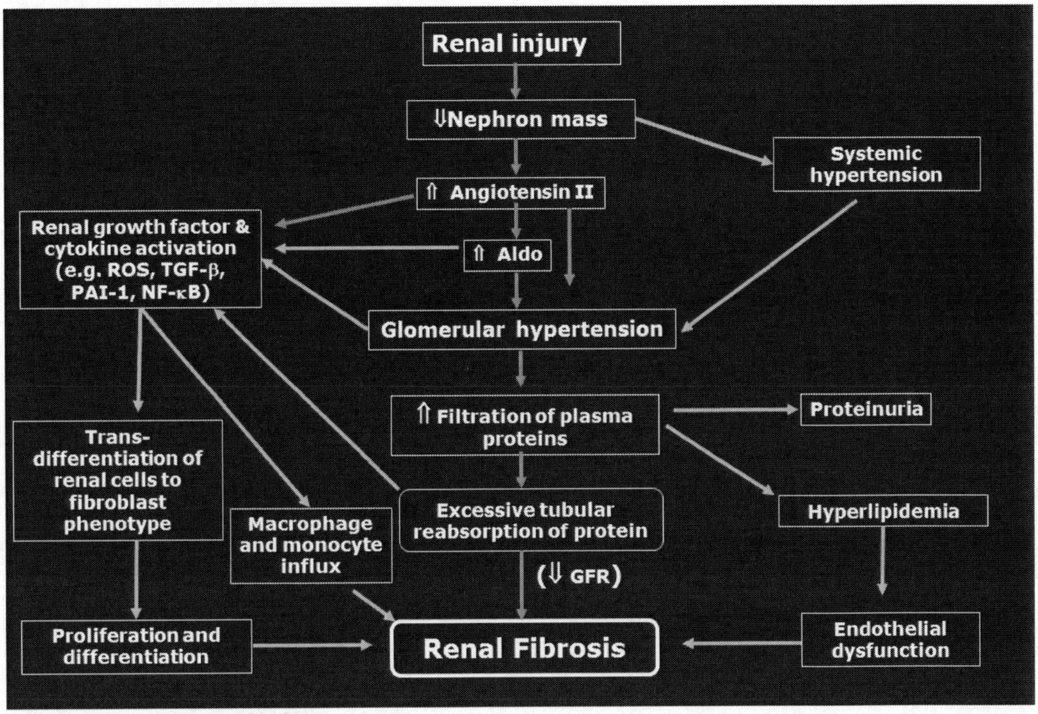

Adapted from reference [119].

Figure 2. Algorithm for hypertension treatment in African Americans with CKD.

Present blood pressure target goals in uncomplicated hypertension based on clinical trial data is <140/90mmHg in all racial groups. A lower target (<130/80mmHg) should be considered in cases of CKD with proteinuria, although the evidence is less consistent [Table 3]; these recommendations apply to African Americans and extend to other patient subgroups as well. The International Society on Hypertension in Blacks consensus statement, recommended a BP target of <130/80mmHg in blacks with elevated blood pressure and target organ damage [121], though others suggest the data to support a BP goal below 140/90 mmHg is insufficient [122].

A recent review recommended diuretic and/or renin–angiotensin inhibition as initial therapy for blood pressure control in African American patients with CKD (most of whom have a protein-to-creatinine ratio >0.22) with a target blood pressure goal <130/80mmHg to enhance the likelihood of patients achieving an actual blood pressure <140/90mmHg, and because AASK found a benefit in the subgroup of patients with protein-to-creatinine ratio >0.22 [119, 123]. These recommendations are consisted with the KDIGO recommendations.

Looking forward, the NIH-funded Systolic Blood Pressure Intervention Trial (SPRINT) trial which will randomize over 7500 patients including significant numbers of patients over 75 years of age, African Americans and patients with CKD to systolic blood pressure targets of <140mmHg or <120mmHg over a period of 9 years, commencing in 2010 and followed up for cardiovascular, cognitive and kidney end points deliberately, should yield additional evidence for optimizing blood pressure treatment guidelines for African Americans and many other high-risk patient groups [124].

Key Points

- Recent guidelines suggest that inhibition of the renin–angiotensin system should be the initial therapy for hypertension in all patients with chronic kidney disease (CKD) and/or proteinuria; a diuretic and at least one other agent is usually also required to achieve the blood-pressure goal ≤140/90mmHg and preferably ≤130/80 mmHg
- Ethnicity is associated with many biologic and sociocultural variations that might influence the level of blood pressure elevation, blood-pressure control, and the risk and progression of CKD and other end organ complications
- African Americans with hypertension have a much higher risk of developing CKD progression to end-stage renal disease (ESRD) than white patients with hypertension
- Some studies have reported that African Americans have a lesser response to the blood pressure lower effects of angiotensin converting enzyme inhibitors than whites
- Angiotensin converting enzyme inhibitors have yielded similar or better outcomes than other pharmacologic therapies in both hypertension clinical trials and CKD clinical trials with no evidence of ethnic differences in clinical outcomes; however the paucity of data for African Americans and other minorities reinforces the need to achieve greater ethnic diversity in clinical trials
- When treating hypertension in African Americans clinicians should pay detailed attention to potential cultural and socioeconomic issues that influence adherence and other factors that impact outcomes

Acknowledgments

This work was supported in part by P20-MD000182 and DK065455, National Institutes of Health.

Financial Disclosures: None.

REFERENCES

[1] He, J., Whelton, P. Epidemiology and prevention of hypertension. *Med. Clin. North Am.* 1997;81(5):1077-1097.

[2] Joint National Committee on prevention Detection, Evaluation, and Treatment of High Blood Pressure. The seventh report of the joint National Committee on Prevention, Detection, Evaluation and Treatment of High Blood Pressure. *JAMA* 2003; 289:2560-2572.

[3] Go, A. S., Mozaffarian, D., Roger, V. L., Benjamin, E. J., Berry, J. D., Borden, W. B., Bravata, D. M., Dai, S., Ford, E. S., Fox, C. S., Franco, S., Fullerton, H. J., Gillespie, C., Hailpern, S. M., Heit, J. A., Howard, V. J., Huffman, M. D., Kissela, B. M., Kittner, S. J., Lackland, D. T., Lichtman, J. H., Lisabeth, L. D., Magid, D., Marcus, G. M., Marelli, A., Matchar, D. B., McGuire, D. K., Mohler, E. R., Moy, C. S., Mussolino, M. E., Nichol, G., Paynter, N. P., Schreiner, P. J., Sorlie, P. D., Stein, J., Turan, T. N., Virani, S. S., Wong, N. D., Woo, D., Turner, M. B.; American Heart Association Statistics Committee and Stroke Statistics Subcommittee. Heart disease and stroke statistics--2013 update: a report from the American Heart Association. *Circulation.* 2013 Jan. 1;127(1):e6-e245.

[4] Ong, K. L., Cheung, B. M., Man, Y. B., Lau, C. P., Lam, K. S. Prevalence, awareness, treatment, and control of hypertension among United States adults 1999-2004. *Hypertension.* 2007 Jan;49(1):69-75.

[5] Egan, B. M., Zhao, Y., Axon, R. N. US Trends in Prevalence, Awareness, Treatment, and Control of Hypertension, 1988-2008. *JAMA* 2010;303(20):2043-2050.

[6] Kramer, H., Han, C., Post, W., Goff, D., Diez-Roux, A., Cooper, R., Jinagouda, S., Shea, S. Racial/Ethnic differences in hypertension and hypertension treatment and control in the multi-ethnic study of atherosclerosis (MESA). *Am. J. Hypertens.* 2004; 17:963–970.

[7] Materson, B. J., Reda, D. J., Cushman, W. C., Massie, B. M., Freis, E. D., Kochar, M. S., Hamburger, R. J., Fye, C., Lakshman, R., Gottdiener, J., Eli A. Ramirez, William G. Henderson, for The Department of Veterans Affairs Cooperative Study Group on Antihypertensive Agents. Single-drug therapy for hypertension in men. A comparison of six antihypertensive agents with placebo. The Department of Veterans Affairs Cooperative Study Group on Antihypertensive Agents. *N. Engl. J. Med.* 1993; 328(13): 914-21. Erratum in: *N. Engl. J. Med.* 1994; 330(23):1689.

[8] National Kidney Foundation. K/DOQI clinical practice guidelines for chronic kidney disease: evaluation, classification, and stratification. *Am. J. Kidney Dis.* 2002 Feb;39(2 Suppl. 1):S1-266.

[9] US Renal Data System. USRDS 2012 annual data report: atlas of end-stage renal disease in the United States: National Institutes of Health, National Institute of Diabetes and Digestive and Kidney Disease. Bethesda, MD; 2012.

[10] Coresh, J., Selvin, E., Stevens, L. A., Manzi, J., Kusek, J. W., Eggers, P., Van Lente, F., Levey, A. S. Prevalence of chronic kidney disease in the United States. *JAMA.* 2007; 298(17):2038-2047.

[11] Eckardt, K. U., Coresh, J., Devuyst, O., Johnson, R. J., Köttgen, A., Levey, A. S., Levin, A. Evolving importance of kidney disease: from subspecialty to global health burden. *Lancet*. 2013 Jul. 13;382(9887):158-69.

[12] Hsu, C. Y., Lin, F., Vittinghoff, E., Shlipak, M. G. Racial differences in the progression from chronic renal insufficiency to end-stage renal disease in the United States. *J. Am. Soc. Nephrol.* 2003 Nov;14(11):2902-2907.

[13] Li, S. MD, Liu, J., Li, S., Collins, A. J. Differences between blacks and whites in the incidence of end-stage renal disease and associated risk factors. *Adv. Ren. Replace Ther.* 2004;1:05-13.

[14] Feehally, J. Ethnicity and renal disease. *Kidney Int.* 2005;68(1):414-24.

[15] Muntner, P., Anderson, A., Charleston, J., Chen, Z., Ford, V., Makos, G., O'Connor, A., Perumal, K., Rahman, M., Steigerwalt, S., Teal, V., Townsend, R., Weir, M., Wright, J. T. Jr; Chronic Renal Insufficiency Cohort (CRIC) Study Investigators. Hypertension awareness, treatment, and control in adults with CKD: results from the Chronic Renal Insufficiency Cohort (CRIC) Study. *Am. J. Kidney Dis.* 2010; 55(3):441-451.

[16] Crews, D. C., Plantinga, L. C., Miller, E. R., 3rd, Saran, R., Hedgeman, E., Saydah, S. H., Williams, D. E., Powe, N. R.; Centers for Disease Control and Prevention Chronic Kidney Disease Surveillance Team. Prevalence of chronic kidney disease in persons with undiagnosed or prehypertension in the United States. *Hypertension.* 2010 May; 55 (5):1102-9.

[17] Egan, B. M., Zhao, Y., Axon, R. N., Brzezinski, W. A., Ferdinand, K. C. Uncontrolled and apparent treatment resistant hypertension in the United States, 1988 to 2008. *Circulation.* 2011 Aug. 30;124(9):1046-58.

[18] Knight, E. L., Kramer, H. M., Curhan, G. C.: High-normal blood pressure and microalbuminuria. *Am. J. Kidney Dis.* 41(3):588-595, 2003.

[19] Klag, M. J., Whelton, P. K., Randall, B. L., et al.: End-stage renal disease in African-American and white men. 16-year MRFIT findings. *JAMA* 277:1293-1298, 1997.

[20] Stehman-Breen, C. O., Gillen, D., Steffes, M., et al.: Racial differences in early-onset renal disease among young adults: the coronary artery risk development in young adults (CARDIA) study. *J. Am. Soc. Nephrol.* 14(9):2352-7, 2003.

[21] Tarver-Carr, M. E., Powe, N. R., Eberhardt, M. S., et al.: Excess risk of chronic kidney disease among African-American versus white subjects in the United States: A population-based study of potential explanatory factors. *J. Am. Soc. Nephrol.* 13:2363–2370, 2002.

[22] Suthanthiran, M., Li, B., Song, J. O., et al.: Transforming growth factor-beta1 hyperexpression in African-American hypertensives: A novel mediator of hypertension and/or target organ damage. *Proc. Natl. Acad. Sci. US* 97(7):3479-84, 2000.

[23] Norris, K. and Nissenson, A. R. Race, gender, and socioeconomic disparities in CKD in the United States. *J. Am. Soc. Nephrol.* 2008; 19:1261-1270.

[24] Freedman, B. I., Parekh, R. S., Kao, W. H. Genetic basis of nondiabetic end-stage renal disease. *Semin. Nephrol.* 2010 Mar.;30(2):101-10.

[25] Norris, K. C. and Francis, C. K. Gender and ethnic differences and considerations in cardiovascular risk assessment and prevention in African Americans. In: Wong, N., Gardin, J. M. and Black, H. R., *Practical Strategies in Preventing Heart Disease.* McGraw-Hill, New York, 2004. pp 415-440.

[26] Ju, W., Eichinger, F., Bitzer, M., Oh, J., McWeeney, S., Berthier, C. C., Shedden, K., Cohen, C. D., Henger, A., Krick, S., Kopp, J. B., Stoeckert, C. J. Jr, Dikman, S., Schröppel, B., Thomas, D. B., Schlondorff, D., Kretzler, M., Böttinger, E. P. Renal gene and protein expression signatures for prediction of kidney disease progression. *Am. J. Pathol.* 2009 Jun;174(6):2073-85.

[27] Dustan, H. P., Valdes, G., Bravo, E. L., Tarazi, R. C. Excessive Na+ retention as a characteristic of salt-sensitive hypertension. *Am. J. Med. Sci.* 1986;29:67-74.

[28] Campese, V. M., Romoff, M. S., Levitan, D., Saglikes, Y., Friedler, R. M., Massry, S. G.: Abnormal relationship between Na+ intake and sympathetic nervous system activity in salt-sensitive patients with essential hypertension. *Kidney Internat.* 1982;21:371-378.

[29] Weinberger, M. H., Miller, J. Z., Luft, F. C., Grim, C. E., Fineberg, N. S. Definitions and characteristics of Na+ sensitivity and blood pressure resistance. *Hypertension* 1986; 8:II 127- II 134.

[30] Grim, C. E., Miller, J. Z., Luft, F. C., Christian, J. C., Weinberger, M. H.: Genetic influences on renin, aldosterone, and the renal excretion of sodium and potassium following volume expansion and contraction in normal man. *Hypertension* 1979;1:583-590.

[31] Wilson, T. W., Grim, C. E. Biohistory of slavery and blood pressure differences in blacks today. A hypothesis. *Hypertension.* 1991 Jan;17(1 Suppl.):I122-8.

[32] Maseko, M. J., Majane, H. O., Milne, J., Norton, G. R., Woodiwiss, A. J. Salt intake in an urban, developing South African community. *Cardiovasc. J. S. Afr.* 2006 Jul-Aug; 17(4):186-91.

[33] Curtin, P. D. The slavery hypothesis for hypertension among African Americans: the historical evidence. *Am. J. Public Health.* 1992 Dec;82(12):1681-6.

[34] Keane, W. F. Proteinuria: its clinical importance and role in progressive renal disease. *Am. J. Kidney Dis.* 2000 Apr;35(4 Suppl. 1):S97-105.

[35] Sangalli, F., Carrara, F., Gaspari, F., Corna, D., Zoja, C., Botti, L., Remuzzi, G., Remuzzi, A. Effect of ACE inhibition on glomerular permselectivity and tubular albumin concentration in the renal ablation model. *Am. J. Physiol. Renal Physiol.* 2011 Jun;300(6):F1291-300.

[36] Benigni, A., Remuzzi, G. Glomerular protein trafficking and progression of renal disease to terminal uremia. *Semin. Nephrol.* 1996 May;16(3):151-9.

[37] Gorriz, J. L., Martinez-Castelao, A. Proteinuria: detection and role in native renal disease progression. *Transplant. Rev.* (Orlando). 2012 Jan;26(1):3-13.

[38] Gaedeke, J., Noble, N. A., Border, W. A. Angiotensin II and progressive renal insufficiency. *Curr. Hypertens. Rep.* 2002 Oct;4(5):403-7.

[39] Fang, F., Liu, G. C., Kim, C., Yassa, R., Zhou, J., Scholey, J. W. Adiponectin attenuates angiotensin II-induced oxidative stress in renal tubular cells through AMPK and cAMP-Epac signal transduction pathways. *Am. J. Physiol. Renal Physiol.* 2013 Jun. 1;304(11):F1366-74.

[40] Eskildsen, T. V., Jeppesen, P. L., Schneider, M., Nossent, A. Y., Sandberg, M. B., Hansen, P. B., Jensen, C. H., Hansen, M. L., Marcussen, N., Rasmussen, L. M., Bie, P., Andersen, D. C., Sheikh, S. P. Angiotensin II Regulates microRNA-132/-212 in Hypertensive Rats and Humans. *Int. J. Mol. Sci.* 2013 May 27;14(6):11190-207.

[41] Hayakawa, H. C. K., Raij, L. Endothelial dysfunction and cardiorenal injury in experimental salt-sensitive hypertension: effects of antihypertensive therapy. *Circulation* 1997; 7:2407-13.

[42] Norris, K. C., Tareen, N., Martins, D., Vaziri, N. Implications of ethnicity for the treatment of hypertensive kidney disease, with an emphasis on African Americans. *Nat. Clin. Pract. Nephrol.* 2008; 4(10):538-49.

[43] Sever, P. S., Gordon, D., Peart, W. S., Beighton, P. Blood-pressure and its correlates in urban and tribal Africa. *Lancet.* 1980 Jul. 12;2(8185):60-4.

[44] Luft, F. C., Grim, C. E., Fineberg, N. S., Weinberger, M. C. Effects of volume expansion and contraction in normotensive whites, blacks, and subjects of different ages. *Circulation.* 1979;59:643–650.

[45] Laffer, C. L., Elijovich, F. Essential hypertension of Caribbean Hispanics: sodium, renin, and response to therapy. *J. Clin. Hypertens.* (Greenwich). 2002 Jul-Aug;4(4): 266-73.

[46] Vaziri, N. D., Bai, Y., Ni, Z., Quiroz, Y., Pandian, R., Rodriguez-Iturbe, B. Intra-renal angiotensin II/AT1 receptor, oxidative stress, inflammation, and progressive injury in renal mass reduction. *J. Pharmacol. Exp. Ther.* 2007 Oct;323(1):85-93).

[47] Vio, C. P., Jeanneret, V. A. Local induction of angiotensin-converting enzyme in the kidney as a mechanism of progressive renal diseases. *Kidney Int.* Suppl. 2003 Oct;(86): S57-S63.

[48] Kobori, H., Nangaku, M., Navar, L. G., Nishiyama, A. The intrarenal renin-angiotensin system: from physiology to the pathobiology of hypertension and kidney disease. *Pharmacol. Rev.* 2007 Sep;59(3):251-87.

[49] Kim, H. J., Sato, T., Rodriguez-Iturbe, B., Vaziri, N. D. Role of intrarenal angiotensin system activation, oxidative stress, inflammation, and impaired nuclear factor-erythroid-2-related factor 2 activity in the progression of focal glomerulosclerosis. *J. Pharmacol. Exp. Ther.* 2011 Jun;337(3):583-90.

[50] Rodríguez-Iturbe, B., Vaziri, N. D., Herrera-Acosta, J., Johnson, R. J. Oxidative stress, renal infiltration of immune cells, and salt-sensitive hypertension: all for one and one for all. *Am. J. Physiol. Renal Physiol.* 2004 Apr;286(4):F606-16.

[51] Vaziri, N. D., Rodriguez-Itrube, B. Mechanisms of Disease: oxidative stress and inflammation in the patogenesis of hypertension. *Nature, Reviews Nephrol.* 2:582-593, 2006.

[52] Kobori, H. N. A., Abe, Y., Navar, L. G. Enhancement of intrarenal angiotensinogen in Dahl salt-sensitive rats on high salt diet. *Hypertension.* 2003;41(3):592-7.

[53] Chandramohan, G., Bai, Y., Norris, K., Rodriguez-Iturbe, B., Vaziri, N. D. Effects of Dietary Salt on Intrarenal Angiotensin System, NAD(P)H Oxidase, COX-2, MCP-1 and PAI-1 Expressions and NF-kappaB Activity in Salt-Sensitive and -Resistant Rat Kidneys. *Am. J. Nephrol.* 2007 Oct. 19;28(1):158-167.

[54] Hayakawa, H. C. K., Raij, L. Endothelial dysfunction and cardiorenal injury in experimental salt-sensitive hypertension: effects of antihypertensive therapy. *Circulation.* 1997;7:2407-13.

[55] Vaziri, N. D., Xu, Z. G., Shahkarami, A., Huang, K. T., Rodríguez-Iturbe, B., Natarajan, R. Role of AT-1 receptor in regulation of vascular MCP-1, IL-6, PAI-1, MAP kinase, and matrix expressions in obesity. *Kidney Int.* 2005 Dec;68(6):2787-93.

[56] Xu, Z. G., Lanting, L., Vaziri, N. D., Li, Z., Sepassi, L., Rodriguez-Iturbe, B., Natarajan, R. Upregulation of angiotensin II type 1 receptor, inflammatory mediators, and enzymes of arachidonate metabolism in obese Zucker rat kidney: reversal by angiotensin II type 1 receptor blockade. *Circulation*. 2005 Apr. 19;111(15):1962-9.

[57] Wolak, T., Kim, H-J., Ren, Y., Kim, J., Vaziri, N.D., Nicholas, S.B. Osteopontin modulates angiotensin II–induced inflammation, oxidative stress, and fibrosis of the kidney. *Kidney International* (2009) 76, 32–43.

[58] Yu, X. Q., Wu, L. L., Huang, X. R., Yang, N., Gilbert, R. E., Cooper, M. E., Johnson, R. J., Lai, K. N., Lan, H. Y. Osteopontin expression in progressive renal injury in remnant kidney: role of angiotensin II. *Kidney Int*. 2000 Oct;58(4):1469-80.

[59] Bianchi, G., Tripodi, M. D., Casari, G., Torielli, L., Cusi, D., Barlassina, C., Stella, P., Zagato, L., Barber, B. R.: Alpha adducing may control blood pressure in both rats and humans. *Clin. Exp. Pharmacol. Physiol*. 1995;1:S7–S9.

[60] Barlassina, C., Norton, G. R., Samani, N. J., Woodwiss, A. J., Candy, G. C., Radevski, I., Citterio, L., Bianchi, G., Cusi, D. Alpha-adducin polymorphism in hypertensives of South African ancestry. *Am. J. Hypertens*. 2000 Jun;13(6 Pt 1):719-23.

[61] Tiago, A. D., Nkeh, B., Candy, G. P., Badenhorst, D., Defterios, D., Brooksbank, R., Nejthardt, M., Luker, F., Milne, J., Woodiwiss, A. J., Norton, G. R. Association study of eight candidate genes with renin status in mild-to-moderate hypertension in patients of African ancestry. *Cardiovasc. J. S. Afr*. 2001 Apr-May;12(2):75-80.

[62] Schork, N. J., Chakravarti, A., Thiel, B., Fornage, M., Jacob, H. J., Cai, R., Rotimi, C. N., Cooper, R. S., Weder, A. B. Lack of association between a biallelic polymorphism in the adducin gene and blood pressure in whites and African Americans. *Am. J. Hypertens*. 2000 Jun;13(6 Pt 1):693-8.

[63] Liu, K., Liu, J., Huang, Y., Liu, Y., Lou, Y., Wang, Z., Zhang, H., Yan, S., Li, Z., Wen, S. Alpha-adducin Gly460Trp polymorphism and hypertension risk: a meta-analysis of 22 studies including 14303 cases and 15961 controls. *PLoS* One. 2010 Sep. 28;5(9).

[64] Martins, D. S., Norris, K. C. Diagnosis and treatment of secondary hypertension. In: Crawford, M. H. and DiMarco, J. P. *International Textbook of Cardiology*. Mosby International Limited. 2003, Section 3, pp. 553-562.

[65] Beeks, E., Kessels, A. G., Kroon, A. A., van der Klauw, M. M., de Leeuw, P. W. Genetic predisposition to salt-sensitivity: a systematic review. *J. Hypertens*. 2004 Jul; 22(7):1243-9.

[66] Tiago, A. D., Samani, N. J., Candy, G. P., Brooksbank, R., Libhaber, E. N., Sareli, P., Woodiwiss, A. J., Norton, G. R. Angiotensinogen gene promoter region variant modifies body size-ambulatory blood pressure relations in hypertension. *Circulation*. 2002 Sep. 17;106(12):1483-7.

[67] Woodiwiss, A. J., Nkeh, B., Samani, N. J., Badenhorst, D., Maseko, M., Tiago, A. D., Candy, G. P., Libhaber, E., Sareli, P., Brooksbank, R., Norton, G. R. Functional variants of the angiotensinogen gene determine antihypertensive responses to angiotensin-converting enzyme inhibitors in subjects of African origin. *J. Hypertens*. 2006 Jun;24(6):1057-64.

[68] Bhatnagar, V., O'Connor, D. T., Schork, N. J., Salem, R. M., Nievergelt, C. M., Rana, B. K., Smith, D. W., Bakris, G. L., Middleton, J. P., Norris, K. C., Wright, J. T., Cheek, D., Hiremath, L., Contreras, G., Appel, L. J., Lipkowitz, M. S. Angiotensin-converting enzyme gene polymorphism predicts the time-course of blood pressure response to

angiotensin converting enzyme inhibition in the AASK trial. *J. Hypertens*. 2007;25(10): 2082-2092.

[69] Norris, K. C., Agodoa, L. Y. Unraveling the racial disparities associated with kidney disease. *Kidney Int*. 2005; 68:914–924.

[70] Powe, N. R.: To have and have not: Health and health care disparities in chronic kidney disease. *Kidney Int*. 2003; 64:763-772.

[71] Genovese, G., Friedman, D. J., Ross, M. D., Lecordier, L., Uzureau, P., Freedman, B. I., Bowden, D. W., Langefeld, C. D., Oleksyk, T. K., Uscinski Knob, A. L., Bernhardy, A. J., Hicks, P. J., Nelson, G. W., Vanhollebeke, B., Winkler, C. A., Kopp, J. B., Pays, E., Pollak, M. R. Association of trypanolytic ApoL1 variants with kidney disease in African Americans. *Science* 2010; 13;329(5993):841-5.

[72] W. H. L. Kao, M. J. Klag, L. A. Meoni, D. Reich, Y. Berthier-Schaad, M. Li, J. Coresh, N. Patterson, N. R. Powe, N. E. Fink, J. Sadler, M. Weir, S. Adler, J. Divers, S. Iyengar, B. I. Freedman, K. Kamp, K. Leehey, S. B. Nicholas, M. Pahl, J. Schelling, J. R. Sedor, D. Thornley-Brown, C. Winkler, M. W. Smith, and R. S. Parekh. MYH9 is associated with nondiabetic end-stage renal disease in African Americans. *Nat. Genet*. 2008; 40: 1185–1192.

[73] Freedman, B. I., Kopp, J. B., Langefeld, C. D., Genovese, G., Friedman, D. J., Nelson, G. W., Winkler, C. A., Bowden, D. W., Pollak, M. R. The apolipoprotein L1 (APOL1) gene and nondiabetic nephropathy in African Americans. *J. Am. Soc. Nephrol*. 2010; 21 (9):1422-1426.

[74] Ko, W. Y., Rajan, P., Gomez, F., Scheinfeldt, L., An, P., Winkler, C. A., Froment, A., Nyambo, T. B., Omar, S. A., Wambebe, C., Ranciaro, A., Hirbo, J. B., Tishkoff, S. A. Identifying Darwinian Selection Acting on Different Human APOL1 Variants among Diverse African Populations. *Am. J. Hum. Genet*. 2013 Jul. 11;93(1):54-66. doi: 10. 1016/j.ajhg.2013.05.014. Epub. 2013 Jun. 13.

[75] Hebert, L. A., Kusek, J. W., Greene, T., Agodoa, L. Y., Jones, C. A., Levey, A. S., Breyer, J. A., Faubert, P., Rolin, H. A., Wang, S. R. Effects of blood pressure control on progressive renal disease in blacks and whites. Modification of Diet in Renal Disease Study Group. *Hypertension*. 1997 Sep;30(3 Pt 1):428-35.

[76] EJ, Hunsicker, L. G., Bain, R. P., et al.: The effect of angiotensin-converting-enzyme inhibition on diabetic nephropathy. The Collaborative Study Group. *N. Engl. J. Med*. 329:1456-62, 1993.

[77] The GISEN Group (Gruppo Italiano di Studi Epidemiologici in Nefrologia): Randomised placebo-controlled trial of effect of ramipril on decline in glomerular filtration rate and risk of terminal renal failure in proteinuric, non-diabetic nephropathy. *Lancet*. 349:1857-63, 1997.

[78] Mann, J. F. E., Gerstein, H. C., Pogue, J., Bosch, J., Yusuf, S. for the HOPE Investigators. Renal Insufficiency as a Predictor of Cardiovascular Outcomes and the Impact of Ramipril: The HOPE Randomized Trial. *Ann. Intern. Med*. 2001;134:629-636.

[79] Whelton, P. K., Lee, J. Y., Kusek, J. W., Charleston, J., Debruge, J., Douglas, M., Faulkner, M., Greene, P., Jones, C., Keefer, S., Kirk Katherine, Lovell, B., Norris, K., Peng, S., Powers, S., Retta, T., Smith, D., and Ward, H. for the AASK Pilot Study Investigators: Recruitment experience in the African-American Study of Kidney

Disease and Hypertension (AASK) Pilot Study. *Controlled Clinical Trials* 1996; 16: 17S-33S.

[80] Wright, J. T. Jr, Bakris, G., Greene, T., Agodoa, L. Y., Appel, L. J., Charleston, J., Cheek, D., Douglas-Baltimore, J. G., Gassman, J., Glassock, R., Hebert, L., Jamerson, K., Lewis, J., Phillips, R. A., Toto, R. D., Middleton, J. P., Rostand, S. G.; African Effect of blood pressure lowering and antihypertensive drug class on progression of hypertensive kidney disease: results from the AASK trial. *JAMA*. 2002 Nov. 20;288(19):2421-31. Erratum in: *JAMA*. 2006 Jun. 21;295(23):2726.

[81] Agodoa, L. Y., Appel, L., Bakris, G. L., et al. for the African American Study of Kidney Disease and Hypertension (AASK) Study Group: Effect of ramipril vs amlodipine on renal outcomes in hypertensive nephrosclerosis: a randomized controlled trial. *JAMA* 285(21):2719-28, 2001.

[82] Wright, J. T. Jr, Agodoa, L., Contreras, G., Greene, T., Douglas, J. G., Lash, J., Randall, O., Rogers, N., Smith, M. C., Massry, S.; African Successful blood pressure control in the African American Study of Kidney Disease and Hypertension. *Arch. Intern. Med.* 2002 Jul. 22;162(14):1636-43.

[83] Norris, K., Bourgoigne, J., Gassman, J., Hebert, L., Middleton, J., Phillips, R., Randall, O., Rostand, S., Sherer, S., Toto, R., Wright, J., Wang, X., Greene, T., Appel, L., Lewis, J.; for the African American Study of Kidney Disease and Hypertension (AASK) Study Group. Cardiovascular Outcomes in the African American Study of Kidney Disease and Hypertension (AASK) Trial. *Am. J. Kidney Dis.* 2006 Nov;48(5): 739-51.

[84] Shulman, N. B., Ford, C. E., Hall, W. D., Blaufox, M. D., Simon, D., Langford, H. G., Schneider, K. A. Prognostic value of serum creatinine and effect of treatment of hypertension on renal function. Results from the hypertension detection and follow-up program. The Hypertension Detection and Follow-up Program Cooperative Group. *Hypertension*. 1989;13:I80-I93.

[85] Leenen, F. H., Nwachuku, C. E., Black, H. R., Cushman, W. C., Davis, B. R., Simpson, L. M., Alderman, M. H., Atlas, S. A., Basile, J. N., Cuyjet, A. B., Dart, R., Felicetta, J. V., Grimm, R. H., Haywood, L. J., Jafri, S. Z., Proschan, M. A., Thadani, U., Whelton, P. K., Wright, J. T.; Antihypertensive and Lipid-Lowering Treatment to Prevent Heart Attack Trial Collaborative Research Group. Clinical events in high-risk hypertensive patients randomly assigned to calcium channel blocker versus angiotensin-converting enzyme inhibitor in the antihypertensive and lipid-lowering treatment to prevent heart attack trial. *Hypertension*. 2006 Sep;48(3):374-84.

[86] Gibbs, C. R., Lip, G. Y., Beevers, D. G.: Angioedema due to ACE inhibitors: increased risk in patients of African origin. *Br. J. Clin. Pharmacol.* 48:861-865, 1999.

[87] Elliott, W. J. Higher incidence of discontinuation of angiotensin converting enzyme inhibitors due to cough in black subjects. *Clin. Pharmacol. Ther.* 1996 Nov;60(5):582-8.

[88] Woo, K. S., Nicholls, M. G. High prevalence of persistent cough with angiotensin converting enzyme inhibitors in Chinese. *Br. J. Clin. Pharmacol.* 1995 Aug;40(2):141-4.

[89] Lewis, E. J., Hunsicker, L. G., Clarke, W. R., et al.: Renoprotective effect of the angiotensin-receptor antagonist irbesartan in patients with nephropathy due to type 2 diabetes. *N. Engl. J. Med.* 345:851-60, 2001.

[90] Brenner, B. M., Cooper, M. E., de Zeeuw, D., et al.: Effects of losartan on renal and cardiovascular outcomes in patients with type 2 diabetes and nephropathy. *N. Engl. J. Med.* 345:861-9, 2001.

[91] De Zeeuw, D., Ramjit, D., Zhang, Z., Ribeiro, A. B., Kurokawa, K., Lash, J. P., Chan, J., Remuzzi, G., Brenner, B. M., Shahinfar, S. Renal risk and renoprotection among ethnic groups with type 2 diabetic nephropathy: a post hoc analysis of RENAAL. *Kidney Int.* 2006; 69(9):1675-82.

[92] ALLHAT Officers and Coordinators for the ALLHAT Collaborative Research Group. The Antihypertensive and Lipid-Lowering Treatment to Prevent Heart Attack Trial. Major outcomes in high-risk hypertensive patients randomized to angiotensin-converting enzyme inhibitor or calcium channel blocker vs diuretic: The Antihypertensive and Lipid-Lowering Treatment to Prevent Heart Attack Trial (ALLHAT). *JAMA*. 2002 Dec. 18;288(23):2981-97. Erratum in: *JAMA* 2003 Jan. 8;289 (2):178. *JAMA*. 2004 May 12;291(18):2196.

[93] Messerli, F. H., Grossman, E. Doxazosin arm of the ALLHAT study discontinued: how equal are antihypertensive drugs? Antihypertensive and Lipid Lowering Treatment to Prevent Heart Attack Trial. *Curr. Hypertens. Rep.* 2000 Jun;2(3):241-2.

[94] Wright, J. T. Jr, Dunn, J. K., Cutler, J. A., Davis, B. R., Cushman, W. C., Ford Outcomes in hypertensive black and nonblack patients treated with chlorthalidone, amlodipine, and lisinopril. *JAMA*. 2005 Apr. 6;293(13):1595-608.

[95] Rahman, M., Pressel, S., Davis, B. R., Nwachuku, C., Wright, J. T. Jr, Whelton, P. K., Barzilay, J., Batuman, V., Eckfeldt, J. H., Farber, M., Henriquez, M., Kopyt, N., Louis, G. T., Saklayen, M., Stanford, C., Walworth, C., Ward, H., Wiegmann, T. Renal outcomes in high-risk hypertensive patients treated with an angiotensin-converting enzyme inhibitor or a calcium channel blocker vs a diuretic: a report from the Antihypertensive and Lipid-Lowering Treatment to Prevent Heart Attack Trial (ALLHAT). *Arch. Intern. Med.* 2005 Apr. 25;165(8):936-46.

[96] Yusuf, S., Teo, K. K., Pogue, J., et al.; ONTARGET investigators. Telmisartan, ramipril, or both in patients at high risk for vascular events. *N. Engl. J. Med.* 2008 Apr. 10; 358(15):1547-59.

[97] Mann, J. F., Schmieder, R. E., McQueen, M., et al.; ONTARGET investigators. Renal outcomes with telmisartan, ramipril, or both, in people at high vascular risk (the ONTARGET study): a multicentre, randomised, double-blind, controlled trial. *Lancet*. 2008 Aug. 16;372(9638):547-53.

[98] Lambers Heerspink, H. J, de Zeeuw, D. ONTARGET still OFF-TARGET? *Circulation* 2011; 123: 1049–1051.

[99] Parving, H. H., Brenner, B. M., McMurray, J. J., et al. Baseline characteristics in the Aliskiren Trial in Type 2 Diabetes Using Cardio-Renal Endpoints (ALTITUDE). *J. Renin. Angiotensin Aldosterone Syst.* 2012; 13: 387–393.

[100] US Food and Drug Administration. FDA drug safety communication: New warning and contraindication for blood pressure medicines containing aliskiren (Tekturna). Accessed 7-22-13 at http://www.fda.gov/Drugs/DrugSafety/ucm300889.htm - posted 02/15/2013.

[101] Balamuthusamy, S., Srinivasan, L., Verma, M., et al. Renin angiotensin system blockade and cardiovascular outcomes in patients with chronic kidney disease and proteinuria: a meta-analysis. *Am. Heart J.* 2008; 155: 791–805.

[102] Cushman, W. C., Evans, G. W., Byington, R. P., et al. Effects of intensive blood pressure control in type 2 diabetes mellitus. *N Engl. J. Med.* 2010; 362: 1575–1585.

[103] Upadhyay, A., Earley, A., Haynes, S. M., Uhlig, K. Systematic review: blood pressure target in chronic kidney disease and proteinuria as an effect modifier. *Ann. Intern. Med.* 2011 Apr. 19;154(8):541-8.

[104] Appel, L. J., Wright, J. T. Jr, Greene, T., et al. AASK Collaborative Research Group. Intensive blood-pressure control in hypertensive chronic kidney disease. *N. Engl. J. Med.* 2010; 363(10):918-29.

[105] Lea, J., Greene, T., Hebert, L., Lipkowitz, M., Massry, S., Middleton, J., Rostand, S. G., Miller, E., Smith, W., Bakris, G. L. The relationship between magnitude of proteinuria reduction and risk of end-stage renal disease: results of the African American study of kidney disease and hypertension. *Arch. Intern. Med.* 2005 Apr. 25; 165(8):947-53.

[106] KDIGO Blood Pressure Work Group. KDIGO clinical practice guideline for the management of blood pressure in chronic kidney disease. *Kidney Int.* 2012; 2(Suppl.): 337–414.

[107] Wheeler, D. C., Becker, G. J. Summary of KDIGO guideline. What do we really know about management of blood pressure in patients with chronic kidney disease? *Kidney Int.* 2013 Jan. 16. doi: 10.1038/ki.2012.425. [Epub. ahead of print].

[108] Leenen, F. H., Nwachuku, C. E., Black, H. R., Cushman, W. C., Davis, B. R., Simpson, L. M., Alderman, M. H., Atlas, S. A., Basile, J. N., Cuyjet, A. B., Dart, R., Felicetta, J. V., Grimm, R. H., Haywood, L. J., Jafri, S. Z., Proschan, M. A., Thadani, U., Whelton, P. K., Wright, J. T.; Antihypertensive and Lipid-Lowering Treatment to Prevent Heart Attack Trial Collaborative Research Group. Clinical events in high-risk hypertensive patients randomly assigned to calcium channel blocker versus angiotensin-converting enzyme inhibitor in the antihypertensive and lipid-lowering treatment to prevent heart attack trial. *Hypertension.* 2006 Sep;48(3):374-84.

[109] Gibbs, C. R., Lip, G. Y., Beevers, D. G.: Angioedema due to ACE inhibitors: increased risk in patients of African origin. *Br. J. Clin. Pharmacol.* 48:861-865, 1999.

[110] Elliott, W. J. Higher incidence of discontinuation of angiotensin converting enzyme inhibitors due to cough in black subjects. *Clin. Pharmacol. Ther.* 1996 Nov;60(5):582-8.

[111] Woo, K. S., Nicholls, M. G. High prevalence of persistent cough with angiotensin converting enzyme inhibitors in Chinese. *Br. J. Clin. Pharmacol.* 1995 Aug;40(2):141-4.

[112] Holtkamp, F. A., de Zeeuw, D., Thomas, M. C., et al. An acute fall in estimated glomerular filtration rate during treatment with losartan predicts a slower decrease in long-term renal function. *Kidney Int.* 2011; 80: 282–287.

[113] Weir, M. R. Acute fall in glomerular filtration rate with renin-angiotensin system inhibition: a biomeasure of therapeutic success? *Kidney Int.* 2011; 80: 235–237.

[114] Srivastava, S., Beevers, D. G. Angioplasty for atheromatous renal artery stenosis: current knowledge and trial results awaited. *J. Hum. Hypertens.* 2007 Jul;21(7):507-8.

[115] Mistry, S., Ives, N., Harding, J., Fitzpatrick-Ellis, K., Lipkin, G., Kalra, P. A., Moss, J., Wheatley, K. Angioplasty and STent for Renal Artery Lesions (ASTRAL trial): rationale, methods and results so far. *J. Hum. Hypertens.* 2007 Jul;21(7):511-5.

[116] Rocha-Singh, K., Jaff, M. R., Rosenfield, K.; ASPIRE-2 Trial Investigators. Evaluation of the safety and effectiveness of renal artery stenting after unsuccessful balloon angioplasty: the ASPIRE-2 study. *J. Am. Coll. Cardiol.* 2005 Sep. 6;46(5):776-83.

[117] Veterans Administration Cooperative Study Group on Antihypertensive Agents: Comparison of propanolol and hydrochlorothiazide for the initial treatment of hypertension: I, Results of short-term titration with emphasis on racial differences in response. *JAMA* 1982;248:1996-2003.

[118] Sehgal, A. R. Overlap between whites and blacks in response to antihypertensive drugs. *Hypertension.* 2004 Mar;43(3):566-72.

[119] Martins, D., Agodoa, L., Norris, K. Hypertensive chronic kidney disease in African Americans: Strategies for improving care. *Cleve Clin. J. Med.* 2012 Oct;79(10):726-734.

[120] Martins, D., Norris, K. Hypertension treatment in African Americans: physiology is less important than sociology. *Cleve Clin. J. Med.* 2004 Sep;71(9):735-43.

[121] Flack, J. M., Sica, D. A., Bakris, G., Brown, A. L., Ferdinand, K. C., Grimm, R. H. Jr, Hall, W. D., Jones, W. E., Kountz, D. S., Lea, J. P., Nasser, S., Nesbitt, S. D., Saunders, E., Scisney-Matlock, M., Jamerson, K. A.; International Society on Hypertension in Blacks. Management of high blood pressure in Blacks: an update of the International Society on Hypertension in Blacks consensus statement. *Hypertension* 2010; 56(5):780-800.

[122] Wright, J. T. Jr, Agodoa, L. Y., Appel, L., Cushman, W. C., Taylor, A. L., Obegdegbe, G. G., Osei, K., Reed, J. New recommendations for treating hypertension in black patients: evidence and/or consensus? *Hypertension* 2010; 56(5):801-3.

[123] Nicholas, S. B., Vaziri, N. D. and Norris, K. C. What Should Be The Blood Pressure Target For Patients With Chronic Kidney Disease? *Curr. Opin. Cardiol.* 2013 Jul;28 (4):439-45.

[124] National Heart Lung and Blood Institute. NIH launches multicenter clinical trial to test blood pressure strategy. http://public.nhlbi.nih.gov/newsroom/home/GetPressRelease.aspx?id=2667. (accessed 7-12-13).

[125] Norris, K. C., Vaughn, C. The Role of Renin-Angiotensin-Aldosterone System Inhibition in Chronic Kidney Disease. *Expert Rev. Cardiovasc. Ther.* 2003;1(1):51-63.

[126] Efficacy of atenolol and captopril in reducing risk of macrovascular and microvascular complications in type 2 diabetes: UKPDS 39. UK Prospective Diabetes Study Group. *BMJ.* 1998 Sep. 12;317(7160):713-20.

[127] Jafar, T. H., Schmid, C. H., Landa, M., Giatras, I., Toto, R., Remuzzi, G., Maschio, G., Brenner, B. M., Kamper, A., Zucchelli, P., Becker, G., Himmelmann, A., Bannister, K., Landais, P., Shahinfar, S., de Jong, P. E., de Zeeuw, D., Lau, J., Levey, A. S. Angiotensin-converting enzyme inhibitors and progression of nondiabetic renal disease. A meta-analysis of patient-level data. *Ann. Intern. Med.* 2001 Jul. 17;135(2):73-87. Erratum in: *Ann. Intern. Med.* 2002 Aug. 20;137(4):299.

[128] Nakao, N., Yoshimura, A., Morita, H., Takada, M., Kayano, T., Ideura, T. Combination treatment of angiotensin-II receptor blocker and angiotensin-converting-enzyme inhibitor in non-diabetic renal disease (COOPERATE): a randomised controlled trial. *Lancet.* 2003 Jan. 11;361(9352):117-24. Erratum in: *Lancet.* 2003 Apr. 5;361(9364): 1230.

[129] Rahman, M., Pressel, S., Davis, B. R., Nwachuku, C., Wright, J. T. Jr, Whelton, P. K., Barzilay, J., Batuman, V., Eckfeldt, J. H., Farber, M. A., Franklin, S., Henriquez, M., Kopyt, N., Louis, G. T., Saklayen, M., Stanford, C., Walworth, C., Ward, H., Wiegmann, T.; ALLHAT Collaborative Research Group. Cardiovascular Outcomes in High-Risk Hypertensive Patients Stratified by Baseline Glomerular Filtration Rate. *Ann. Intern. Med.* 2006;144:172-180.

[130] Bakris, G. L., Ruilope, L., Locatelli, F., Ptaszynska, A., Pieske, B., de Champlain, J., Weber, M. A., Raz, I. Treatment of microalbuminuria in hypertensive subjects with elevated cardiovascular risk: results of the IMPROVE trial. *Kidney Int.* 2007 Oct; 72 (7):879-85.

In: ACE Inhibitors. Volume 2
Editor: Macaulay Amechi Onuigbo
ISBN: 978-1-62948-422-8

Chapter 3

Angiotensin-Converting Enzyme Inhibitors: A Seattle Internist's Perspective

Ngozi Janet Achebe, MD*
Capital Medical Center, Olympia, WA, US

Abstract

Angiotensin converting enzyme inhibitors (ACEIs) were introduced into clinical medicine following the pioneering work started by Squibb Laboratory scientists in 1971. Captopril, the first orally effective ACE inhibitor was discovered by the Squibb Laboratory in 1977 as an antihypertensive agent. This chapter is a reflection of a Seattle Internist's perspective of the use, role and place of ACEIs and ARBs in modern day medicine.

Introduction

Following the innovative work of Squibb Laboratory scientists in the early 1970s, angiotensin-converting enzyme inhibitors (ACEIs) came into widespread use beginning in the late 80's as antihypertensive agents [1, 2]. Subsequent studies including randomized clinical trials (RCTs) on ACEIs that had highlighted the efficacy of this group of drugs in hypertensive and normotensive diabetics was greeted with a great deal of excitement. These trials, completed in the late 1980's and early 1990's demonstrated that ACEIs had the potential of halting, delaying and even reversing the nephropathic effects of diabetes on kidney tissue, beyond blood pressure lowering [3-7].

* Corresponding author: Ngozi Janet Achebe MD, E-mail: ngoziachebe@hotmail.com.

Role of ACE Inhibition in Hypertension Control and in Renoprotection

The renin-angiotensin-aldosterone system (RAAS) plays a major physiologic role in the regulation of blood pressure in the human body. Angiotensin converting enzyme (ACE) enables the conversion of the biologically inactive angiotensin I to the active moiety, angiotensin II. Angiotensin II then increases blood pressure by its action as a vasoconstrictor and also by promoting sodium and water retention in the body by stimulating the production of aldosterone, together with other effects on the renal and cardiovascular systems. Furthermore, ACE also inactivates bradykinin which lowers blood pressure by a vasodilatory effect on the circulation achieved by stimulating the production of prostaglandins and nitric oxide. Further details of this cascade are described in the introductory chapter of this book. From the foregoing, the blockade of the RAAS by ACEIs leads to a lowering of blood pressure. Moreover, in type II diabetic patients, ACEIs also reduce monocyte migration and differentiation to macrophages; since macrophages are responsible through production of certain cytokines, for extracellular matrix production and tubulointerstitial fibrosis, blocking RAAS leads to a slowing down or even reversal of diabetic nephropathy [8]. Besides, studies had also shown that ACEIs slowed down the progression of microalbuminuria and diabetic nephropathy with preservation of glomerular filtration rate in normotensive patients with insulin dependent diabetes and microalbuminuria [3-7, 9]. It must be acknowledged here that in the US, diabetic nephropathy accounts for about 40% of new cases of ESRD, and in 1997, the cost for treatment of diabetic patients with ESRD was in excess of $15.6 billion and climbing [10]. Therefore, drugs that target both microalbuminuria and hypertension, both of which have deleterious effects on the diabetic kidney, would thus constitute an important part of the armamentarium of pharmaceutical agents at the disposal of the physician in the fight against diabetic nephropathy and end stage kidney disease. ACEIs fit into this niche.

ACE Inhibition and Insulin Sensitivity

Besides, some studies have suggested that ACEIs may increase tissue insulin sensitivity. This is a modest effect of insulin-mediated glucose disposal probably as a result of increased muscle blood flow, local renin-angiotensin system blockade, and elevated kinin levels [11]. Additionally, ACEIs with a sulphydryl group seem to have a more potent action on insulin sensitivity than those without [12]. As hyperinsulinemia and increased insulin resistance are both risk factors for cardiovascular disease, the importance of this effect, albeit modest, cannot be over emphasized.

ACE Inhibition and Cardioprotection

The HOPE trial (Heart Outcomes Prevention Evaluation), a landmark study published in 2000 was the most important study that helped solidify the position of ACEIs as a group by extending the indications for their use into the arena of cardiovascular disease prophylaxis [13].

The HOPE study was the culmination of accumulating epidemiologic data that suggested that the RAAS played a strong role in increasing the risk of myocardial infarction. Ramipril, the ACEI used in the HOPE trial significantly reduced the rates of death, myocardial infarction, and stroke in a broad range of high-risk patients, including diabetics, who are not known to have a low ejection fraction or heart failure [13]. The SOLVD and SAVE trials found a significant reduction in subsequent acute coronary events in patients on ACEIs [14, 15].

In the Studies Of Left Ventricular Dysfunction (SOLVD) trial, the angiotensin-converting-enzyme inhibitor, Enalapril, significantly reduced the incidence of heart failure and the rate of related hospitalizations, as compared with the rates in the group given placebo, among patients with asymptomatic left ventricular dysfunction [14]. The Survival And Ventricular Enlargement (SAVE) trial randomized patients with acute MI and left ventricular dysfunction (left ventricular ejection fraction [LVEF] $\leq$40%) to receive the ACE inhibitor captopril or placebo and demonstrated that ACE inhibitor therapy was associated with reductions in the risk of death, the development of heart failure, and recurrent MI [15].

From the foregoing evidence-base, it is the general consensus that ACE inhibitors which blocked the conversion of angiotensin I to angiotensin II could indeed slow down the process and/or progression of atherosclerosis. To the contrary, in the HOPE trial vitamin E, an antioxidant, was compared with Ramipril, an ACEI [13]. An antioxidant, theoretically could potentially delay the pro-atherogenic processes on which atherosclerotic disease depends upon by inhibiting the oxidation of lipids. However, while the vitamin E arm showed no significant benefit, the Ramipril/placebo arm of the study was stopped early because of indisputable evidence of a reduction in strokes, heart attacks, heart failure and overall cardiovascular deaths by Ramipril [13]. In addition, coronary artery bypass graft surgery, and other revascularization procedures were significantly reduced in the ACEI patients [13].

ACE Inhibition and Renoprotection in Non-Diabetic Proteinuric Nephropathy

In addition to the renoprotection afforded to diabetic nephropathy with proteinuria, there is evidence for the extension of this effect of ACEIs in non-diabetic nephropathy with proteinuria as demonstrated in the REIN trials [16].

ACEIs as First-Line Antihypertensive Agents and Other Indications

ACEIs have become included in first line anti-hypertensive therapy by several regional, national and professional organizations including the American Heart Association, the Joint National Committee (US) on Prevention, Diagnosis and Management of Hypertension and the European and European Society of Hypertension in conjunction to the European Society of Cardiology (ESH/ESC), for the positive benefits indicated in patients with persistent left ventricular dysfunction and also in patients who show signs of early heart failure during an acute coronary syndrome [17-19].

ACE inhibitors may also be used in African Americans successfully, although higher doses and adding a diuretic may be necessary to optimize treatment. Therefore the current main indications for ACEIs are as first-line therapy in hypertensive patients with type 1 diabetes mellitus with proteinuria, in type II diabetics with proteinuria, in heart failure patients, with diastolic and/or systolic dysfunction, and in the post-MI patients with systolic dysfunction.

Do ACEIs Represent the Magic Bullet in Cardiovascular Pharmacology?

With all these beneficial effects of ACEIs, cited above, it is no wonder that an editorialist had once proclaimed that soon there would be a "pril for every ill". Indeed, in a 2001 editorial in the journal *Circulation*, Lip had surmised that the ACE inhibitors seem to be a "pill for every ill"; their use is well-established for the treatment of hypertension, heart failure, left ventricular systolic dysfunction, and perhaps for all patients with myocardial infarction, diabetic nephropathy, diabetic retinopathy, and possibly even diabetic neuropathy [20]. We pause here – a word of caution is necessary.

Side Effects of ACE Inhibition with Particular Reference to Kidney Dysfunction

Nonetheless, the great success story of the introduction and widespread use of ACEIs into clinical medicine has not come without a price. ACEIs may cause a syndrome of "functional renal insufficiency" and hyperkalemia that commonly develops shortly after initiation of ACE inhibitor therapy but can also occur after years of therapy. Preexisting hypotension and low cardiac filling pressures predict an adverse outcome of the use of ACEIs and so does volume depletion, bilateral renal artery stenosis, or stenosis of a dominant or single kidney, as in a renal transplant recipient [22].

Such reports of renal failure associated with ACEI have been reported since the 1990s [23-34]. However, there is this consensus among practicing physicians including nephrologists, that such renal failure associated with concomitant angiotensin inhibition is short-lived, predictable, and usually reversible upon drug discontinuation [23-34].

To the contrary, in a recent letter to the British Medical Journal in February 2013, Onuigbo et al. had postulated that the exponential increase in the observed incidence of acute kidney injury in chronic kidney disease (CKD) patients, both here in the US and around the world, in the past decade or so, could at least partly be blamed on the use of ACEIs (and angiotensin receptor blockers or ARBs) in the elderly patients with later stages (3-5) CKD [35].

Onuigbo et al. in another chapter in this book have discussed in detail, a related topic, the syndrome of late onset renal failure from angiotensin blockade (LORFFAB), first described in 2005 [36]. Indeed, Descombes and Fellay had described iatrogenic irreversible ESRD complicating angiotensin inhibition as far back as 2000 [37].

In yet another related chapter in this book, Fournier has highlighted the need for increased pharmacovigilance given their recent finding of infrequent serum creatinine testing in CKD patients on concurrent angiotensin inhibition, NSAIDs and diuretics, the so-called "triple whammy", in a large French database [38]. In still another chapter of this book, we have also described the syndrome of "quadruple whammy", a new syndrome that describes the increased AKI risk associated with patients on "triple whammy" combination medications who undergo major cardiovascular or other surgical procedures [39].

In summary, ACEIs represent a very important drug class that internists have used in the last two or more decades to treat hypertension, in the management of heart failure, for renoprotection in diabetic and non-diabetic nephropathies, and for cardiac remodeling following acute myocardial infarction. They remain very useful agents, but there is the need for caution, especially in the older (>65 year old) CKD patient with later stage (>3) CKD. In such patients, there is the need to "start low, and go slow" with the dose titration of angiotensin inhibition [40]. Moreover, the monitoring of serum creatinine – pharmacovigilance - must be strictly adhered to, following drug initiation, following angiotensin inhibition dose increases, and must be continued routinely and indefinitely as long as a patient is on an ACEI and/or an ARB, since renal failure could occur at any time in the continuum of angiotensin inhibition [35, 36, 38-43]. Finally, at any point in time, the treating internist must be ready to discontinue ACEI (and/or ARB) whenever there is observed any otherwise unexplained worsening of AKI on CKD I such patients [35, 36, 38-43].

REFERENCES

[1] Ondetti, M. A., Williams, N. J., Sabo, E. F., Pluscec, J., Weaver, E. R., Kocy, O. Angiotensin-converting enzyme inhibitors from the venom of Bothrops jararaca. Isolation, elucidation of structure, and synthesis. *Biochemistry.* 1971;10(22):4033-9.

[2] Ondetti, M. A., Rubin, B., Cushman, D. W. Design of specific inhibitors of angiotensin-converting enzyme: new class of orally active antihypertensive agents. *Science.* 1977; 196(4288):441-4.

[3] Bjorck, S., Mulec, H., Johnsen, S. A., et al. Renal protective effect of enalapril in diabetic nephropathy. *Br. Med. J.* 1992;304:339-43.

[4] Lewis, E. J., Hunsicker, L. G., Bain, R. P., et al. The effect of angiotensinconverting enzyme inhibitors on diabetic nephropathy. *N. Engl. J. Med.* 1993;329:1456-62.

[5] Bakris, G. L. Angiotensin-converting enzyme inhibitors and progression of diabetic nephropathy. [editorial] *Ann. Int. Med.* 1993;18:643-4.

[6] Mathiesen, E. R., Hommel, E., Giese, J., et al. Efficacy of captopril postponing nephropathy in normotensive insulin dependent diabetic patients with microalbuminuria. *Br. Med. J.* 1991;303:81-7.

[7] Remuzzi, G., Ruggenenti, P. Slowing the progression of diabetic nephropathy. *N. Engl. J. Med.* 1993 Nov. 11;329(20):1496-7.

[8] Amann, B., Tinzmann, R., Angelkort, B. ACE inhibitors improve diabetic nephropathy through suppression of renal MCP-1. *Diabetes Care.* 2003 Aug;26(8):2421-5.

[9] Mathiesen, E. R., Hommel, E., Hansen, H. P., Smidt, U. M., Parving, H. H. Randomised controlled trial of long term efficacy of captopril on preservation of kidney function in normotensive patients with insulin dependent diabetes and microalbuminuria. *BMJ.* 1999;319(7201):24-5.

[10] American Diabetes Association. Diabetes 2001 Vital Statistics. Alexandria, VA, ADA, 2001.

[11] Donnelly, R. Angiotensin-converting enzyme inhibitors and insulin sensitivity: metabolic effects in hypertension, diabetes, and heart failure. *J. Cardiovasc. Pharmacol.* 1992;20 Suppl. 11:S38-44.

[12] Uehara, M., Kishikawa, H., Isami, S., Kisanuki, K., Ohkubo, Y., et al. Effect on insulin sensitivity of angiotensin converting enzyme inhibitors with or without a sulphydryl group: bradykinin may improve insulin resistance in dogs and humans. *Diabetologia.* 1994;37(3):300-7.

[13] Yusuf, S., Sleight, P., Pogue, J., et al. Effects of an Angiotensin-Converting–Enzyme Inhibitor, Ramipril, on Cardiovascular Events in High-Risk Patients: The Heart Outcomes Prevention Evaluation Study. *N. Engl. J. Med.* 2000 Jan. 20;342(3):145-53. Erratum in: *N. Engl. J. Med.* 2000 Mar. 9;342(10):748. 2000 May 4;342(18):1376.

[14] Effect of enalapril on mortality and the development of heart failure in asymptomatic patients with reduced left ventricular ejection fractions. The SOLVD Investigators. *N. Engl. J. Med.* 327(10):685-691, 1992. Erratum in: *N. Engl. J. Med.* 1992; 327(24):1768.

[15] Pfeffer, M. A., Braunwald, E., Moyé, L. A., Basta, L., Brown, E. J., Cuddy, T. E., Davis, B. R., Geltman, E. M., Goldman, S., Flaker, G. C., Klein, M., Lamas, G. A., Packer, M., Rouleau, J., Rouleau, J. L., Rutherford, J., Wertheimer, J. H., Hawkins, C. M., on behalf of the SAVE Investigators. Effect of captopril on mortality and morbidity in patients with left ventricular dysfunction after myocardial infarction: results of the Survival And Ventricular Enlargement trial. *N. Engl. J. Med.* 1992; 327: 669–677.

[16] Ruggenenti, P., Perna, A., Remuzzi, G., Gruppo Italiano di Studi Epidemiologici in Nefrologia. ACE inhibitors to prevent end-stage renal disease: when to start and why possibly never to stop: a post hoc analysis of the REIN trial results. Ramipril Efficacy in Nephropathy. *J. Am. Soc. Nephrol.* 2001 Dec;12(12):2832-7.

[17] Chobanian, A. V., Bakris, G. L., Black, H. R., Cushman, W. C., Green, L. A., Izzo, J. L. Jr, Jones, D. W., Materson, B. J., Oparil, S., Wright, J. T. Jr, Roccella, E. J.; National Heart, Lung, and Blood Institute Joint National Committee on Prevention, Detection, Evaluation, and Treatment of High Blood Pressure; National High Blood Pressure Education Program Coordinating Committee: The Seventh Report of the Joint National Committee on Prevention, Detection, Evaluation and Treatment of High Blood Pressure: The JNC 7 Report. *JAMA* 2003;289: 2560 –2571.

[18] Guidelines Committee: 2003 European Society of Hypertension–European Society of Cardiology Guidelines for the management of arterial hypertension. *J. Hypertens.* 2003; 21:1011 –1053.

[19] Mancia, G., Grassi, G.; European Society of Hypertension; European Society of Cardiology. Joint National Committee VII and European Society of Hypertension/ European Society of Cardiology guidelines for evaluating and treating hypertension: a two-way road? *J. Am. Soc. Nephrol.* 2005;16 Suppl. 1:S74-7.

[20] Lip, G. Y. Regression of left ventricular hypertrophy and improved prognosis. *Circulation.* 2001;104:1582–1584.

[21] Swan, L. A pill for every ill. *Circulation*. 2002 Apr. 9;105(14):e82; author reply e82.
[22] Schoolwerth, A. C., Sica, D. A., Ballermann, B. J., Wilcox, C. S.; Council on the Kidney in Cardiovascular Disease and the Council for High Blood Pressure Research of the American Heart Association. Renal considerations in angiotensin converting enzyme inhibitor therapy: a statement for healthcare professionals from the Council on the Kidney in Cardiovascular Disease and the Council for High Blood Pressure Research of the American Heart Association. *Circulation*. 2001 Oct. 16;104(16):1985-91.
[23] Silas, J. H., Klenka, Z., Solomon, S. A. Captopril induced reversible renal failure: A marker of renal artery stenosis affecting a solitary kidney. *Br. Med. J.* (Clin. Res. Ed.). 1983;286(6379):1702–1703.
[24] Murphy, B. F., Whitworth, J. A., Kincaid-Smith, P. Renal insufficiency with combinations of angiotensin converting enzyme inhibitors and diuretics. *Br. Med. J.* (Clin. Res. Ed.). 1984;288(6420):844–845.
[25] Jackson, B., McGrath, B. P., Matthews, P. G., et al. Differential renal function during angiotensin converting enzyme inhibition in renovascular hypertension. *Hypertension*. 1986;8:650–654.
[26] Kalra, P. A., Mamtora, H., Holmes, A. M., et al. Renovascular disease and renal complications of angiotensin-converting enzyme inhibitor therapy. *QJM* 1990;7 (282): 1013–1018.
[27] Devoy, M. A. B., Tomson, C. R., Edmunds, M. E., et al. Deterioration in renal function associated with angiotensin converting enzyme inhibitor therapy is not always reversible. *J. Intern. Med.* 1992;232(6):493–498.
[28] Thomas, M. C. Diuretics, ACE inhibitors and NSAIDs—the triple whammy. *Med. J.* Aust. 2000;172(4):184–185.
[29] Boyd, I. W., Mathew, T. H., Thomas, M. C. Cox-2 inhibitors and renal failure: The triple whammy revisited. *Med. J. Aust.* 2000;173:274.
[30] Vachharajani, T. J., Dacie, J. E., Yaqoob, M. M., et al. Detection of occult renovascular disease in unexplained chronic kidney disease. *Int. Urol. Nephrol.* 2005; 37(4):793–796.
[31] Schalekamp, M. A. D. H., Wenting, G. J. Angiotensin converting enzyme inhibition in renovascular hypertension: Failure of the stenotic kidney. *Lancet*. 1984;1(8374):464.
[32] Hricik, D. E., Browning, P. J., Kopelman, R., et al. Captopril-induced functional renal insufficiency in patients with bilateral renal-artery stenosis or renal-artery stenosis in a solitary kidney. *N. Eng. J. Med.* 1983;308(7):373–376.
[33] Wenting, G. J., Tan-Tjiong, H. L., Derkx, F. H., et al. Split renal function after captopril in unilateral renal artery stenosis. *Br. Med. J.* (Clin. Res. Ed.). 1984:288(6421):886–890.
[34] Jackson, B., Matthews, P. G., McGrath, B. P., et al. Angiotensin converting enzyme inhibition in renovascular hypertension: Frequency of reversible renal failure. *Lancet*. 1984;1(8370): 225–226.
[35] Onuigbo, M. A. The nephrotoxic "triple whammy" of combining diuretics, ACE inhibitors, and NSAIDs [corrected]. *BMJ*. 2013 Feb. 19;346:f678. doi: 10.1136/bmj.f678. Erratum in BMJ. 2013;346:f1221.

[36] Onuigbo, M. A., Onuigbo, N. T. Late onset renal failure from angiotensin blockade (LORFFAB): a prospective thirty-month Mayo Health System clinic experience. *Med. Sci. Monit.* 2005;11(10):CR462-9. Epub. 2005 Sep. 26.

[37] Descombes, E., Fellay, G. End-stage renal failure after irbesartan prescription in a diabetic patient with previously stable chronic renal insufficiency. *Ren. Fail.* 2000;22 (6):815–821.

[38] Fournier, J. P., Lapeyre-Mestre, M., Sommet, A., Dupouy, J., Poutrain, J. C., Montastruc, J. L. Laboratory monitoring of patients treated with antihypertensive drugs and newly exposed to non steroidal anti-inflammatory drugs: a cohort study. *PLoS One.* 2012;7(3):e34187. doi: 10.1371/journal.pone.0034187. Epub. 2012 Mar. 27.

[39] Onuigbo, M. A., Onuigbo, N. T. "Quadruple Whammy", a new syndrome of potentially preventable yet iatrogenic acute kidney injury in the ICU. *BMJ 2013: Rapid Response,* Published online February 25, 2013. http://www.bmj.com/content/346/bmj.f678/rr/632570.

[40] Onuigbo, M. A. C. Reno-prevention vs. reno-protection: a critical re-appraisal of the evidence-base from the large RAAS blockade trials after ONTARGET — a call for more circumspection. *Q. Med. J.* 2009; 102: 155-1.

[41] Onuigbo, M. A., Onuigbo, N. T. Late-onset renal failure from angiotensin blockade (LORFFAB) in 100 CKD patients. *Int. Urol. Nephrol.* 2008;40(1):233-9. Epub. 2008 Jan. 15.

[42] Onuigbo, M. A., Onuigbo, N. T. Late onset azotemia from RAAS blockade in CKD patients with normal renal arteries and no precipitating risk factors. *Ren. Fail.* 2008; 30 (1):73-80.

[43] Onuigbo, M. A., Onuigbo, N. In: *Chronic Kidney Disease and RAAS Blockade: A New View of Renoprotection.* London, England: Lambert Academic Publishing GmbH 11 and Co. KG; 2011.

In: ACE Inhibitors. Volume 2
Editor: Macaulay Amechi Onuigbo

ISBN: 978-1-62948-422-8

Chapter 4

ACEIs in Cardiovascular Medicine: A 21st Century Caribbean Perspective

Pradip Kumar Karmakar, MD, FACC, Dainia Baugh, MD, Felix Nunura, MD, Noel Crooks, MD and Ernest C. Madu, MD, FACC, FRCP***

Heart Institute of the Caribbean, Kingston, Jamaica

Abstract

There is strong evidence in the literature to support the universal acceptance of ACE inhibitors (ACEIs) in the treatment of cardiovascular disease worldwide. ACEIs alter the balance between the vasoconstrictive, salt-retention and hypertrophic properties of angiotensin II and the vasodilatory and natriuretic properties of bradykinin and alter the metabolism of a number of other vasoactive substances. ACEIs differ in the chemical structure of their active moieties, in potency, in bioavailability, in plasma half-life, in route of elimination, in their distribution and affinity for tissue-bound ACE, and in whether they are administered as prodrugs. ACEIs decrease systemic vascular resistance without increasing heart rate and promote natriuresis. ACEIs decrease mortality in congestive heart failure and left ventricular dysfunction after myocardial infarction, delay the progression of diabetic nephropathy in some patients and have proved effective in the treatment of hypertension. Ongoing studies will elucidate the effect of ACEIs on cardiovascular mortality in essential hypertension, the role of ACEIs in patients without left ventricular systolic dysfunction after myocardial infarction, and the role of ACE inhibitors compared with newly available angiotensin AT_1 receptor antagonists. Patients vary widely in their response to drugs. Having an understanding of the pharmacokinetic, pharmacogenomic and pharmacodynamic properties of various medications is important when assessing ethnic differences in drug response. This is particularly relevant in the Caribbean where we have very diverse multiethnic populations. Genetic factors can account for 20 to 95 percent of patient variability. Genetic polymorphisms for many drug-metabolizing enzymes and drug targets (e.g., receptors) have been identified. Although currently limited to a few pathways, pharmacogenetic testing may enable

* Corresponding author: Ernest C. Madu MD, FACC, FRCP; E-mail: emadu@caribbeanheart.com.

physicians better understand why patients react differently to various drugs and inform better decisions about therapy. Ultimately, this understanding may shift the medical paradigm to highly individualized therapeutic regimens. ACEIs enjoy a wide usage and acceptance in the Caribbean. In a recently conducted island-wide study in Antigua evaluating the use of antihypertensive drugs, ACEIs were the most commonly used class of antihypertensive drugs (63.6%) in 281 patients studied. In addition to Hypertension, utilization of ACE inhibitors in heart failure has been closely evaluated in the Caribbean population, in relation with their beneficial effects on mortality and morbidity. The etiology of heart failure in the Caribbean tends to be different from that seen in more developed countries where CAD accounts for most cases. Several studies in the Caribbean point to systemic hypertension as the primary culprit as opposed to ischemic heart disease. This probably reflects the much higher prevalence and severity of hypertension in our population and may contribute to better tolerability of ACEIs, and their combination, hence the higher percentage use of these medications in the Caribbean. Further studies in this area are required. In this chapter, we explore the current and potential role of angiotensin converting enzyme inhibitors (ACEIs) in cardiovascular medicine in the Caribbean, examine the data on ethnic variations in response to ACEIs and finally propose general recommendations for the appropriate use of ACEIs in the Caribbean community.

INTRODUCTION

The Caribbean, long referred to as the West Indies includes more than 7,000 islands. Many countries within the Caribbean are members of the Caribbean Community (CARICOM) and share similar demographic and pathological patterns. The region is multi-racial, multi-lingual, stratified, and multi-cultural. Although people of African descent constitute the majority in terms of population, the Caribbean is home to an ethnically diverse group including people with Native American, European, and Asian (Chinese and Indian) heritages.

The Caribbean region has experienced an epidemiological transition over the past sixty years, evident in the shift from communicable disease predominance to a rising prevalence of non-communicable diseases, particularly cardiovascular diseases (CVD). CVDs now constitute a significant health challenge in the region. To address the rising prevalence of cardiovascular diseases in the Caribbean, a systematic evaluation of the drivers of CVDs and treatment modalities must be part of a unified strategy to combat the epidemic. Essential to the treatment of CVDs is the use of ACEIs, the subject of our review. ACE inhibitors have achieved widespread usage in the treatment of cardiovascular and renal disease. ACE inhibitors alter the balance between the vasoconstrictive, salt-retentive, and hypertrophic properties of angiotensin II (Ang II) and the vasodilatory and natriuretic properties of bradykinin. They also alter the metabolism of a number of other vasoactive substances. ACE inhibitors differ in the chemical structure of their active moieties, in potency, in bioavailability, in plasma half-life, in route of elimination, in their distribution and affinity for tissue-bound ACE, and in whether they are administered as prodrugs. ACE inhibitors decrease systemic vascular resistance without increasing heart rate and promote natriuresis. ACEIs have an established role in the treatment of patients across the cardiovascular disease continuum [1]. They are effective in the treatment of hypertension (HTN), decrease mortality in congestive heart failure (CHF) and in patients with left ventricular dysfunction after myocardial infarction (MI) and are believed to delay the progression of diabetic nephropathy. Ongoing studies will elucidate the effect of ACE inhibitors on cardiovascular mortality in essential hypertension, the role of ACE inhibitors in patients without ventricular dysfunction after myocardial infarction, and the role of ACE inhibitors compared with newly available angiotensin AT_1 receptor antagonists.

RISK FACTORS AND CARDIOVASCULAR PATHOLOGY IN THE CARIBBEAN

Globally and in the Caribbean, cardiovascular diseases are on the rise. Certain biological factors such as high blood pressure, obesity, high blood sugar, and high blood cholesterol increase risk of cardiovascular diseases in the population, particularly in those who are genetically predisposed. These biological risk factors are influenced by lifestyle-related, socially determined characteristics such as unhealthy diet, physical inactivity and tobacco use. While lifestyle or health behaviors are important as risk or protective factors for cardiovascular diseases, these are heavily influenced by social determinants, such as availability/pricing of healthy and unhealthy foods, taxes, the built environment, security and safety considerations, advertising and marketing of unhealthy foods and products. These external determinants assume a more significant role in low resource environments like the Caribbean basin. Access to medical care through effective, efficient health services is fundamental to the management of chronic diseases and their complications [2]. The burden of non-communicable diseases and injury has escalated in the Caribbean partly as a result of demographic and epidemiological transitions. The four leading causes of death in the Caribbean in 2000 were all NCDs — heart disease, cancer, stroke, and diabetes. These four conditions accounted for 47 per cent of deaths in 1980 and 51 per cent in 2000, the most recent year for which relatively complete mortality data is available. The major NCDs in the Caribbean share common underlying risk factors, namely unhealthy eating habits, physical inactivity, obesity, tobacco and alcohol use and inadequate utilization of preventive health services [3]. Cardiovascular disease (stroke, coronary artery disease and diabetes) was the principal cause of death in the Caribbean in 2006. Raised blood pressure is the leading single cause of cardiovascular disease, accounting for 62% of strokes and 49% of coronary heart disease. Available data for 2007-2008 from the British Virgin Islands (BVI), Dominica and St. Kitts, show hypertension rates of approximately 35%, with marked increases in prevalence with advancing age. It is estimated that there is a 90% lifetime likelihood of developing hypertension in the Caribbean population [4]. A comparison of data from the two lifestyle surveys conducted in Jamaica in 2000/01 and 2007/08 revealed that there was a statistically significant increase in the prevalence of such chronic non-communicable disease risk factors as hypertension (20.9% to 25.2%) and obesity (19.7% to 25.3%). The estimated prevalence of diabetes mellitus in 2007/08 was also higher than in 2000/01 (7.2% to 7.9%). With regards to physical activity levels, almost twice as many persons reported being inactive in 2007/08 compared to 2000/01 (30% vs. 17%) and the proportion of persons engaging in high activity had decreased significantly with 33% reporting high activity in 2007/08 compared to 47% in 2000/01. On a positive note, there was a small decrease in the use of cigarettes comparing 2007/08 to 2000/01 (18.5% to 14.5%) [5].

Substantial ethnic differences in cardiovascular mortality have been noted in several studies. For example, compared to whites, Afro-Caribbean and other people of African descent have a higher incidence of stroke and end stage renal failure, whereas coronary artery disease is less common. Conversely, South Asians (defined as people originating from the Indian subcontinent and East Africa) have a higher incidence of coronary heart disease. There is increased prevalence of left ventricular hypertrophy (LVH) in Afro-Caribbeans. This is thought to be, in part, due to their higher nighttime blood pressure with smaller degrees of nocturnal blood pressure dip. LVH is an independent predictor of morbidity and mortality. Ethnic differences in morbidity and mortality may also in part, be explained by differences in other cardiovascular risk factors. Both diabetes mellitus and obesity are common in ethnic minority groups, with a high prevalence among Afro-Caribbean females. Plasma lipid concentrations, however, show a different pattern with South Asians having higher concentrations than whites and Afro-Caribbeans having lower values. This may, in part, explain why, despite a high prevalence of hypertension and type 2 diabetes mellitus, coronary heart disease is less common in the Afro-Caribbean than the other two ethnic groups [6].

ACEIs in Essential Hypertension and Hypertensive Heart Disease

ACE inhibitors effectively lower the mean, systolic, and diastolic pressures in hypertensive patients as well as in salt-depleted normotensive subjects [7-9]. The acute change in blood pressure correlates with pretreatment plasma renin-angiotensin (PRA) and angiotensin levels, such that the greatest reductions in blood pressure are seen in patients with the highest PRA [10-13]. However, with long-term therapy, a greater percentage of patients achieve a decrease in blood pressure, and the antihypertensive effect no longer correlates with pretreatment PRA [11-13]. The mechanism for this increased efficacy with chronic administration is not clear but may involve the kallikrein-kinin system or production of vasodilatory prostaglandins [14]. The effects of ACE inhibitors on smooth muscle cell growth and proliferation, fibrinolysis, and thrombogenesis, as well as endothelial apoptosis, may result in anti-atherothrombotic benefits in excess of those expected from blood pressure lowering alone [15]. Although ACE inhibitors are generally effective in reducing blood pressure, they appear to be less potent in hypertensive blacks than whites. In a 2002 study in 89 Caribbean Hispanic hypertensive patients who participated in six double-blind, randomized trials of antihypertensive agents blood pressure reductions by calcium channel blockers, HCTZ, and ACE inhibitor/HCTZ combinations were significantly greater than that with placebo, while those of ACE inhibitors and β blockers as monotherapy were not. The authors concluded that essential hypertension of Caribbean Hispanics is associated with multiple risk factors and is largely of the low-renin type. Responses to therapy are consistent with those observed in the Afro-Caribbean and other populations with the low-renin phenotype and suggest salt-sensitivity of blood pressure in this population. In Afro-Caribbeans, the traditional approach has been to start treatment with diuretics or calcium antagonists, as the beta-blockers or ACE inhibitors (or angiotensin receptor blockers (ARBs) tend to be less effective at blood pressure lowering, in view of the low renin state in this ethnic group.

Generally, when used as initial monotherapy, beta-blockers, ACE inhibitors and ARBs are less effective at lowering blood pressure in people of African descent when compared to white patients, due to the intrinsically low renin state in this ethnic group [17, 18]. Despite these observations, a descriptive, cross-sectional survey conducted at 22 primary healthcare facilities across Trinidad using a de novo, pilot-tested questionnaire between June 2006 and August 2006, showed that ACEIs, particularly enalapril, were the most commonly prescribed class of antihypertensive drugs in 63.6% of patients. ß-blockers, thiazide diuretics and calcium channel blockers were prescribed in 29.2%, 25.8% and 12.0% of patients respectively [19]. In a Veterans Administration Cooperative Study Group trial, captopril reduced blood pressure significantly more in white patients with mild to moderate hypertension than in black patients at 7 weeks [20]. Similar studies have also shown ACE inhibitors and β-blockers to be less effective than calcium channel blockers in young and elderly black men [21]. Cumulative data reinforced the observation that hypertensive blacks tend to have low renin levels more often than do whites [22-24]. This view is supported by the abolition of racial differences in response to ACEI therapy by co-administration of drugs that increase PRA such as diuretics [25]. Weir et al. have suggested that the mechanism through which ACE inhibitors lower blood pressure differs in blacks and whites [26]. This group observed the dissociation between the potency of ACE inhibitors for decreasing plasma ACE activity and their antihypertensive potency in blacks. However, in some dose groups, baseline ACE activity was higher in the blacks than in the whites studied. Nevertheless, this study underscores the need to use higher doses of ACE inhibitors in black patients whether in the Caribbean or elsewhere.

Current and Potential Role of ACEIs in High Risk Caribbean Population: The Hypertensive - Diabetic Patient

The Jamaica Survey, 2002-2007, of living conditions, showed consistent increase in the prevalence rates of diabetes mellitus and hypertension [27]. Similar trends are seen in other Caribbean Islands including Barbados and Trinidad. Diabetes occurs in 17% of Barbadians over age 40 and in 17% of Jamaicans over age 25. The combination of a rapid increase in calorie intake and a decrease in physical activity, against a background of cultural traditions that favor female obesity are thought to play a role in the rising prevalence of diabetes and hypertension in the Caribbean [28]. In addition to the high burden of diabetes, there is also a high burden of complications. In Barbados, the incidence of diabetic foot complications has been found to be second only to a population of Native Americans in Navajo. The Barbados Eye Study revealed that among persons 40-84 years old in Barbados, 28.5% had evidence of diabetic retinopathy on fundus photographs. With regards to renal complications, the Caribbean Renal Registry reports that diabetes is the leading cause of end stage renal disease in the Caribbean, accounting for 28% of patients on long term renal replacement therapy. Among persons with diabetes attending primary care clinic in Tobago, 12% of males and 24% of females had chronic kidney disease [29]. Available data from Jamaica showed that 54% of patients admitted with diabetes at the University Hospital of West Indies had some form of cardiovascular disease with higher prevalence in females [30].

The renin-angiotensin-system (RAS) and increased glomerular capillary pressure have been implicated in the progression of renal dysfunction due to a number of renal diseases, including diabetic nephropathy [31]. ACE inhibitors decrease glomerular capillary pressure by decreasing arterial pressure and by selectively dilating efferent arterioles [32]. In addition, Angiotensin II causes mesangial cell growth and matrix production [33, 34]. Numerous animal studies and small clinical trials have suggested that ACE inhibitors significantly slow down the progression of loss of kidney function in diabetic nephropathy [35]. ACE inhibitors prevent progression of microalbuminuria to overt proteinuria [36]. A large, prospective, placebo-controlled study has now shown that captopril slows the progression of nephropathy in patients with insulin-dependent diabetes mellitus, as measured by the rate of decline in creatinine clearance and the combined end points of dialysis, transplantation, and death [37]. A second large-scale, prospective, double-blind study extended these observations by showing a protective effect of ACE inhibitors in patients with a variety of renal diseases, including glomerulopathies, interstitial nephritis, nephrosclerosis, and diabetic nephropathy [38]. The exception was polycystic kidney disease. Importantly, the protective effect of ACE inhibition was independent of the severity of renal insufficiency. Ongoing studies will determine whether ACE inhibitors other than captopril are also effective in slowing progression of nephropathy and will also clarify the value of ACE inhibitors in slowing progression of renal disease in patients with non–insulin-dependent diabetes mellitus. This is particularly relevant when one considers that, whereas 89% of the patients in the captopril trial were white, [39], non–insulin-dependent diabetes mellitus is two times more prevalent among blacks than whites [40]. We must consider several factors for chronic kidney disease (CKD) prognostication with a need to individualize CKD management. Onuigbo has called attention to the misgiving and the pitfalls of the "one size fits all" approach to CKD management in general and to diabetic nephropathy in particular [41]. Further research is clearly needed in these areas, because several questions remain unanswered for example, because black patients are less responsive to the antihypertensive effects of ACE inhibitors, it remains to be determined whether there are ethnic differences in the renal protective effects of ACE inhibitors.

Potential Role of the ACEIs in Caribbean Patients with Diabetes

Experimental and epidemiological data suggest that activation of the renin-angiotensin-aldosterone system plays an important role in increasing the micro- and macrovascular complications in patients with diabetes mellitus.

Not only are ACE inhibitors potent antihypertensive agents but, while controversial, there is a growing body of data suggesting that they also potentially have a specific 'organ-protective' effect. For the same degree of blood pressure control, compared with other antihypertensive agents, ACE inhibitors are presumed to demonstrate functional and tissue protection of considered organs. ACE inhibitors have been reported to improve kidney, heart, and to a lesser extent, eye and peripheral nerve function of patients with diabetes mellitus. These favorable effects are the result of inhibition of both hemodynamic and tissue effects of angiotensin II.

In light of these observations, there are a growing number of investigators favoring the use of ACE inhibitors very early in patients with diabetes mellitus [42]. The 2008 NICE clinical guideline for patients with type 2 diabetes recommended that the first-line blood-pressure-lowering therapy for a person of African-Caribbean descent with type 2 diabetes mellitus should be an ACE inhibitor plus either a diuretic or a generic calcium-channel blocker [43]. In the previously noted descriptive, cross-sectional survey of primary healthcare facilities across Trinidad, there was a high prevalence of diabetes mellitus (57.6%). Angiotensin converting enzyme inhibitors (as monotherapy or in combination with other drug classes) were more likely to be prescribed in diabetic hypertensive patients [19]. The apparent advantage of ACEIs over other agents includes a protective effect on the kidney against the development of microalbuminuria, which is a major risk factor for CV events and death in this population [44].

Current and Potential Role of ACEIs in Coronary Heart Disease (CHD)

Coronary heart disease (CHD) is the single largest cause of death in developed countries and is one of the leading causes of disease burden in developing countries. In 2001, there were 7.3 million deaths due to CHD worldwide. Three-fourths of global deaths due to CHD occurred in the low and middle-income countries. The rapid rise in CHD burden in most of the low and middle and income countries is due to socio-economic changes, increase in life span and acquisition of lifestyle related risk factors. The CHD death rate, however, varies dramatically across the developing countries. The varying incidence, prevalence, and mortality rates reflect the different levels of risk factors, other competing causes of death, availability of resources to combat CHD, and the stage of epidemiologic transition that each country or region finds itself. The economic burden of CHD is equally large but solutions exist to manage this growing burden. The WHO Global Burden of Disease study ranked CHD as the single leading cause of mortality in the Latin America and Caribbean region, estimating it to be 11% of all deaths in 2001. The approach to treatment of CHD events is more conservative in the region. In terms of secondary prevention after CHD events, data from the WHO PREMISE study found the use of angiotensin enzyme (ACE) inhibitors at around 50% [45]. While data is lacking on the use of ACEIs for cardio-protection in the Caribbean, there is a vast amount of literature confirming the beneficial cardio-protective effects of ACEIs large randomized controlled trials. By inference, these data have largely informed practice patterns in the Caribbean. Certain ACE inhibitors have been compellingly demonstrated to decrease the frequency of ischemic events in patients with stable coronary artery disease. These benefits presumably are based at least in part on drug-mediated effects that have been demonstrated experimentally, including retardation of atherosclerosis development, reversal of endothelial dysfunction, and favorable alteration of fibrinolytic balance; effects that are presumed to involve inhibiting both angiotensin II (Ang II) and bradykinin (BK) pathways [46-49]. These pharmacological effects formed the basis for large trials of ACE inhibitors in atherosclerotic vascular disease. These include the HOPE trial, in patients at high risk of CV events, which showed that ramipril at a dose of 10 mg daily decreased the risk of stroke, MI, and death by 22% in comparison with placebo ($P < 0.001$) [50].

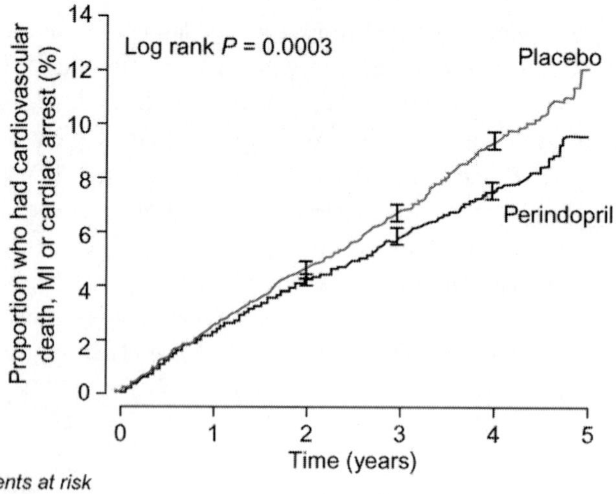

Patients at risk

Placebo	6108	5943	5781	5598	4450	71
Perindopril	6110	5957	5612	5653	4515	64

Reproduced with permission from Figure 2 [51].
MI, myocardial infarction.

Figure 1. Time to the first occurrence of the primary endpoint after perindopril treatment of patients with stable coronary artery disease: the European Trial on Reduction of Cardiac Events with Perindopril among Patients with Stable Coronary Artery Disease (EUROPA). The primary endpoint was a composite of cardiovascular death, MI, or cardiac arrest. Error bars depict standard error.

The European Trial on Reduction of Cardiac Events with Perindopril among Patients with Stable Coronary Artery Disease (EUROPA) trial, [51], aimed at a population with stable CAD and somewhat less evidence of risk than the HOPE population, confirmed and extended the findings of HOPE (Figure 1). Treatment with perindopril 8 mg daily on a background of now-standard preventive therapy (antiplatelet drugs, lipid-lowering agents, and beta-blockers if MI had occurred) reduced risk of cardiac death, non-fatal MI, or resuscitated cardiac arrest by 20% in comparison with placebo (P = 0.0003) [51].

The Prevention of Events with ACE Inhibition (PEACE) trial failed to show the benefit of trandolapril in patients with stable CHD [52]. This finding may relate to the dose selected for study (4 mg) or to intrinsic differences in the pharmacological profile of this ACE inhibitor vs. ramipril and perindopril. Nonetheless, the usefulness of ACE inhibitors, as a group, for secondary prevention in patients with established, stable CHD has been demonstrated by results of meta-analyses of all relevant trials [53]. These results have been recognized by the European Society of Cardiology and the American College of Cardiology/ American Heart Association.

Current and Potential Role of ACEIs in Heart Failure and Cardiomyopathy

The incidence of hypertension and diabetes mellitus among the largely African and East Indian Caribbean populations is high. Both of these chronic non-communicable diseases predispose patients to the development of cardiac disease.

McSwain et al. [54] showed that in Antigua and Barbuda, the prevalence of Congestive Heart Failure (CHF) in the general population was 1% in the 40 to 65 year age-group, and 4% in those over 65 years-of-age. ACEIs were part of the treatment strategy in 78% of the reviewed cases.

It has been reported that congestive cardiac failure with LV hypertrophy is the most frequent finding in this Afro-Caribbean population, with LV systolic dysfunction occurring in only 35% of patients. These findings are consistent with possible diastolic LV dysfunction due to hypertension as the primary cause of cardiac failure in this population. In many populations heart failure patients predominantly present with left ventricular systolic dysfunction, which is associated with a reduced ejection fraction (HF-REF). In the Caribbean however, a significant number of patients are found to have either normal or no significant reduction in left ventricular ejection fraction – so-called preserved ejection fraction (HF-PEF).

It is thought that most HF-PEF patients have left ventricular diastolic dysfunction. Patients with HF-PEF tend to be older, more often female and obese, less likely to have coronary artery disease but more likely to have hypertension and atrial fibrillation. This classification is important because management of these underlying conditions in addition to symptomatic management of heart failure is an important aspect of overall care and informs decision making in the treatment of these patients in the Caribbean. Most clinical trials in heart failure have focused on patients with HF-REF, therefore current treatment guidelines relate mainly to this group of patients. ACEIs are essential for the treatment of these patients in the Caribbean. ACEIs inhibit the renin-angiotensin-aldosterone system (RAAS), by blocking the conversion of angiotensin I to angiotensin II. They have been shown to reduce death, hospitalization or myocardial infarction, compared with placebo, in several randomized controlled trials (RCTs) undertaken in patients with clinical heart failure or significant left ventricular dysfunction.

Beneficial effects on mortality are observed rapidly within a few weeks of starting treatment, increase with duration of treatment and are independent of age, sex and baseline use of diuretics, aspirin and β-blockers. They are reported to have a modest effect on LV remodeling. Therapy should be initiated at a low dose and slowly titrated upwards to optimal response. Anticipated side effects include symptomatic hypotension, hyperkalemia, cough and renal dysfunction but in general these are not life-threatening and are usually reversible upon stopping the drug or reducing the dose. Several large, prospective, randomized, placebo-controlled clinical trials have demonstrated that treatment with several different ACE inhibitors reduces mortality rates in patients who have HF associated with systolic dysfunction.

In the Cooperative North Scandinavian Enalapril Survival Study I (CONSENSUS I), substantial mortality benefit was conferred by administration of enalapril when compared with placebo, when administered to patients with severe HF (Figure 2) [55]. The Studies of Left Ventricular Dysfunction (SOLVD) extended these benefits to a broader range of patients, including not only those with symptomatic HF but also those with LV dysfunction who were asymptomatic ('Functional Class 0' HF) [56]. The Vasodilator-Heart Failure Trial II (V-HeFT II) compared enalapril with hydralazine plus nitrates, a combination that improved outcome vs. placebo in the earlier Vasodilator-Heart Failure Trial I (V-HeFT I), and demonstrated significantly enhanced survival with ACE inhibition [57].

As a result of these and other parallel studies, ACE inhibitors have been recommended for indefinite administration to patients with chronic HF and systolic dysfunction, both to minimize symptoms and to prolong survival. These recommendations enjoy wide acceptance in the Caribbean and are uniformly applicable in clinical practice in the region.

Although, as of yet, less compellingly demonstrated, HF associated primarily with diastolic dysfunction may respond to ACE inhibitor. This putative benefit may result from drug-mediated cardiac remodeling, with reduction of myocardial mass, fibrosis (possibly a direct effect of ACE inhibitors, as discussed subsequently), and stiffness. Consistent with this hypothesis, a meta-analysis of studies of anti-hypertensive drugs has found ACE inhibitors to be the most effective of these agents in reversing LV hypertrophy [58]. More importantly, in a study of the ACE inhibitor, perindopril [Perindopril in Elderly People with Chronic Heart Failure (PEP-CHF)], among patients with HF and diastolic dysfunction, benefit was suggested, although not conclusively proven [59]. Although the study lost its randomization power after 1 year, relative risk reduction was 31% for the primary outcome (all-cause mortality or unplanned HF hospitalization) when perindopril was administered rather than placebo (P=0.055). Symptomatic improvement, including more normal functional class (P=0.030) and enhanced 6-min walk distance (P=0.011), was also noted. Studies in heart failure patients of Afro-Caribbean (black) origin reveal a high prevalence (up to 30%) of myocardial trabeculations and raise the potential diagnosis of left ventricular non-compaction (LVNC) [60]. It is unclear whether the myocardial morphology is representative of LVNC or whether it represents an ethnicity related epiphenomenon to increased cardiac preload.

Possible Beneficial Effects of the ACEIs in the Caribbean Rheumatic Heart Disease and HIV-Related Heart Disease

In developing countries, rheumatic fever (RF) is the most frequent cause of heart disease in the 5-13-year-old group, causing 25-40 percent of all cardiovascular diseases and 33-50 percent of all hospital admissions. An estimated 12 million people are currently affected by rheumatic fever and rheumatic heart diseases (RHD) of which 2/3 are children between 5 and 15 years of age. Of the estimated 12 million with RF/RHD, at least 3 million had congestive heart failure (CHF), which required hospitalization. A large proportion with CHF required cardiac valve surgery within 5-10 years [61]. Human immunodeficiency virus (HIV) disease is recognized as an important cause of dilated cardiomyopathy. Myocarditis and myocardial infection with HIV-1 are the best-studied causes of cardiomyopathy in HIV disease. Co-infection with other viruses (usually, coxsackievirus B3 and cytomegalovirus) may also play an important etiopathogenetic role. The introduction of highly active antiretroviral therapy (HAART) has significantly reduced the incidence of myocarditis in HIV-infected patients living in developed countries.

By contrast, in developing countries, where the availability of HAART is scanty and greater is the pathogenetic role of nutritional factors, the incidence of HIV-associated myocarditis and cardiomyopathy is increasing with a high mortality rate for congestive heart failure [62]. While it is common practice in the Caribbean to use ACEIs in the treatment of rheumatic cardiomyopathy and HIV associated myocarditis and cardiomyopathy, data supporting its efficacy and effectiveness is lacking.

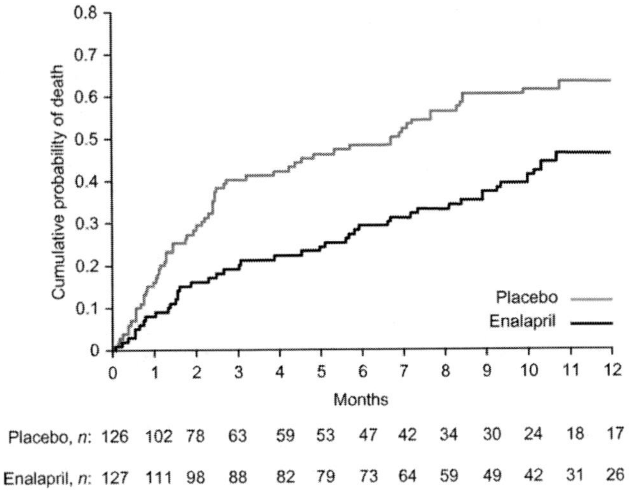

Reproduced with permission [55].

Figure 2. Cumulative probability of death in the placebo and enalapril groups: the Cooperative North Scandinavian Enalapril Survival Study I (CONSENSUS I) trial of patients with severe heart failure.

ADVERSE EFFECTS OF ACEI INHIBITORS

The adverse effects of ACE inhibitors can be divided into those that are specific to the entire class and those that are related to chemical structure (specifically, related to the presence of a sulfhydryl group). Like all antihypertensive agents, ACE inhibitors can cause hypotension. The frequency of hypotension is greater in renin-dependent states, such as during low sodium intake and diuretic use [63].

It is recommended that lower starting doses be used under these conditions. ACE inhibitors can cause hyperkalemia because of a decrease in aldosterone· This effect is usually not significant in patients with normal renal function.

However, in patients with impaired kidney function or in patients who are taking potassium supplements (including salt substitutes) or potassium-sparing diuretics, hyperkalemia can occur [64, 65].

Angioedema is a rare but potentially life-threatening side effect of ACE inhibitors. It is characterized by localized swelling of the lips, tongue, mouth, throat, nose, or other parts of the face [66]. The mechanism appears to involve bradykinin or one of its metabolites. The rate of angioedema has been reported to be 1 to 2 per 1000 in primarily white populations, but appears to be increased in blacks [67].

Although the rate of angioedema is highest within the first month of ACE inhibitor use, angioedema may occur years after the initiation of therapy. In a report reviewing six years experience of angioedema at the University Hospital of the West Indies (Kingston-Jamaica), ACEIs were related to 60% of admissions for angioedema. Lip and tongue swelling were the most common manifestation [68].

ACEIs and Pharmacogenomic Data, New Trends and Greatest Challenges in the Caribbean Region

Ethnic Variations

Antihypertensive drugs were the first cardiovascular therapies for which there was wide recognition of clinical differences in response based on ethnicity. The Fourth Report of the Joint National Committee (JNC-IV) on the Detection, Evaluation and Treatment of High Blood Pressure, published in 1988, was the first to recommend consideration of race/ethnicity in selection of antihypertensive therapy and the three subsequent sets of JNC guidelines have contained similar recommendations.

The most notable differences are in response to β-blockers, ACE inhibitors and angiotensin receptor blockers (ARBs). The widespread clinical recognition of such differences followed the 1982 VA Cooperative Study Group finding that 62% of whites and 54% of blacks achieved blood pressure goal with propanolol, while such goal was attained with hydrochlorothiazide (HCTZ) in 55% of whites and 71% of blacks. Another VA cooperative study, a decade later, similarly found that, particularly in older blacks, atenolol and captopril were less effective at blood pressure lowering than HCTZ and diltiazem. A meta-analysis, published in 2004, evaluated 15 clinical trials published between 1984 and 1998 that reported differences in antihypertensive response between blacks and whites, and met other specified criteria. Their analysis highlights that blacks generally respond more favorably to diuretics or calcium channel blockers, while whites tend to respond similarly to all the drug classes. In comparisons between groups, blacks respond slightly better than whites to diuretics and CCBs, while whites respond slightly better than blacks to ACE inhibitors and β-blockers. More recent data on lisinopril, quinapril and losartan support the differences with ACE inhibitors and ARBs suggested by the meta-analysis. Ethnic differences in response to ACE inhibitors were also suggested by the investigators in the V-HeFT trials [57].

However, it is not clear the data support this contention. Specifically, the manuscript does not report statistical comparisons of mortality in enalapril-treated blacks and whites, and while mortality was numerically lower in whites than blacks, it seems unlikely that this difference was statistically significant. In a matched cohort analysis of blacks and whites from the Studies of Left Ventricular Dysfunction (SOLVD) Prevention and Treatment trials, investigators found that enalapril was associated with a significant 49% adjusted risk reduction in heart failure hospitalization in whites, and a nonsignificant 14% adjusted risk reduction in blacks, for a significant treatment ethnicity interaction (p=0.005) [56]. They did not however observe differences in mortality reduction between ethnic groups. In both the V-HeFT II and SOLVD analyses, whites had greater BP reduction with enalapril than blacks, which may have contributed to the observed differences in outcomes. A subsequent analysis that only involved the SOLVD Prevention Trial, did not observe any differences between blacks and whites in the risk reduction associated with enalapril in progression to symptomatic heart failure [69].

Finally, a meta-analysis did not suggest any differences in ACE inhibitor efficacy in reducing adverse cardiovascular outcomes in heart failure between blacks and non-blacks in heart failure.

Ethnic Variations and Genetic Polymorphisms

The literature does not provide much insight regarding genetic polymorphisms and response. Despite the fact that there have been many studies evaluating the associations of numerous candidate genes with ACE inhibitor or ARB response, none has been consistently associated. Most studied is the ACE gene, and most of the studies with this gene have focused on an insertion/deletion (I/D) polymorphism, with equivocal data. The most convincing study in this area is the pharmacogenetic sub study of ALLHAT, called GenHAT. This study tested the association of various outcomes in ALLHAT with the I/D polymorphism in 37,939 patients. They found no association between this polymorphism and BP lowering (with lisinopril or any other study drugs), nor with any of the study outcomes, when considered combined or stratified by drug therapy [70].

Ethnic differences in linkage disequilibrium between blacks and whites may be diminishing the ability to document associations with this gene, since the I/D is not believed to be the functional polymorphism. While this gene remains one of interest, any polymorphism that influences the ACE inhibitor or ARB response remains to be identified. Another gene that has been widely studied relative to the ACE inhibitor and ARB response is the gene for the angiotensin type 1 receptor, AGTR1. Similar to ACE, there have been no consistent findings with this gene and as so far been reported, there is no proven association with blood pressure response to trandolapril in whites, blacks or Hispanics.

There are also clear ethnic differences in the risk for angioedema from ACE inhibitors, with blacks being at greater risk, but there are no pharmacogenetic studies to provide insight into these differences. The contribution of bradykinin to the hemodynamic effects of ACE inhibitors in humans is uncertain. ACE inhibitors potentiate the hypotensive effects of intravenous bradykinin in humans [71]. However, endogenous bradykinin is difficult to measure because of its short half-life, and investigators have reported that bradykinin levels are either increased or unchanged during ACE inhibition. Similarly, prostaglandin levels have been reported to be increased or unchanged in patients treated with ACE inhibitors [72-74].

The recent availability of specific bradykinin (B_2) receptor antagonists has begun to shed light on the contribution of bradykinin to the actions of ACE inhibitors [75]. In animal models, co-administration of a bradykinin antagonist attenuates the antihypertensive effect of ACE inhibitors.

Recent data suggest that B_2 antagonism blunts the hypotensive effects and reduces the endothelium-dependent vasodilator effects in humans as well [76]. Vascular reactivity to bradykinin and the endothelium-independent vasodilator SNP is decreased in normotensive blacks compared with whites, consistent with attenuated vascular smooth muscle reactivity. The data suggest that genetic variation at the ACE gene locus interacts with ethnicity to impact the vascular response to bradykinin [77].

Collectively, these data suggest that the roles of AGT and AGTR1 differences may warrant further investigation, whereas the evidence for a meaningful ACE (ID)/ACE inhibitor interaction has grown perhaps more tenuous, a view supported by recent gene-expression studies of ACE [78]. While the pharmacogenetics of hypertension treatment remains a priority area because of the pandemic distribution of the disease and its associated renal and cardiovascular co-morbidities, progress towards identification of the genes that contribute to variable treatment response has been slow. Translation of findings into clinical practice remains a distant goal.

Progress in the future will depend upon our ability to launch large studies using high-fidelity phenotyping with multiple drugs and multiple ethnic groups [79].

Discussion, Conclusion and Recommendations: ACEIs in the Caribbean Population

Ethnic differences in responses to cardiovascular drugs have been recognized for several decades, and in some cases ethnicity is used in drug therapy decision-making. It is intuitively attractive to speculate that pharmacogenetics may contribute to our understanding of ethnic differences in drug responses, and some of the examples cited herein support that pharmacogenetics may contribute to such differences. However, there are certain challenges to defining the role of pharmacogenetics in ethnic differences in drug response that must be recognized.

First, the heritable contribution to drug response variability is rarely defined experimentally, but if one assumes that it is approximately the same as the heritable contribution to the diseases the drug treats, then on average, this would represent 30-60% of variability that has a genetic basis, with the remaining being environmental or demographic. Additionally, it is expected that for most drug responses, the genetic underpinnings will be explained by a variety of genes, thus making any calculation of the role of pharmacogenetics in ethnic differences in response more challenging. It is possible that the examples provided herein are ones for which the genetic contribution from a single gene is larger than normal, thus making the potential contribution of that gene to ethnic differences in response more evident.

Additionally, as genetic studies move toward a tag SNP approach, where the functional polymorphism is unknown, differences in linkage disequilibrium between ancestral populations will add to the challenge of defining an association across different ethnic groups, and defining the role of that polymorphism in ethnic differences in response. This has been clearly evident with warfarin and the VKORC1 SNPs. The contribution of environmental factors to drug response, particularly diet for many of the cardiovascular drugs, and how this may confound the search for the genetic underpinnings of ethnic differences in response remains to be clarified.

Finally, there are the challenges associated with translation of any finding or technology to practice. This includes accumulating sufficient data that the genetic (and probably other) information is predictive enough to be useful clinically, followed by the education required of clinicians for adoption to practice.

Despite these many challenges, it appears that in at least some cases, pharmacogenetic findings may help to explain ethnic differences in response. As the goals of personalized medicine begin to be realized, it is possible that the use of genetic and other patient-specific information, including environmental factors, will be superior to use of ethnic information and will help guide drug-therapy decisions for certain drugs.

CONCLUSION AND RECOMMENDATIONS: ACEIS IN THE CARIBBEAN POPULATION

1 ACE inhibitors merit consideration, along with other antihypertensive drug classes, as initial drug therapy for the Caribbean population.
2 In addition, in the Afro-Caribbean with CHF, ACE inhibitor therapy should constitute a key part of the pharmacotherapy.
3 In special conditions, such as in the setting of coexisting diseases (e.g. diabetes), ACEIs, should be considered when selecting first-line monotherapy considering its favorable effect on outcomes.
4 It appears that the RAA system may be of greater importance than previously assumed in the expression of the excessive hypertension and BP-related target-organ damage in Afro-Caribbean population.
5 It remains to be clarified how much of the ACE inhibitor-mediated target-organ protection may be potentially useful in conditions such rheumatic heart disease and HIV cardiomyopathy.
6 ACE inhibitors are viable therapeutic options for the Caribbean population with high cardiovascular risk or established cardiovascular conditions like hypertensive, diabetic, or ischemic heart disease and heart failure from different causes, because, when appropriately prescribed, (as monotherapy or combination therapy), they are cost effective and the results are clinically beneficial.

In Conclusion: Almost three decades after their introduction into clinical use, ACE inhibitors have become recognized therapeutic choices throughout the entire spectrum of CV diseases. Newer ACE inhibitors with pharmacological profiles differing from those of older agents have added to the ease of application and relative safety of these drugs both for reduction of symptoms and for improvement of outcomes. Although other agents modulating RAS (ARBs and Renin Inhibitors) can provide some overlapping pharmacological effects and important clinical benefits, ACE inhibitors remain unique in the range of their proven benefits, justifying their central role in the armamentarium of the Cardiovascular Specialist and occupy an important place in the therapeutic management of cardiovascular disorders in the Caribbean.

REFERENCES

[1] Ferrari, R. Do ACE inhibitors differ, and in which way? –ACE Inhibition as a cornerstone of hypertension treatment - *Medicographia*. 2009;31 (1): 24-31.
[2] Working Document for the Summit of CARICOM Heads of Government on the Chronic Non-communicable Diseases. Stemming the tide of Non-communicable diseases in the Caribbean. February, 2007.
[3] Caribbean Commission on Health and Development Report of the Caribbean Commission on Health and Development. PAO/WHO, CARICOM. Produced in Jamaica, 2006 www.ianrandlepublishers.com.

[4] The Caribbean Community (CARICOM) Secretariat/Pan American Health Organization/World Health Organization January 2011, www.caricom.org.

[5] Ferguson, T. S., Tulloch-Reid, M. K., Cunningham-Myrie, C. A., Davidson-Sadler, T., Copeland, S., E. Lewis-Fuller, E., Wilks, R. J. Chronic disease in the Caribbean: strategies to respond to the public health challenge in the region. What can we learn from Jamaica's experience?. *West Indian Med. J.* 2011 Jul;60(4):397-411.

[6] Khan, J. M., Beevers, D. G. Management of hypertension in ethnic minorities. Heart. 2005; 91(8): 1105–1109.

[7] Vidt, D. G., Bravo, E. L., Fouad, F. M. Captopril. *N. Engl. J. Med.* 1982;306:214–219.

[8] Todd, P. A., Heel, R. C. Enalapril: a review of its pharmacodynamic and pharmacokinetic properties, and therapeutic use in hypertension and congestive heart failure. *Drugs.* 1986;31:198–248.

[9] Pool, J. L., Gennari, J., Goldstein, R., Kochar, M. S., Lewin, A. J., Maxwell, M. H., McChesney, J. A., Mehta, J., Nash, D. T., Nelson, E. B., Rastogi, S., Rofman, B., Weinberger, M. Controlled multicenter study of antihypertensive effects of lisinopril, hydrochlorothiazide, and lisinopril plus hydrochlorothiazide in the treatment of 394 patients with mild to moderate essential hypertension. *J. Cardiovasc. Pharmacol.* 1987; 3:S36–S42.

[10] Case, D. B., Atlas, S. A., Laragh, J. H., Sullivan, P. A., Sealey, J. E. Use of first-dose response or plasma renin activity to predict the long-term effect of captopril: identification of triphasic pattern of blood pressure response. *J. Cardiovasc. Pharmacol.* 1980;2:339–346.

[11] Given, B. D., Taylor, T., Hollenberg, N. K., Williams, G. H. Duration of action and short-term hormonal responses to enalapril (MK-421) in normal subjects. *J. Cardiovasc. Pharmacol.* 1984;6: 436–441.

[12] Waeber, B., Gavras, I., Brunner, H. R., Cook, C. A., Charocopos, F., Gavras, H. P. Prediction of sustained antihypertensive efficacy of chronic captopril therapy: relationships to immediate blood pressure response and control plasma renin activity. *Am. Heart J.* 1982;103:384–390.

[13] Waeber, B., Brunner, H. R., Brunner, D. B., Curtet, A. L., Turini, C. A., Gavras, H. Discrepancy between antihypertensive effect and angiotensin converting enzyme inhibition by captopril. *Hypertension.* 1980;2:236–242.

[14] Ujhelyi, M. R., Ferguson, R. J., Vlasses, P. H. Angiotensin-converting enzyme inhibitors: mechanistic controversies. *Pharmacotherapy.* 1989;9:351–362.

[15] Pepine, C. J., Pleiotropic effects of ACE inhibitors. *Medicographia.* 2009;31:9-15.

[16] Laffer, C. L., Elijovich, F. Essential Hypertension of Caribbean Hispanics: Sodium, Renin, and Response to Therapy. *J. Clin. Hypertens.* 2002;4:266–273.

[17] Douglas, J. G., Bakris, G. L., Epstein, M., Ferdinand, K. C., Ferrario, C., et al. Management of high blood pressure in African Americans: consensus statement of the Hypertension in African Americans Working Group of the International Society on Hypertension in Blacks. *Arch. Intern. Med.* 2003; 163(5):525-41.

[18] *NICE clinical guideline 127.* Hypertension. Clinical management of hypertension in adults. The National Institute for Health and Clinical Excellence, 2011.

[19] Clement, Y. N., Ali, S. Drug prescribing for hypertension at primary health care facilities in Trinidad. *West Indian Med. J.* 2012; 61 (1).

[20] Veterans Administration Co-operative Study Group of Antihypertensive Agents. Racial differences in response to low-dose captopril are abolished by the addition of hydrochlorothiazide. *Br. J. Clin. Pharmacol.* 1982;14:97S–101S.

[21] Materson, B. J., Reda, D. J., Cushman, W. C., Massie, B. M., Freis, E. D., Kochar, M. S., Hamburger, R. J., Fye, C., Lakshman, R., Gottdiener, J., Ramirez, E. A., Henderson, W. G. Single drug therapy for hypertension in men: a comparison of six antihypertensive agents with placebo. *N. Engl. J. Med.* 1993;328:914–921.

[22] Freis, E. D., Materson, B. J., Flamenbaum, W. Comparison of propanolol or hydrochlorothiazide alone for treatment of hypertension, III: evaluation of the renin-angiotensin system. *Am. J. Med.* 1983;74:1029–1041.

[23] Creditor, M., Loschky, U. Plasma Renin Activity in hypertension. *Am. J. Med.* 1967;43: 371–382.

[24] Wisenbaugh, P. E., Garst, J. B., Hull, C., Freedman, R. J., Matthews, D. N., Haddy, M. Renin, aldosterone, sodium and hypertension. *Am. J. Med.* 1972;52:175–186.

[25] Veterans Administration Co-operative Study Group of Antihypertensive Agents. Racial differences in response to low-dose captopril are abolished by the addition of hydrochlorothiazide. *Br. J. Clin. Pharmacol.* 1982;14:97S–101S.

[26] Weir, M. R., Gray, J. M., Paster, R., Saunders, E. Differing mechanisms of action of angiotensin-converting enzyme inhibition in black and white hypertensive patients. *Hypertension.* 1995;26:124–130.

[27] Gati, S., Bourne, P., McDaniel, S. The changing faces of diabetes, hypertension and arthritis in a Caribbean population N. Am. J. Med. Sci. 2010 May; 2(5): 221–229.

[28] Fraser, H. S. The dilemma of diabetes: health care crisis in the Caribbean Rev Panam Salud Publica/Pan. *Am. J. Public Health* 9(2), 2001

[29] Sosin, M. Heart failure - the importance of ethnicity. *Eur. J. Heart Fail.* (2004) 6 (7): 831-843.

[30] Ferguson, T. S., Tulloch-Reid, M. K., Wilks, R. J. The epidemiology of diabetes mellitus in Jamaica and the Caribbean: a historical review. *West Indian Med. J.* 2010; 59 (3).

[31] Ichikawa, I., Brenner, B. M. Glomerular actions of angiotensin II. *Am. J. Med.* 1984; 76:43–49.

[32] Anderson, S. G., Rennke, H. G., Brenner, B. M. Therapeutic advantage of converting enzyme inhibitors in arresting progressive renal disease associated with systemic hypertension in rat. *J. Clin. Invest.* 1986;77:1993–2000.

[33] Fogo, A., Yoshida, Y., Yared, A., Ichikawa, I. Importance of angiogenic action of angiotensin II in the glomerular growth of maturing kidneys. *Kidney Int.* 1990;38:1068–1074.

[34] Ruiz-Ortega, M., Gomez-Garre, D., Alcazar, R., Palacios, I., Bustos, C., Gonzalez, S., Plaza, J. J., Gonzalez, E., Egido, J. Involvement of angiotensin II and endothelin in matrix protein production and renal sclerosis. *J. Hypertens.* 1994;12:S51–S58.

[35] Hoelscher, D. D., Weir, M. R., Bakris, G. L. Hypertension in diabetic patients: an update of interventional studies to preserve renal function. *J. Clin. Pharmacol.* 1995;35: 73–80.

[36] Ravid, M., Lang, R., Rachmani, R., Lishner, M. Long-term renoprotective effect of angiotensin-converting enzyme inhibition in non-insulin-dependent diabetes mellitus: a 7-year follow-up study. *Arch. Intern. Med.* 1996;156:286–289.

[37] Lewis, E. J., Hunsicker, L. G., Bain, R. P., Rohde, R. D. The effect of angiotensin-converting-enzyme inhibition on diabetic nephropathy. *N. Engl. J. Med.* 1993;329: 1456–1462.
[38] Maschio, G., Alberti, D., Janin, G., Locatelli, F., Mann, J. F., Motolese, M., Ponticelli, C., Ritz, E., Zucchelli, P. Effect of the angiotensin-converting-enzyme inhibitor benazepril on the progression of chronic renal insufficiency: the Angiotensin-Converting-Enzyme Inhibition in Progressive Renal Insufficiency Study Group. *N. Engl. J. Med.* 1996;334:939–945.
[39] Lewis, E. J., Hunsicker, L. G., Bain, R. P., Rohde, R. D. The effect of angiotensin-converting-enzyme inhibition on diabetic nephropathy. *N. Engl. J. Med.* 1993;329: 1456–1462.
[40] Cowie, C. C., Harris, M. I., Silverman, R. E., Johnson, E. W., Rust, K. F. Effect of multiple risk factors on differences between blacks and whites in the prevalence of non-insulin-dependent diabetes mellitus in the United States. *Am. J. Epidemiol.* 1993;137: 719–732.
[41] Onuigbo, M. A. C. Natural history of Chronic Kidney Disease revisited-A 72 month Mayo Health System Hypertension Clinic Practice Based research network prospective report on End-Stage Renal Disease and death rates in 100 high risk CKD patients: a call for circumspection. *Adv. Perit. Dial.* 2009;25:85-8.
[42] Cordonnier, D. J., Zaoui, P., Halimi, S. Role of ACE inhibitors in patients with diabetes mellitus. *Drugs.* 2001;61(13):1883-92.
[43] National Institute for Health and Clinical Excellence, 2008 www.nice.org.uk.
[44] Remuzzi, G., Macia, M., Ruggenenti, P. Prevention and Treatment of Diabetic Renal Disease in Type 2 Diabetes: The BENEDICT Study. *JASN* April 2006 vol. 17 no. 4 suppl. 2 S90-S97.
[45] Gaziano, T. Growing Epidemic of Coronary Heart Disease in Low- and Middle-Income Countries. Curr. Probl. Cardiol. 2010 February; 35(2): 72–115.
[46] Zusman, R. M. Effects of converting-enzyme inhibitors on the renin-angiotensin-aldosterone, bradykinin, and arachidonic acid-prostaglandin systems: correlation of chemical structure and biologic activity. *Am. J. Kidney Dis.* 1987;10:13–23.
[47] Mira, M. L., Silva, M. M., Manso, C. F. The scavenging of oxygen free radicals by angiotensin converting enzyme inhibitors: the importance of the sulfhydryl group in the chemical structure of the compounds. *Ann. N Y Acad. Sci.* 1994;723:439–441.
[48] Fabris, B., Jackson, B., Cubela, R., Mendelsohn, F. A. O., Johnston, C. I. Angiotensin converting enzyme in the rat heart: studies of its inhibition in vitro and ex vivo. *Clin. Exp. Pharmacol. Physiol.* 1989;16:309–313.
[49] Cohen, M. L., Kurz, K. D. Angiotensin converting enzyme inhibition in tissues from spontaneously hypertensive rats after treatment with captopril or MK-421. *J. Pharmacol. Exp. Ther.* 1982;220:63–69.
[50] Yusuf, S., Sleight, P., Pogue, J., Bosch, J., Davies, R., Dagenais, G. Effects of an angiotensin-converting-enzyme inhibitor, ramipril, on cardiovascular events in high-risk patients. The Heart Outcomes Prevention Evaluation Study Investigators. *N. Engl. J. Med.* 2000 Jan. 20;342(3):145-53.
[51] Fox, K. M., European trial on reduction of cardiac events with Perindopril in stable coronary artery disease Investigators. Efficacy of perindopril in reduction of cardiovascular events among patients with stable coronary artery disease: randomised,

double-blind, placebo-controlled, multicenter trial (the EUROPA study). *Lancet.* 2003 Sep. 6;362(9386):782-8.

[52] Braunwald, E., Domanski, M. J., Fowler, S. E., Geller, N. L., Gersh, B. J., Hsia, J., Pfeffer, M. A., Rice, M. M., Rosenberg, Y. D., Rouleau, J. L., PEACE Trial Investigators. Angiotensin-converting-enzyme inhibition in stable coronary artery disease. *N. Engl. J. Med.* 2004;351(20):2058-68. Epub. 2004 Nov. 7.

[53] Al-Mallah, M. H., Tieyjeh, I. M., Abdel-Latif, L. A., Weaver, W. D. Angiotensin-converting enzyme inhibitors in coronary artery disease and preserved left ventricular systolic function: a systematic review and meta-analysis of randomized controlled trials. *J. Am. Coll. Cardiol.* 2006 Apr. 18;47(8):1576-83.

[54] Mc Swain, M., Martin, T. C. M-mode echocardiographic findings in a contemporary Afro-Caribbean population referred for evaluation of congestive cardiac failure. *West Indian Med. J.* 2002 Jun;51(2):93-6.

[55] The Consensus Study Trial group. Effects of Enalapril on Mortality in Severe Congestive Heart Failure. *N. Engl. J. Med.* 1987; 316:1429-1435.

[56] The SOLVD Investigators. Effect of enalapril on survival in patients with reduced left ventricular ejection fractions and congestive heart failure. *N Engl. J. Med.* 1991; 325 (5):293-302.

[57] Cohn, J. N., Archibald, D. G., Ziesche, S., Franciosa, J. A., Harston, W. E., Tristani, F. E., Dunkman, W. B., Jacobs, W., Francis, G. S., Flohr, K. H. Effect of vasodilator therapy on mortality in chronic congestive heart failure. Results of a Veterans Administration Cooperative Study. *N. Engl. J. Med.* 1986;314(24): 1547-52.

[58] Björn, D., Pennert, K., Hansson, L. Reversal of Left Ventricular Hypertrophy in Hypertensive Patients. A Metaanalysis of 109 treatment studies. *Am. J. Hypertens.* (1992) 5 (2): 95-110.

[59] Cleland, J. G., Tendera, M., Adamus, J., Freemantle, N., Polonski, L., Taylor, J. The perindopril in elderly people with chronic heart failure (PEP-CHF) study. *Eur. Heart J.* 2006; 27(19):2338-45.

[60] Gati, S., K. Melchiorre, M. Papadakis. Increased left ventricular trabeculation in afro-caribbean individuals: and inherited cardiomyopathy or a physiological response to increased cardiac preload. *Heart* 2013;99.

[61] International Cardiovascular Disease Statistics. 2004. American Heart Association. 2004, americanheart.org.

[62] Barbaro, G. HIV- associated cardiomyopathy etiopathogenesis and clinical aspects. *Herz.* 2005 Sep;30(6):486-92.

[63] Hodsman, G. P., Isles, C. G., Murray, G. D., Usherwood, T. P., Webb, I., Robertson, J. I. Factors related to first dose hypotensive effect of captopril: prediction and treatment. *BMJ.* 1983;286:832–834.

[64] Warren, S. E., O'Connor, D. T. Hyperkalemia resulting from captopril administration. *JAMA.* 1980;244:2551–2552.

[65] Textor, S. C., Bravo, E. L., Fouad, F. M., Tarazi, R. C. Hyperkalemia in azotemic patients during angiotensin-converting enzyme inhibition and aldosterone reduction with captopril. *Am. J. Med.* 1982;73:719–725.

[66] Israili, Z. H., Hall, W. D. Cough and angioneurotic edema associated with angiotensin-converting enzyme inhibitor therapy. *Ann. Intern. Med.* 1992;117:234–242.

[67] Brown, N. J., Ray, W. A., Griffin, M. R. Black Americans have an increased rate of angiotensin converting enzyme inhibitor-associated angioedema. *Clin. Pharmacol. Ther.* 1996;60:8–13.

[68] Williams-Johnson, J. A., Hemmings, S., Williams, E. W., Channer, G., McDonald, A. H. Six years experience of angioedema at the University Hospital of the West Indies. *West Indian Med. J.* 2007; 56 (3).

[69] The Solvd investigators. Effect of Enalapril on Mortality and the Development of Heart Failure in Asymptomatic Patients with Reduced Left Ventricular Ejection Fraction. *N. Engl. J. Med.* 1992; 327:685-691.

[70] D. K. Arnett, E. Boerwinkle, B. R. Davis, J. Eckfeldt, C. E. Ford and H. Black. Pharmacogenetic approaches to hypertension therapy: design and rationale for the Genetics of Hypertension Associated Treatment (GenHAT) study. *The Pharmacogenomics Journal* (2002) 2, 309–317.

[71] Hornig, B., Kohler, C., Drexler, H. Role of bradykinin in mediating vascular effects of angiotensin-converting enzyme inhibitors in humans. *Circulation.* 1997;95:1115–1118.

[72] Stanek, B., Silberbauer, K. Acute and chronic effects of captopril on bicyclo-PGEm, the stable bicyclic end product of prostaglandin E_2 in essential hypertension. *Nephron.* 1986;44:40–45.

[73] Vlasses, P. H., Ferguson, R. K., Smith, J. B., Rotmensch, H. H., Swanson, B. N. Urinary excretion of prostacyclin and thromboxane A_2 metabolites after angiotensin converting enzyme inhibition in hypertensive patients. *Prostaglandins Leukot. Med.* 1983;11:143–150.

[74] Witzgall, H., Scherer, B., Weber, P. C. Involvement of prostaglandins in the actions of captopril. *Clin. Sci.* 1982;63:265S–267S.

[75] Linz, W., Scholkens, B. A. A specific B_2-bradykinin receptor antagonist HOE 140 abolishes the antihypertrophic effect of ramipril. *Br. J. Pharmacol.* 1992;105:771–772.

[76] Bouaziz, H., Joulin, Y., Safar, M., Benetos, A. Effects of bradykinin B_2 receptor antagonism on the hypotensive effects of ACE inhibition. *Br. J. Pharmacol.* 1994;113: 717–722.

[77] Gainer, J. V., Stein, C. M., Neal, T., Vaughnan, D. E., Brown, N. J. Interactive Effect of Ethnicity and ACE Insertion/Deletion Polymorphism on Vascular Reactivity. *Hypertension.* 2001; 37: 46-51.

[78] Johnson, A. D., Gong, Y., Wang, D., et al.: Promoter polymorphisms in ACE associated with clinical outcomes in hypertension. *Clin. Pharmacol. Ther.* 2009;85:36-44.

[79] Donna K. Arnett, Steven, A. Cl Pharmacogenetics of Antihypertensive Treatment: Detailing Disciplinary Dissonance. *Pharmacogenomics.* 2009;10(8):1295-1307.

In: ACE Inhibitors. Volume 2
Editor: Macaulay Amechi Onuigbo

ISBN: 978-1-62948-422-8

Chapter 5

ACEIs as Antihypertensives: A Nigerian CKD Clinic Experience

Ifeoma I. Ulasi, MD[1,2*], Chinwuba K. Ijoma, MD[1], Benedict C. Anisiuba, MD[3] and Ngozi A. Ifebunandu, MD[2,4]

[1]Renal Unit, Department of Medicine, College of Medicine, University of Nigeria Teaching Hospital, Ituku-Ozalla, Enugu, Nigeria
[2]Department of Medicine, Federal Teaching Hospital Abakaliki, Ebonyi State, Nigeria
[3]Cardiology Unit, Dept of Medicine, College of Medicine, University of Nigeria Teaching Hospital, Ituku-Ozalla, Enugu, Nigeria
[4]Department of Internal Medicine, College of Health Sciences, Ebonyi State University, Ebonyi State, Nigeria

Abstract

The incidence and prevalence of chronic kidney disease (CKD) have been increasing worldwide. The overall world prevalence of CKD is difficult to determine because of under-diagnosis and lack of or poor registries in many parts of the world. In Nigeria, CKD accounts for 8-10% of hospital admissions. Cardiovascular disease is the commonest complication of CKD and accounts for the greatest mortality in CKD. Most patients with CKD are on angiotensin converting enzyme inhibitors (ACEIs) for various indications, including control of hypertension, left ventricular dysfunction/hypertrophy, treatment of CCF, and as reno-protective agent in diabetic and non-diabetic CKD with significant proteinuria. Some clinical practice guidelines including JNC VII recommend use of ACEIs as compelling indication in some of these diseases. ACEIs have also been shown to improve outcome in both pre-dialysis and dialysis patients. This improved outcome in patients is independent of blood pressure and other clinical and demographic variables. ACEIs have been reported to be less effective antihypertensive agents in black patients as compared to white patients when used as monotherapy. This has been generally attributed to the fact that blacks have low renin essential hypertension as against high renin essential hypertension seen in white patients. One of the most important side effects of ACEIs is a dry cough which occurs in about 5-20% of patients.

* Corresponding author: Ifeoma I Ulasi MD; Email: ifeomaulasi@yahoo.co.uk

A less common but significant side effect of ACEIs is angioedema which occurs in 1 to 2 per 1000 patients in Caucasians and about double this rate in blacks. Other side effects of this class of drugs include a reversible decline in renal function especially in the setting of decreased renal perfusion. The side effects appear to be commoner in women than men; 26% versus 21 % in one study. The local experience of ACEIs in CKD in Nigeria will be reported in this chapter, the results of an on-going retrospective study of the prescription pattern of ACEIs in CKD in University of Nigeria Teaching Hospital, Enugu, in Southeastern Nigeria, from 2008 - 2012. This study will provide information on the use of ACEIs in CKD locally, the various indications for their use, their efficacy and the side-effect profile. ACEIs are important agents in management of CKD patients with considerable improvement in mortality. The controversy relating to the discrepancy in efficacy and side effect profile between black and white patients may partially be settled from the on-going retrospective study.

1. Introduction and Background

1.1. Epidemiology of CKD in Nigeria and Africa

Literature from all regions of the world suggests increasing prevalence of chronic kidney disease [1, 2]. Across Africa, reports document that the rates of end-stage renal disease (ESRD) increased by 75% between 2000 and 2004 [3]. Chronic kidney disease (CKD) accounts for nearly 10% of hospital admissions [4, 5] and renal outpatient visits represent nearly 25% of all medical outpatient attendance while deaths from renal disease account for over 20% of all medical deaths [6].

Burden of Hypertension and Other Non-Communicable Diseases (NCDs) as Risk Factors for CKD

The world's disease trend is changing even in the developing world and chronic diseases are increasingly being the prevalent cause of morbidity and mortality in the world [2, 7]. Chronic diseases cause about 60% of all deaths. Non-communicable diseases (NCDs) have supplanted communicable diseases as the most common causes of ill health and premature death globally [8, 9]. The economic impact of NCDs worldwide is enormous and approximately half of the total economic burden is accounted for by cardiovascular disease. This implies that cardiovascular diseases (such as stroke, ischemic heart disease, and peripheral vascular disease) cause more deaths than communicable diseases (such as HIV/AIDS, malaria, and tuberculosis) combined [8, 9]. The extent of the burden is such that it is extrapolated that by 2015, two diseases - cardiovascular disease and diabetes – could reduce global gross domestic product by 5% [10].

CVDs account for approximately 17 million deaths yearly, and this amounts to about a third of all global deaths [11, 12]. Hypertension and its associated complications account for about 9.4 million deaths every year [13], amounting to over half of cardiovascular deaths. The World Health Report 2002 identified hypertension as the third ranked factor for disability-adjusted life years [14]. The latest global burden of disease published in 2012 lists hypertension as the leading risk factor for global disease burden, standing at 7.0% of global DALYs [13]. Hypertension and cardiovascular diseases are currently noted to disproportionately affect people in low- and middle-income countries [12, 15]. In Nigeria, hypertension has prevalence that range from 20% to over 40% depending on populations assessed [16, 17]. For example, a study in a market population in Enugu, South-east Nigeria documented a prevalence of about 43% [17]. Presently, 80% of deaths due to cardiovascular disease occur in low- and middle-income countries (LMICs), where the health systems can least afford the social and economic burden of ill health [11, 12]. The chance of dying from a non-communicable disease in populations between the ages of 30 and 70 years is highest in sub-Saharan Africa, Eastern Europe and parts of Asia [15]. The importance of adequate control of hypertension cannot be over emphasized; evidence shows that just as for stroke and ischemic heart disease, the risk of renal failure occurs as a continuum, therefore it is not just restricted to populations with high levels of blood pressure [18, 19].

These disease trends informed the World Health Assembly's decision to endorse a Global Action Plan for NCD prevention and control in 2008 [20]. Although kidney disease is not one of the four NCDs identified in the current Action Plan for NCDs, convincing evidence indicate that kidney disease is an important determinant of the poor health outcomes for major NCDs [7, 21]. The World Health Organization (WHO) has reiterated the need to include prevention of kidney disease in national NCD programs, especially at the primary-care level [7, 21].

The increase in prevalence of non-communicable diseases will inevitably be accompanied by increases in rates of ESRD [22]. Unfortunately, in addition to the threat of non-communicable diseases, the LMICs still have significant rates of chronic kidney disease (CKD) from infectious causes such as HIV, tuberculosis, bacterial infections, hepatitis B and C, etc., which prompted the WHO to raise to the fore the double burden of diseases in developing countries [22]. Other non-infectious diseases such as sickle cell anaemia, prevalent use of herbal medications, environmental pollution from hydrocarbons such as petroleum products, lead, etc., all contribute to the high burden of CKD [22, 23]. Also, low socioeconomic status per se has been associated with higher rates of ESRD [24]. Socioeconomic differentials in health have been widely recognized as an important determinant of NCDs; individuals of lower socioeconomic status (SES) are known to have a higher risk for mortality and morbidity compared with those of higher SES [12]. Fundamentally, the level of education determines one's socioeconomic status; invariably people in low socio-economic cadre have less education. Bello et al, 2008 [25] used the UK Index of Multiple Deprivation (IMD) Score 2000 to measure residential area deprivation, as an indicator of SES. They observed a greater risk for CKD in patients who live in areas with low SES. Another study in the UK demonstrated that incidence of diagnosed and referred CKD is more in deprived areas, and is associated with poorer prognosis and decreased survival [26]. Similarly, in the US, some national surveys have shown trends of prevalent CKD in people with low SES and this relationship was predominant among the African-American groups [24]. Ulasi et al, 2013 [27], working in South-east Nigeria demonstrated that CKD correlated with low level of education and low-income occupation among other factors identified in the rural and semi-urban population they studied.

1.2. Evidence for ACEIs in Chronic Kidney Disease

Experimental studies have shown that proteins filtered into the Bowman's capsule in the setting of renal diseases are actively reabsorbed by proximal tubular cells through receptor-mediated endocytosis, and then degraded by lysosomes [28, 29]. Therefore when protein concentration increases in the proximal cell tubular lumen, there is increased synthesis of vasoactive and pro-inflammatory substances - angiotensin, endothelin-1, transforming growth factor beta, etc. [30]. These substances stimulate the migration of macrophages and T lymphocytes into the interstitium; hence cellular infiltrates are typically observed in renal biopsies of patients with proteinuric renal diseases. These interstitial infiltrates continue to produce the pro-inflammatory and profibrotic factors that culminate in gradual transformation from an infiltrative process to a diffuse and irreversible fibrosis [29]. The severity of tubulo-interstitial changes is more predictive of the prognosis than the glomerular changes [31]. Several clinical studies have established that proteinuria is one of the most important risk factors for progressive renal function loss in both diabetic and non-diabetic renal diseases [32, 33]. Therapeutic strategies that reduce the level of proteinuria will ameliorate or stop renal function loss. The salutary effect of ACEIs on urinary protein loss is well established in literature. ACEIs have been shown to decrease proteinuria more effectively than other anti-hypertensives; this antiproteinuric effect is thought to be independent of the underlying renal disease, and is mediated by other mechanisms. Wapstra, Navis, de Jong, de Zeeuw (2000) [34] showed that the anti-proteinuric effect of ACE inhibition was mainly related to reduction of angiotensin II and independent of the bradykinin pathway. The anti-proteinuric effect of ACEIs leads to reduced progression of renal disease and this effect is greater in patients with higher urine protein excretion at the onset of treatment. Furthermore, other phenomena associated with urinary protein loss for example hypoalbuminemia and hyperlipidaemia/dyslipidaemia, also improve during ACEI treatment [35, 36].

Data from a meta-analysis of randomized control trials (RCTs) demonstrated that patients treated with regimens which included ACEIs had slower progression of kidney disease than those who received treatment regimens without ACEIs. The studies include Collaborative Study Group (CSG) Captopril Trial [37], for diabetic kidney disease and Ramipril in non-diabetic renal failure (REIN) [38], Angiotensin-converting-enzyme Inhibition on Progressive Renal Insufficiency (AIPRI) Study [39], for non-diabetic kidney disease. The AASK study to date is the largest study on CKD involving persons of African descent [40]. It compared ACEIs with CCBs in patients with hypertension induced CKD. The information from the various large RCTs that mold or influence the recommendations of the guidelines will be discussed in a later section of this chapter.

1.3. What the Guidelines Say on Use of ACEIs in Hypertension and Chronic Kidney Disease

The guidelines depend on evidence from clinical trials to make recommendations. Guidelines have different ways of grading the level of evidence. The National Institute for Health and Clinical Excellence (NICE) [41], Renal Association of UK [42] and Caring for Australasians with Renal Impairment (CARI) Guidelines [43] use the traditional levels of evidence employed in clinical trials. The KDOQI assessed the quality of the evidence and the strength of recommendations using the Grading of Recommendation Assessment, Development, and Evaluation (GRADE) approach which grades evidence depending on how confident they are that the true effect lies close to the estimated effect, and they range from the highest – A to D – the lowest [44].

Recommendations from the major guidelines are discussed below:

KDOQI Guidelines

The KDOQI Guidelines 1, 8 and 9 [45] endorsed ACEIs and ARBs as favored agents for diabetic kidney disease and non-diabetic kidney diseases with proteinuria. The guidelines acknowledge that ample evidence shows that they lower blood pressure, reduce proteinuria, slow the progression of kidney disease, and likely reduce CVD risk in these diseases by other mechanisms in addition to lowering the blood pressure. Therefore these older guidelines recommended the use of ACEIs and ARBs even when there is no hypertension. The KDOQI Update of 2012 came out strongly against use of ACEIs or ARBs for the primary prevention of diabetic kidney in normotensive normo-albuminuric patients [44]. But they upheld the use of ACEIs or ARBs in normotensive patients with diabetes and albuminuria levels >30 mg/g who are at high risk of diabetic kidney disease or its progression.

The other recommendations from KDOQI 8 and 9 are as follows:

- Target blood pressure in diabetic and non-diabetic kidney diseases should be <130/80 mm Hg.
- Patients with diabetic and non-diabetic kidney diseases whose spot urine total protein to creatinine ratio ≥200 mg/g, with or without hypertension, should be treated with an ACEI or ARB.

KDOQI Guideline 11 [45] details how and when to use angiotensin-converting enzyme inhibitors and angiotensin receptor blockers in CKD:

- ACEIs and ARBs should be used at moderate to high doses and as indicated in clinical trials.
- ACEIs and ARBs could be used as alternatives to each other, in situations where the preferred class cannot be used.
- ACEIs and ARBs may be used in combination to lower blood pressure or reduce proteinuria if necessary.

Patients on ACEIs or ARBs treatments should be monitored for hypotension, decreased GFR and hyperkalemia; the schedule for monitoring should depend on baseline levels. Generally, the ACEI or ARB can be continued if:

a) GFR decline over 4 months is <30% from baseline value
b) Serum potassium is ≤5.5 mEq/L.

Caring for Australasians with Renal Impairment (CARI) Guidelines

The CARI 2005 guidelines stated that:

For non-diabetic kidney [43]:

a) Regimens that contain ACEIs are more effective at slowing progression of kidney disease than those that do not include ACEIs.
b) Combination therapy of ACEIs and ARBs are more effective at slowing progression of non-diabetic kidney disease than either single agent.

c) ACEIs seem more effective at slowing progressive kidney disease than beta-blockers and dihydropyridine calcium channel blockers.

The guidelines further suggested that in clinical care, ACEIs should be used with caution in patients with renal impairment. For such patients plasma electrolytes and renal function should be monitored closely during therapy.

For Diabetic Kidney Disease [46]:

Patients who have type 2 diabetes mellitus and microalbuminuria or macroalbuminuria, should receive ARBs or ACEIs to protect against progression of kidney disease. Their blood pressure should be tightly controlled within target range using ARBs or ACEIs as first choice antihypertensive agents. Multi-drug therapy could be used as necessary to achieve target blood pressure. Patients should be informed about the consequences of some lifestyle habits, for example smoking increases the risk of chronic kidney disease.

National Institute for Health and Clinical Excellence (NICE)

The NICE guidelines [41] indicated in their choice of antihypertensive agents:

- For angiotensin system blockade, ACEIs should be used first, if not well tolerated then an ARB could be introduced.
- For patients with diabetes mellitus: ACEIs/ARBs could be given irrespective of presence of hypertension when albumin creatinine ratio (ACR) is >2.5mg/mmol for men and >3.5mg/mmol for women.
- For patients without diabetes mellitus: ACEIs/ARBs could be given to those with CKD and hypertension who have ACR ≥30 mg/mmol or urinary protein excretion ≥0.5gm/24 hours. Those who have non-diabetic kidney disease and ACR ≥70 mg/mmol with or without hypertension or cardiovascular disease should be offered ACEIs/ARBs. For patients who have non-diabetic kidney disease and hypertension whose ACR < 30 mg/mmol; the choice of anti-hypertensive treatment should be in accordance with the NICE guidance on hypertension to prevent or ameliorate progression of CKD.
- ACEIs/ARBs should be titrated to the maximum tolerated therapeutic dose before considering a second-line agent.
- Patients on ACEIs/ARBs should be informed about the importance of achieving the optimal tolerated dose of ACEI/ARB, and the need to monitor eGFR and serum potassium.
- CKD patients commencing on ACEIs/ARBs should have measurements of serum potassium concentrations and estimated GFR before starting therapy; measurements should be repeated after 1 and 2 weeks following commencement of therapy and thereafter with each dose increase.
- NICE guidelines further highlighted recommendations related to serum potassium levels and hyperkalaemia and when there is decreased eGFR or increased serum creatinine following treatment. These will be discussed in the subsection on complications and side effects of ACEI therapy.

UK Renal Association Guidelines

The guideline [42] discussed aspects of treatment of CKD patients with hypertension or raised blood pressure from sub-sections 2.1 – 2.4. The UK RA guidelines recommended that:

- For most CKD patients, systolic blood pressure should be reduced to <140 mmHg with target range of 120-139 mmHg while the diastolic blood pressure should be lowered to <90 mmHg. For patients with diabetes or proteinuria of 1g/24 hours or more, the aim is to lower the systolic blood pressure to <130 mmHg with target range 120-129 mmHg and the diastolic blood pressure to <80 mmHg. They emphasized that antihypertensive therapy should be individualized and lowering of the systolic blood pressure to less than 120 mmHg should be avoided.
- Angiotensin-Converting Enzyme Inhibitor or Angiotensin Receptor Blocker treatment should be part of the antihypertensive therapy of patients with CKD and urinary protein excretion of >0.5g/day. And the treatments should be increased to achieve the lowest possible level of proteinuria.
- Patients with diabetes mellitus and microalbuminuria should receive ACEIs or ARBs, titrated to maximum licensed antihypertensive dose if tolerated.

The Nigerian Association of Nephrology (NAN) Guidelines for the Detection and Management of CKD:

The NAN guidelines (2011) [47] emphasized the meticulous control of blood pressure as the most crucial strategy for retarding progression of CKD.

The blood pressure targets recommended are as follows: 130/80mmHg for proteinuria <1gm/24hours, 120/75mmHg if proteinuria is greater than 1gm/24hours and for patients with diabetes mellitus. For children, blood pressure target is <90th percentile for the age, sex and height.

World Health Organization (WHO)/ International Society of Hypertension (ISH) 2003 Guidelines:

The WHO/ISH guidelines [48] noted that decisions about the management of hypertensive patients should consider blood pressure levels, presence of other cardiovascular risk factors, target organ damage, and associated clinical conditions. The Committee stratified patients according to presence and number of risk factors, target organ damage and associated clinical conditions. Patients with kidney disease were defined as: plasma creatinine concentration >1.4mg/dl (120μmol/l) for females and > 1.5mg/dl (133μmol/l) for males, and albuminuria > 300 mg/day. Such patients were grouped as having clear and compelling indications for the use ACEIs if they had type-1 diabetic kidney disease or non-diabetic kidney disease and ARBs if they had type-2 diabetic kidney disease.

The Nigerian Hypertension Society guidelines [49] basically adopted the recommendations of WHO/ISH.

Other guidelines such as the European Society of Hypertension guideline and JNC 7 [50] have also recommended the use of ACEIs or ARBs for those with diabetes. The new ESH/ESC guidelines [51] on hypertension recommended against dual renin-angiotensin system (RAS) blockade using (ARBs, ACE inhibitors, and direct renin inhibitors) in clinical practice because of issues related to hyperkalemia, low blood pressure, and kidney failure.

The meta-analysis reviewing the safety of dual RAS blockade showed increased risk when ARBs and ACEIs were used together. JNC 7 guidelines added that patients with kidney disease must be treated differently from those without and a combination of ACEIs or ARBs with diuretics are preferred for patients with kidney disease. The new JNC 8 guideline(s) is still being expected.

2. Mechanism of Action of ACEIs

2.1. Brief Overview of the Renin-Angiotensin System (RAS)

ACEIs are a group of drugs that inhibit the formation of angiotensin II, a powerful vasoconstrictor that mediates most of the actions of the renin-angiotensin system (RAS). The classical view of the RAS is that angiotensinogen, a plasma protein, is acted upon by a proteolytic enzyme, renin which breaks it down to angiotensin I. Angiotensin converting enzyme (ACE) then breaks down angiotensin I to angiotensin II. Recently, there has been a lot of development in our understanding of the RAS. The simple classical view of the RAS has massively expanded and become complicated. Renin receptors have been discovered. The angiotensin 'family' now has many new members. A new type of ACE, called ACE2 has been discovered. The circulating RAS which has been regarded as an endocrine system is now known to also act as a paracrine and an intracrine system due to the discovery of local RAS. New facts continue to emerge on a regular basis.

2.2. Historical Perspective

History of the RAS dates back to 1898 when Robert Tigerstedt - a Finnish professor of physiology, and Per Bergman, his Swedish student, both working in the Karolinska Institute, Stockholm discovered that renin, a saline extract of the rabbit kidney produced a sustained rise in blood pressure when injected into rabbits [52]. In 1938, Friedman et al were puzzled when they discovered that renin was not effective in vitro [53]. The puzzle was answered two years later by independent researchers from two widely separated laboratories. Page and Helmer in US [54] and Braun-Menendez [55] and his group in Argentina found that renin acted on a substance (peptide) in the plasma to produce the powerful vasoconstriction. Page called this new peptide angiotonin while Braun-Menendez called it hypertensin. Many years later, Page and Braun-Menendez compromised and called it angiotensin [56].

2.3. The Renin-Angiotensin Family

2.3.1. Angiotensinogen

Angiotensinogen is an alpha-2 globulin produced by the liver and released into the circulation. It is a member of the serpin superfamily of protease inhibitors. However it does not inhibit any enzyme unlike most members of this group. It consists of 450 amino acids but it is only the first 12 that are responsible for its activity: Asp-Arg-Val-Tyr-Ile-His-Pro-Phe-His-Leu-Val-Ile-...

2.3.2. Renin

Renin is a proteolytic enzyme produced by the juxtaglomerular cells around the afferent glomerular arteriole. Its precursor has 406 amino acids. The pre-segment contains 20 amino acids while the post- contains 46. In its mature form, renin contains 340 amino acids. It is produced in the kidneys in response to renal sympathetic activity. Other stimulants for renin production include low blood pressure at the afferent arteriole ($\leq$90 mmHg systolic pressure) and low sodium and chloride delivery to the macula densa. Renin acts on the N-terminal of angiotensinogen to produce a decapeptide, called angiotensin I. The first and rate-limiting step in the RAS is the renin action. (57)

2.3.3. Angiotensin I

Angiotensin 1 (Asp-Arg-Val-Tyr-Ile-His-Pro-Phe-His-Leu) is inactive. Its main function is to act as a precursor for angiotensin II.

2.3.4. Angiotensin Converting Enzymes

Angiotensin I is converted to angiotensin II by a variety of enzymes including ACE and chymase

ACE is a bivalent peptidyl dipeptidase. It is present in a membrane-bound form in the brain, endothelial, epithelial and neuroepithelial cells. It is also present in a soluble form in the blood and various body fluids. ACE is not specific for angiotensin I as it cleaves a variety of other peptides such as bradykinin, leutenizing hormone releasing hormone, [58] enkephalins, substance P, etc. The recently-discovered angiotensin converting enzyme 2 (ACE2) catalyses the formation of angiotensin 1-9 from angiotensin I and angiotensin 1-7 from angiotensin II.[59]

2.3.5. Angiotensin II and other Angiotensins

Angiotensin II (Ang 1-8: Asp-Arg-Val-Tyr-Ile-His-Pro-Phe) is the most active member of the angiotensin 'family'. There are two main receptors for angiotensin II – AT1 and AT2 receptors but it is more active at the AT1 receptor subtype.

Activation of the AT1 receptor by angiotensin II stimulates a variety of activities including stimulation of thirst and release of aldosterone and vasopressin, vasoconstriction, amplification of sympathetic nervous outflow, promotion of cell growth and cell migration in the cardiovascular system, stimulation of fibrosis, and pro-inflammatory modulation including atherosclerosis and vascular aging. Angiotensin II stimulation also leads to impaired glucose metabolism through suppression of adiponection – an insulin sensitizer, stimulation of insulin secretion, reduction of gluconeogenesis and consequent reduction of hepatic glucose output. It also leads to increase in plasma triglycerides, cellular apoptosis and generation of free radicals. [60]

When applied to the kidneys, the above actions of angiotensin II will lead to increased intra-glomerular pressure (from systemic hypertension, efferent arteriolar constriction, contraction of mesangial cells, direct stimulation of renal tubular reabsorption and stimulation of aldosterone synthesis by the adrenal cortex). Most of these actions will also lead to increased permeability to macromolecules, activation of fibrogenesis and oxidative stress.

AT2 receptors are usually found in the foetus, injured tissue, and few adult organs such as the brain and adrenal medulla. They mediate actions opposite to those of AT1 receptors, mainly inhibition of cell growth, vasoconstriction and release of nitrous oxide (NO). In addition, stimulation of AT2 receptors has a neurotrophic effect leading to prevention of ischaemic brain damage.

Angiotensin III (angiotensin 2-8 heptapeptide) has similar actions to angiotensin II especially in the secretion of vasopressin. It is cleaved from angiotensin II by aminopeptidase A but it has a very short half-life.

Angiotensin IV (angiotensin 3-8 hexapeptide) is produced from angiotensin III by the action of aminopeptidase M. It has important metabolic functions in cognition, renal metabolism (through vasodilatation and anti-thrombotic properties) and cardiovascular function. The receptor for angiotensin IV is the insulin-regulated amino peptidase receptor (IRAP).

Angiotensin 1-7 heptapeptide is generated from angiotensin II by ACE2. Other peptidases have been found to generate angiotensin 1-7 from angiotensin I or II. It acts on the mas receptor to produce vasodilatation (as well as amplify the vasodilatation caused by bradykinin) and anti-trophic actions. It opposes the actions of angiotensin II.

Angiotensin 1-9 is generated from angiotensin I by carboxypeptidase A and similar enzymes. It has prothrombotic properties similar to angiotensin II in rats, part of which may be due to conversion of angiotensin 1-9 to angiotensin II. [61]

2.3.6. Angiotensin Converting Enzyme Inhibitors (ACEIs)

ACEIs block the formation of angiotensin II and thereby reduce the stimulation of AT1 and AT2 receptors. They antagonise the actions of angiotensin II thus causing arterial and venous dilatation which leads to a reduction in blood pressure, reduction in preload and afterload, down-regulation of sympathetic adrenergic activity in addition to the natriuretic and diuretic effects. The overall result is reduction in blood volume as well as reduction in arterial and venous pressures.

ACEIs inhibit cardiac and arterial remodelling associated with chronic hypertension, heart failure and myocardial infarction. They also inhibit cell migration, proliferation, and hypertrophy caused by angiotensin II. These actions of ACEIs result in reduction of overall CV risk and renal damage.

On the kidneys, ACEIs decrease glomerular capillary pressure head by decreasing arterial pressure and by selectively dilating efferent arterioles with reduction in permselectivity and proteinuria. ACEIs inhibit mesangial cell growth and matrix production, reduce angiotensin II-mediated oxidative stress and promote production of nitrous oxide and vasodilator prostaglandins. ACEIs also block the degradation of bradykinin to inactive moieties leading to the accumulation of bradykinin with enhancement of peripheral and efferent vasodilatation and reduction of aldosterone production.

However, ACEIs do not inhibit the formation of angiotensin I and II from other sources such as chymase. The implication is incomplete blockade of RAS which will result in the attenuation of the actions of ACEIs.

Angiotensin receptor blockers (ARBs) cause more complete blockade of the RAS but they do not lead to the accumulation of bradykinin. The beneficial vasodilatory effect of bradykinin is lost. The inadequate blockade of the RAS by ACEI or ARB alone has made the combined use of both agents more attractive.

2.3.7. Tissue RAS

Many tissues have been found to contain all the components of the RAS. These include the adrenal gland, kidneys, brain, heart, blood vessels, reproductive organs, pancreas and adipose tissue. They may operate independent of the circulating RAS (brain, adrenal gland) or they may operate in a complimentary manner as in the kidneys and the heart. [62]

The tissue RAS exhibits mainly local effects such as cell growth and proliferation, protein synthesis, etc. In the heart, they help in cardiac remodeling after myocardial injury such as myocardial infarction. Tissue RAS also participates in vascular inflammatory processes of atherosclerosis. Growth and fibrosis of glomerular mesangial cells are influenced by tissue RAS. Some activities of the brain (central regulation of BP), the testis (fertility) and those of the adipose tissue (components of the metabolic syndrome such as insulin resistance) are mediated by the tissue RAS [63]

2.3.8. Intracellular RAS

The role of intracellular RAS is unclear but it is reported to be involved in intracellular calcium fluxes and activation of genes. In vivo, intracellular RAS has been reported to cause cardiac hypertrophy in mice. [64]

2.4. Rationale for the Use of ACEIs to slow Progression of CKD

2.4.1. ACEIs Reduce BP

There is slower progression of chronic kidney disease in patients with normal BP. This is supported by the review of 3 studies: MDRD, AASK and REIN. [65] Hypertension worsens the progression of chronic kidney disease and there is strong evidence from the above studies that the use of ACEIs slows this progression (of kidney disease) through the reduction of intraglomerular and systemic BP. However, the beneficial effect of ACEIs in these patients appears greater than would be expected from their antihypertensive effects alone. Other mechanisms must be involved.

2.4.2. ACEIs Reduce Proteinuria

Proteinuria causes a more rapid decline in GFR in CKD patients no matter the aetiology of the CKD and the initial GFR. Inflammation of the interstitium may ensue due to the activation of pro-inflammatory factors by the reabsorbed protein. Studies have also shown a correlation between reduction of proteinuria during antihypertensive therapy and slowing of progression of kidney disease. ACEIs appear to reduce proteinuria preferentially more than other antihypertensive agents and this reduction is by far greater than could be predicted from their antihypertensive effects alone. Other mechanisms by which ACEIs reduce proteinuria include direct improvement in permselectivity of the glomerular capillaries and anti-fibrotic effects. Reduction in proteinuria may also lead to reduction in serum lipid levels and slowing of atherosclerosis in general which improves kidney function.

2.4.3. Class Effect

Some of the beneficial effects of ACEIs in patients with CKD cannot be explained by their antihypertensive and anti-proteinuric effects. Other factors contributing to the slowing of the progression of renal disease include the improvement in mesangial function and reduction of oxidative stress.

3. Clinical Uses of ACEIs with Evidence from Clinical and Outcome Trials

ACEIs have been used effectively in the treatment of hypertension, reduction of mortality in congestive heart failure and left ventricular dysfunction after myocardial infarction; and for renoprotection in patients with a variety of kidney diseases including diabetic nephropathy, glomerulopathies, interstitial nephritis and glomerulosclerosis. These clinical effects are achieved by antagonising the various actions of angiotensin II as discussed in the section on mechanism of action of ACEIs.

ACEIs are effective agents in treatment of mild to moderate hypertension as monotherapy [66, 67] and in severe hypertension as combination with other agents [44, 45]. ACEIs are used extensively to retard the progression of diabetic and non-diabetic kidney disease and proteinuria. Many Clinical Practice Guidelines [41-51] including NKF K/DOQI and KDIGO recommend ACEIs as preferred agents for diabetic and non-diabetic kidney diseases with proteinuria.

3.1. Clinical Indications

3.1.1. Hypertension

Since the introduction of captopril for the treatment of hypertension in 1981, many other ACEIs have been developed. As a group, the ACEIs are effective agents in the treatment of all stages hypertension [66-69]. The blood pressure lowering effect of ACEIs is similar to other classes of antihypertensive drugs as demonstrated by the result of the Antihypertensive and Lipid-Lowering Treatment to Prevent Heart Attack Trial (ALLHAT) Study [70]. ACEIs generally reduce systolic blood pressure by 6-9mmHg and diastolic blood pressure by 4-5mmHg [71]. ACEIs lower blood pressure without affecting heart rate.

The aim of treating hypertension goes beyond control of blood pressure. It also includes reducing the risk of end organ damage and mortality. Use of ACEIs in hypertension is associated with significant reduction in mortality; for example a meta-analysis of randomized clinical trials of renin-angiotensin-aldosterone system inhibitors involving 158,998 patients [72] showed a 10% reduction in all-cause mortality. Recent studies suggest that arterial stiffness which is an independent risk factor for cardiovascular disease is also ameliorated by ACEIs [73, 74].

It is assumed that ACEIs are generally more effective in reducing blood pressure in white than black patients as a result of the conclusions of Veteran Administration Co-operative Study [75]. This study demonstrated that blood pressure was reduced significantly more in white patients with mild to moderate hypertension than in black patients after seven (7) weeks of captopril. This poor response in black patients was explained in part on the basis of lower renin levels in black hypertensive patients than in white patients [76, 77]. To support this hypothesis, addition of agents such as diuretics that increase renin plasma activity, eliminated the racial differences in response to ACEIs. There is need for a major RCT of ACEIs in black patients living in Africa.

3.1.2. Congestive Cardiac Failure and Left Ventricular Dysfunction

ACE inhibitors reduce preload, afterload and systolic wall stress in patients with congestive cardiac failure from systolic dysfuncion. These have been demonstrated convincingly in many studies [78-81]. In addition ACEIs increase salt excretion by increasing renal blood flow and by reducing antidiuretic hormone and aldosterone production. ACEIs are therefore important agents in the management of congestive cardiac failure.

Evidence of reversal of ventricular remodelling through the blockage of the trophic effect of angiotensin II on cardiac myocytes came initially from animal experiments [82].

In clinical practice, left ventricular hypertrophy, one of the manifestations of hypertensive heart disease is effectively regressed by ACE inhibitors. Many studies have demonstrated significant reduction in mortality in patients with CCF from systolic dysfunction with use of ACEI. [83-85]

For example in the CONCENSUS I trial, 253 patients with severe CCF (NYHA Class IV) were randomized to either enalapril or placebo in a double blind study. After 6 months, the crude mortality in the enalapril group was 26 versus 44 in the placebo group achieving a reduction of 40%. [83]. In the SOLVD trial mortality and hospitalization was significantly reduced with the addition of enalapril to conventional therapy in patients with chronic congestive heart failure and reduced ejection fraction [84].

3.1.3. Post Myocardial Infarction

Angiotensin converting enzyme inhibitors reduce cardiovascular mortality and slow the progression to congestive cardiac failure in patients after myocardial infarction. This has been amply demonstrated in some studies [86 - 88]. For example in the AIRE study [89], about 2000 patients with acute MI were recruited from 144 centres in 14 countries. The patients were randomly allocated to either ramipril or placebo in a double blind manner. The results show that mortality was significantly lower in the ramipril group (17%) than in the placebo group (23%). However, the result of the CONCENSUS II study [83, 86] did not give similar favourable result as 'Enalapril therapy started within 24 hours of the onset of acute myocardial infarction did not improve survival during the 180 days after infarction'

3.1.4. Renoprotection in Renal Disease

3.1.4.1. Slowing the Progression of Kidney Disease in Type I and Type 2 Diabetes with ACEIs

Raised glomerular capillary pressure and RAS are responsible for the progression of impaired kidney function in many kidney diseases including diabetes mellitus. By reducing arterial pressure and selectively dilating the efferent arteriole, intraglomerular pressure is reduced thus ameliorationg glomerular hypertension and progression of renal disease. In addition, ACE inhibitors reduce angiotensin II mediated mesangial cell proliferation and matrix formation. There is strong evidence from RCTs [90-91] showing that ACE inhibitors are more effective than other antihypertensive agents in slowing the progression of renal disease in patients with microalbuminuria.

ACE inhibitors reduce albumin excretion, and slow the progression from microalbuminuria to macroalbuminuria in kidney disease caused by type 1 and type 2 diabetes mellitus. This delay in progression from microalbuminuria to overt proteinuria in diabetes has been amply demonstrated in long term follow up studies [91]

3.1.4.2. ACE Inhibitors Delay Progression of Disease in Non-Diabetic Renal Disease

Several large interventional studies have uniformly found that proteinuria is a major risk factor for the progression of renal disease [92 - 95]. Renin-angiotensin-aldosterone system inhibition exerts a renoprotective effect independent of blood pressure reduction [96].

Recently, the African American Study of Kidney Disease and Hypertension (AASK) trial [40, 96] in which a total of 1094 African Americans aged 18 to 70 years with hypertensive renal disease recruited from 21 clinical centers in United States of America and followed up for 3 to 6.4 years were studied, showed that angiotensin-converting enzyme inhibitors were more effective than β-blockers or dihydropyridine calcium channel blockers in slowing the decline of GFR in black patients. [96]

In the REIN study [97], 583 patients with renal insufficiency from various disorders were randomly assigned to receive either benazepril or placebo. The group was studied for 3 years with the primary end point as doubling of basal creatinine or need for dialysis. In the benazepril arm there was significant reduction of risk compared with the placebo arm. It was concluded that benazepril provided protection against progression of renal disease in patients with various kidney disorders [97].

However, the ONTARGET study produced a conflicting result showing that combination therapy significantly increased the risk for kidney dysfunction compared with ramipril or telmisartan alone [98].

4. Adverse Effects of ACEIs

The adverse effects of ACEIs could be due to class effect or be specific to the individual drug. The incidence of adverse effects from ACEIs and ARBs is from 5% to 20% [45]. These may be classified into four main types which include: (a) effects due to interfering with the activity of RAS in maintaining blood pressure and serum potassium; (b) effects due to interfering with the activity of other enzymes and receptors; (c) allergic effects, and (d) effects on the fetus [45].

4.1. Class Effects

4.1.1. Effects Due to ACEIs Interfering with the Activity of RAAS in Maintaining Blood Pressure and Serum Potassium:

They include hypotension, early decrease in glomerular filtration rate (GFR) and hyperkalemia [45, 99].

Hypotension

This is usually most common after initiation of therapy or dose increase. Hypotension follows reduction of blood pressure and it presents with weakness, dizziness or syncope. The first-dose hypotension which may occur at initiation of therapy is more severe in hypovolemic patients with high baseline renin levels [100]. To reduce the occurrence of hypotension, ACEI therapy is avoided in volume-depleted patients, and is initiated 3 to 5 days after discontinuation of diuretics or commenced at a low dose.

Early Decrease in Glomerular Filtration

A modest reduction in kidney function may be observed in some patients who have bilateral renal artery stenosis, hypertensive nephrosclerosis, congestive cardiac failure, polycystic kidney disease and chronic kidney disease [45, 99, 101, 102]. Glomerular filtration rate reduction occurs rapidly within 3-5 days of initiating ACEI therapy. In patients with marked stenotic lesion (>95%), renal artery thrombosis could occur and may result in acute kidney injury (AKI).

Hyperkalemia

Angiotensin II and hyperkalemia are major factors that cause aldosterone release which in turn is a major stimulus for renal potassium excretion. Hence blockage of both systemic angiotensin II and that produced locally by zona glomerulosa of the adrenal cortex results in impaired potassium excretion and hyperkalemia [45, 101, 102]. Hyperkalemia is more marked in patients with renal insufficiency and in concomitant use of potassium sparing diuretics and non-steroidal anti-inflammatory drugs (103). It is also common among the elderly [103].

Most guidelines - KDOQI, NICE etc., emphasize the importance of monitoring serum potassium, creatinine and GFR. The side effects are reduced or avoided if low doses of ACEIs are used or low dose titration is done.

4.1.2. Effects Due to Interfering with the Activity of Other Enzymes and Receptors

Angiotensin converting enzymes degrade bradykinin to inactive moieties [45, 104]. Administration of ACEI therefore results in accumulation of kinins which may induce cough, angioneurotic edema and some allergic reactions [105, 106]. These kinin-related complications are not usually experienced by patients on ARBs.

Cough: usually a dry hacking cough and it may be seen in 10-20% of patients and even up to 40% in patients with congestive cardiac failure [45]. Cough usually starts within 1-2 weeks of initiating ACEI therapy. It is commoner in females than in males [107]. Although Asians have higher incidence than Caucasians, Elliot et al reported a high incidence of cough in black American patients especially the female patients suggesting a race or ethnic related difference [108]. ACEI-induced cough usually resolves within 1-4 days of discontinuation of ACEIs, but it could last up to 4 weeks. It may reoccur with re-challenge. Potential risks for ACEI induced cough include increasing age, female sex, congestive heart failure, East Asian ethnicity, black race, and history of smoking [107 - 109].

4.1.3. Suggested Mechanisms for ACEI-Induced Cough

Cough reflex is mediated by the vagus nerve through the afferent C fiber via the type J receptors in the respiratory tract [45]. Bradykinin and substance P induce the formation of prostaglandin E2, and the accumulation of prostaglandin E2 in the C fiber receptors stimulates cough [45]. Since angiotensin-converting enzyme degrades bradykinin and substance P, the use of ACE inhibitors results in increased levels of bradykinin. In heart-lung transplant patients with denervated cholinergic nerve, ACEI treatment also caused cough. This suggests that there could be local accumulation of bradykinin [45, 104]. Bradykinin and substance P are known to cause broncho-constriction of the human respiratory tract [105].

Though increased local concentration of kinins, substance P, prostaglandins or thromboxane may partially explain ACEI–induced cough, the mechanism of ACEI-induced cough is still not fully known. For example, ARBs block only angiotensin II effects with no effect on kinins, yet they are known to induce cough. Genetic polymorphism has been shown to be a risk factor for cough and angioedema [45].

Treatment of ACEI-induced cough is dose reduction or discontinuation of the ACEI.

4.2. Drug Specific Effects

4.2.1. Captopril

Captopril is associated with severe skin conditions which may include lichenoid eruptions, bullous pemphigus-like rash, rosacea, erythroderma with exfoliative dermatitis, tongue ulcers, necrotizing blepharitis and fatal Steven-Johnson syndrome [110].

Bone marrow suppression has been reported on exposure to captopril and the presentation varies from agranulocytosis, anaemia, thrombocytopenia to pancytopenia [110].

Captopril therapy may result in nephrotic syndrome which presents with intermittent proteinuria with pathological changes suggestive of membranous glomerulonephritis. The nephrotic syndrome may be accompanied by immune-complex neuropathy. Dysguesia has been reported in 6% of patients [45].

Other adverse events though rare and isolated include cholestatic jaundice, toxic hepatitis, pericarditis, Parkinsonism, psychotic reactions, neuropathy and sometimes lupus-like syndrome [110]. Captopril use in pregnancy may result in fetal abnormalities.

4.2.2. Enalapril

Enalapril may cause renal glycosuria. There is also diminished bioavailability when administered with propranolol [110].

4.2.3. Lisinopril

This is a relatively safe drug but it may cause side effects such as joint pain, fever, rash, indigestion, nausea, cramps and lethargy. It may on rare occasions cause intestinal angioedema, head and neck angioedema, laryngeal edema, myocardial infarction, cerebrovascular accident, pleural effusion, acute hepatic failure, toxic epidermal necrolysis and Steven -Johnson Syndrome [109].

5. Drug Interactions

ACEIs may interact with other drugs. Concurrent administration of potassium supplements, potassium-sparing diuretics, or salt substitutes may precipitate hyperkalemia in ACE inhibitor-treated patients in whom aldosterone is suppressed [45]. Patients taking diuretics may be particularly sensitive to the hypotensive effects of ACE inhibitors. Nonsteroidal anti-inflammatory drugs may attenuate the antihypertensive effects of ACEIs; this effect is more prominent in patients with low renin levels [45, 99]. Antacids may reduce the availability of ACEIs.

6. ACEIs in Pregnancy

ACEIs are contraindicated in pregnancy because they are associated with increased incidence of fetal complications [18, 114]. They should be used with caution in women who do not practice contraception. Women of child-bearing potential should be counseled about adverse effects on the fetus. Contraception is advocated; if however the patient on ACEI becomes pregnant, the drug should be discontinued as soon as possible during the first trimester [45, 114]

Bullo et al (2012) [115] in a systematic review of published case reports and case series of intrauterine exposure to ACEIs or to ARBs, observed that the neonatal complications noted were as follows: kidney failure or need for dialysis (23%), anuria (20%), oligohydramnios (19%), death (intrauterine or after birth) or miscarriage (18%), arterial hypotension (17%), intrauterine growth retardation (15%), respiratory distress syndrome (14%), hypocalvaria (8%), limb defects (8%), persistent patent ductus arteriosus (6%), pulmonary hypoplasia (5%), or cerebral complications (4%). The complications were more frequent following exposure to ARBs than ACEIs.

7. Racial or Ethnic Differences in Adverse Reactions

There may be a race or ethnicity related difference in the prevalence of cough attributed to ACEI therapy. A higher incidence of discontinuation of ACEIs due to cough has been reported in black subjects [108, 116]. Woo and associates [107] demonstrated that ACEI-induced cough was more common in Chinese than Caucasian patients in their study.

Elliot [108] analyzing the register of a tertiary hypertension clinic in Chicago, observed that in a group of patients who received their first ever dose of ACEI therapy, the prevalence of cough requiring discontinuation of ACEI therapy was four times commoner in black patients compared to other races[108]. Black subjects had a relative risk of 2.6 (95% Confidence Interval, 1.21 - 4.65; $p = 0.01$) of discontinuation of ACEIs due to cough. There were no significant differences observed across the three most commonly used ACEIs Captopril 6.6% (all black subjects); Enalapril 6.1% (94% blacks subjects) and Lisinopril 7.3% (90% black subjects). Cough was more common in women and they comprised 70% of the subjects in this study [108].

Adigun and Ajayi demonstrated 27% incidence of ACEI-induced cough in a study of 100 Nigerian patients [116]. The prevalence in female patients (43%) was significantly higher than in males (12%) in their study population.

Angioedema was found to be two to four times commoner in blacks than in white populations [108].

8. Local Experience with ACEI in the Nephrology Clinic of University of Nigeria Teaching Hospital (UNTH)

ACEIs are extensively used in UNTH for various indications including management of hypertension, treatment of congestive cardiac failure, post myocardial infarction; and for management of various kidney conditions including diabetic and non-diabetic CKD, proteinuria, glomerulopathies and interstitial nephritis.

A local retrospective study of use of ACEIs in the nephrology clinics from 2008 to 2012 revealed the following results - 120 patients had analysable data.

The number of patients was 120 (male 72 [60%], female 48 [40%]). The mean age (years) for all patients was 50.5±15.3. The male patients were significantly older than the female patients; (male 53.8±14.9, female 45.5±14.6, p=0.003).

Table 1 details the diagnosis of the patients. Only one patient had uncomplicated hypertension. The rest of the patients had a combination of conditions e.g. CKD and hypertension, DM and CKD, DM, HTN and CKD.

Table 1. Diagnosis of patients

Diagnosis	Frequency	Percentage (%)
CKD	20	16.7
DM	2	1.7
HIVAN	6	5.0
Glomerulonephritis	1	0.8
ADPKD	1	0.8
HTN+CKD	32	26.7
HTN+DM	15	12.5
DM+CKD	13	10.8
HTN+CKD+CCF	5	4.2
DM+CKD+CCF	1	0.8
GN+CKD	20	16.7
CKD+CCF	1	0.8
HTN+DM+CKD	3	2.5
TOTAL	120	100

These patients were fairly distributed into various stages of CKD but the majority were in stages 4 and 5 CKD. See Table 2.

Table 2. Stages of CKD of study population

CKD Stage	Frequency	Percentage (%)
Stage 1 eGFR >/=90ml/min	20	17.9
Stage 2 eGFR 60-89ml/ml	18	16.1
Stage 3 eGFR 30-59ml/ml	19	17.0
Stage 4 eGFR 15-29ml/ml	27	24.1
Stage 5 eGFR <15ml/ml	28	25.0
Total	112	100

8.1. Pattern of ACEI Prescription

Table 3 details the prescription pattern of ACEIs during the period under consideration. Lisinopril was the commonest ACEI prescribed for various indications and accounted for 91% of the prescriptions. Ramipril came a distant second accounting for 7% of the prescriptions. The preference for lisinopril is probably due to its relative cheaper cost.

Table 3. ACEI Prescription Pattern

Drug	Frequency	Percentage (%)
Lisinopril	104	91
Ramipril	8	7.0
Enalapril	2	2.0
Total	114	100

8.2. Reasons for Prescribing ACEIs

The major indications for prescribing ACEI are treatment of hypertension, to reduce mortality in CCF and post myocardial infarction and as reno-protection in patients with impaired renal function from diverse aetiologies including diabetic nephropathy. Majority of the patients seen in the CKD clinic received ACEIs for renal protection and control of hypertension.

Analysis of effect of ACEIs on progression of CKD (Tables 4a and 4b) showed that the mean serum creatinine of the patients did not rise with ACEI and in fact decreased by 12 months of use, although the differences did not reach statistical significance. Analysis of the mean eGFR over time showed similar results. It will be correct to infer from this observation that ACEIs alone or in concert with other modalities and drugs slowed the progression of CKD.

Table 4a. Effect of ACEI on Serum creatinine

	Base line vs 3 months N=16	Baseline Vs 6 months N=12	Baseline Vs 12 months N=8
Mean S creatinine (µmol/l)	401.56±69.75 470.38±85.58	354.92±365.6 372.75±303.80	419.00±419.10 202.75±86.58
p-value	0.104	0.908	0.325

Table 4b. Effect of ACEI on eGFR

	Base line vs 3 months N=20	Baseline Vs 6 months N=13	Baseline Vs 12 months N=8
Mean eGFR (ml/min)	32.50±38.68 33.11±36.39	43.43±40.22 40.34.±47.27	57.73±53.97 75.71±41.16
p-value	0.925	0.829	0.514

Use of ACEIs alone or in combination with other antihypertensive agents achieved control of hypertension and this was sustained (Table 5).

Table 5. Effect of antihypertensive agents including ACEI on BP

	Baseline Vs 3 month N=60	Baseline Vs 6 month N=42	Baseline Vs 12 month N=19
Mean SBP	159.90±23.47 138.90±25.57	156.43±25.64 134.00±21.64	153.16±21.36 144.74±29.70
p-value	<0.001	<0.001	0.291
Mean DBP	93.87±12.25 87.50±19.71	92.14±12.20 83.95±12.97	93.16±8.85 87.89±17.18
p-value	0.015	<0.001	0.106

8.3. Side Effect Profile

The ACEIs were well tolerated. There were no major adverse effects and patients did not stop medication on account of the drug

Conclusion

Since ACEIs came into clinical use in the 1980s, they have become popular in the management of many conditions including treatment of hypertension, reduction of mortality in congestive heart failure and left ventricular dysfunction after myocardial infarction, and for renoprotection in patients with a variety of kidney diseases including diabetic nephropathy, glomerulopathies, interstitial nephritis and glomerulosclerosis. These clinical effects are achieved by antagonizing the various actions of angiotensin II. The beneficial effects of ACEIs occur in all racial groups including blacks.

Local experience at the Nephrology clinic of University of Nigeria Teaching Hospital, Enugu, Nigeria where the class of drug is used for the mentioned indications shows that lisinopril is the most popular ACEI and this observed pattern of prescription is thought to be partly because of expediency of cost considerations. The experience is that ACEIs are effective in controlling blood pressure and in delaying the progression renal disease due to diverse causes including diabetic nephropathy.

ACEIs are relatively free of side effects. Cough is the major side effect but the incidence of this in the local population is not frequent. Although angioedema is the most worrisome adverse effect of the drug class, local experience is that this complication is uncommon.

REFERENCES

[1] Yirsaw BD. Chronic kidney disease in sub-Saharan Africa: Hypothesis for research demand. *Annals of African Medicine* 2012, 11; 2: 119 – 120.

[2] Onuigbo MAC (2013). Can ACE Inhibitors and Angiotensin Receptor Blockers Be Detrimental in CKD Patients? *Nephron Clin Pract* 2011; 118: c407–c419 DOI: 10.1159/000324164.

[3] Naicker S: End-stage renal disease in sub-Sa- haran Africa. *Ethn Dis* 2009; 19 (suppl 1) :13- 15.

[4] Akinsola W, Odesanmi WO, Ogunniyi JO, Ladipo GO, Akinsola W, Odesanmi WO, Ogunniyi JO, Ladipo GO: Diseases causing chronic renal failure in Nigerians – a prospective study of 100 cases. *Afr J Med Med Sci* 1989; 18: 131–137.

[5] Adetuyibi A, Akisanya JB, Onadeko BO: Analysis of the causes of death on the medical wards of the University College Hospital, Ibadan, over a 14-year period (1960–1973). *Trans R Soc Trop Med Hyg* 1976; 70: 466–473.

[6] Ulasi II, Ijoma CK: The enormity of chronic kidney disease in Nigeria: the situation in a teaching hospital in South-East Nigeria. *J Trop Med* 2010; 2010: 501957.

[7] Beaglehole R, Yach D. Globalization and the prevention and control of non-communicable disease: The neglected chronic diseases of adults. *Lancet* 2003; 362; 9387: 903 – 908.

[8] El Nahas M. The global challenge of chronic kidney disease. *Kidney Int* 2005; 68: 2918–2929.

[9] Zhang QL, Rothenbacher D. Prevalence of chronic kidney disease in population-based studies: systematic review. *BMC Public Health* 2008; 8: 117.

[10] World Health Organization. Preventing chronic diseases: a vital investment: WHO global report. Geneva: WHO, 2005.

[11] World Health Organization. Causes of death 2008: data sources and methods. Geneva: WHO, 2011.

[12] World Health Organization. Global status report on non-communicable diseases 2010. Geneva: WHO, 2011.

[13] Lim SS, Vos T, Flaxman AD, Danaei G, Shibuya K, Adair-Rohani H, et al. A comparative risk assessment of burden of disease and injury attributable to 67 risk factors and risk factor clusters in 21 regions, 1990–2010: a systematic analysis for the Global Burden of Disease Study 2010. *Lancet.* 2012; 380(9859):2224–2260.

[14] Chockalingam A, Campbell NR, Fodor JG Worldwide epidemic of hypertension. *Can J Cardiol.* 2006 May; 22(7): 553–555. PMCID: PMC2560860

[15] Mendis S. Hypertension: a silent contributor to the global cardiovascular epidemic. *Regional Health Forum* 2013– Volume 17, Number 1, 2013: 1 – 5.

[16] Ogah O.S., Okpechi i., Innocent I Chukwuonye I. I., Akinyemi J. O., Onwubere B. J. C., Falase A. O., Stewart S., Sliwa K. Blood pressure, prevalence of hypertension and hypertension related complications in Nigerian Africans: A review. *World J. Cardiol.* 2012, 4(12): 327–340.

[17] Ulasi II, Ijoma CK, Onwubere BJ, Arodiwe E, Onodugo O, Okafor C. High prevalence and low awareness of hypertension in a market population in Enugu, Nigeria. *Int J Hypertens.* 2011; 2011:869675

[18] World Health Organization, International Society of Hypertension Writing Group. 2003 World Health Organization (WHO)/International Society of Hypertension (ISH) statement on management of hypertension. *J Hypertens,* 2003, 21:1983–1992.

[19] WHO. World Health Report 2002: Chapter 4 – Quantifying selected major risks to Health. Geneva: World Health Organization 2002.

[20] World Health Organization. 2008–2013 Action plan for the global strategy for the prevention and control of non-communicable diseases: prevent and control cardiovascular diseases, cancers, chronic respiratory diseases and diabetes. Geneva: *World Health Organization* 2008.

[21] Couser G. C., Remuzzi G., Mendis S., Tonelli M. The Contribution of Chronic Kidney Disease to the Global Burden of Major Noncommunicable Diseases. *Kidney Int.* 2011; 80(12): 1258-1270

[22] White SL, Chadban SJ, Jan S, Chapman JR, Cass A (2008).How can we achieve global equity in provision of renal replacement therapy? *Bulletin of the World Health Organization,* 86, 3: 161-240. Available from: http://www.who.int/ bulletin/ volumes/86/3/07-041715/en/ (Accessed: 5th July 2013).

[23] Barsoum R. End-stage renal disease in North Africa. *Kidney Int Suppl.* 2003;63(S83):111–4. doi: 10.1046/j.1523-1755.63.s83.23.x.

[24] Young EW, Mauger EA, Jiang KH, Port FK, Wolfe RA. Socioeconomic status and end-stage renal disease in the United States. *Kidney Int* 1994; 45: 907-11.

[25] Bello A. K., Peters J., Rigby J., Rahman A. A., El Nahas M. Socioeconomic Status and Chronic Kidney Disease at Presentation to a Renal Service in the United Kingdom. *Clin J Am Soc Nephrol.* 2008, 3(5): 1316–1323. doi: 10.2215/CJN.00680208 PMCID: PMC2518794

[26] Drey N, Roderick P, Mullee M, Rogerson M: A population-based study of the incidence and outcomes of diagnosed chronic kidney disease. *Am J Kidney Dis* 2003, 42: 677–684. PubMed: 14520617.

[27] Ulasi I. I., Ijoma C. K., Onodugo O. D., Arodiwe E.B., Ifebunandu N. A., Okoye J. U. Towards prevention of chronic kidney disease in Nigeria: a community-based study in Southeast Nigeria. *Kidney Int. Suppl.* 2013, 3: 195–201; doi:10.1038/kisup.2013.13

[28] Burton C. J., Harper S. J., Bailey E., et al. Turnover of human tubular cells exposed to proteins in vivo and in vitro. *Kidney Int.* 2001, 59: 507–514.

[29] Praga M. Therapeutic measures in proteinuric nephropathy. *Kidney Int.* 2005, 68, Suppl 99: S137–S141

[30] Eddy A: Molecular insights into renal interstitial fibrosis. *J Am Soc Nephrol* 1996, 7: 2495–2508.

[31] Bennett WM, Walker RG, Kincaid-Smith P. Renal cortical interstitial volume in mesangial IgA nephropathy. Dissociation from creatinine clearance in serially biopsied patients. *Lab Invest* 1982, 47: 330 – 335.

[32] De Zeeuw D, Remuzzi G, Parving H-H, et al: Proteinuria, a target for renoprotection in patients with type 2 diabetic nephropathy: Lessons from RENAAL. *Kidney Int.* 2004, 65: 2309 –2320.

[33] Jafar T.H., Stark P.C., Schmid C.H., Landa M., Maschio G., Marcantoni C., De Jong P. E., De Zeeuw D, Shahinfar S., Ruggenenti P., Remuzzi G., Levey A. S. and for the AIPRD Study Group. Proteinuria as a modifiable risk factor for the progression of non-diabetic renal diseases. *Kidney Int.* 2001, 60: 1131–1140.

[34] Wapstra F. H., Navis G., de Jong P. E., de Zeeuw D. Chronic Angiotensin II Infusion But Not Bradykinin Blockade Abolishes the Antiproteinuric Response to Angiotensin-Converting Enzyme Inhibition in Established Adriamycin Nephrosis. *J Am Soc Nephrol.* 2000, 11: 490–496.

[35] Gansevoort RT, de Zeeuw D, de Jong PE. ACE inhibitors and proteinuria. *Pharm World Sci.* 1996, 18(6): 204 – 210.

[36] Bakris G. L., Smith A. C., D J Richardson D. J., Hung E., Preston R., Goldberg R., Epstein M. Impact of an ACE inhibitor and calcium antagonist on microalbuminuria and lipid subfractions in type 2 diabetes: a randomised, multi-centre pilot study. *Journal of Human Hypertension* 2002, 16, 185-191. DOI: 10.1038/sj/jhh/1001315.

[37] Lewis E. J., Hunsicker L. G., Bain R. P., Rohde R. D. The effect of angiotensin-converting-enzyme inhibition on diabetic nephropathy. The Collaborative Study Group. *N Engl J Med.* 1993, 329 (20):1456-62.

[38] The GISEN Group. Randomised placebo-controlled trial of effect of ramipril on decline in glomerular filtration rate and risk of terminal renal failure in proteinuric, non-diabetic nephropathy. *The Lancet* 1997, 349 (9069): 1857 – 1863. Doi:10.1016/S0140-6736(96)11445-8.

[39] Maschio G, Alberti D, Locatelli F, Mann JF, Motolese M, Ponticelli C, Ritz E, Janin G, Zucchelli P. Angiotensin-converting enzyme inhibitors and kidney protection: the AIPRI trial. The ACE Inhibition in Progressive Renal Insufficiency (AIPRI) Study Group. *J Cardiovasc Pharmacol.* 1999, 33 Suppl 1:S16-20.

[40] Rahman M. Initial Findings of The AASK: African Americans with hypertensive kidney disease benefit from an ACE inhibitor. Cleveland Clinic Journal of Medicine 2003, 70 (4): 304 – 312.

[41] National Institute for Health and Clinical Excellence (NICE). NICE Clinical Guideline 73: Chronic kidney disease Early identification and management of chronic kidney disease in adults in primary and secondary care. 2008. London: National Institute for Health and Clinical Excellence 2008. [Online] Available from: http://www.nice.org.uk/nicemedia/live/12069/42117/42117.pdf (Accessed: 1st July 2013).

[42] MacGregor M. S., Taal M. W. Clinical Practice Guidelines: Detection, Monitoring and Care of Patients with CKD. UK Renal Association 5th Edition, 2009-2011. London: UK Renal Association 2011.

[43] Gilian A. Prevention of Progression of Kidney Disease: Blood Pressure Control – role of specific antihypertensives. The CARI Guidelines – Caring for Australasians with Renal Impairment. 2006. [Online] Available from: http://www.cari.org.au/CKD_Prevent_List_Published/Blood_pressure_Control_role_of_specific_antihypertensive.pdf (Accessed: 4th July 2013)

[44] National Kidney Foundation (2012). KDOQI Clinical Practice Guideline for Diabetes and CKD: 2012 update. Am J Kidney Dis. 2012, 60(5): 850-886. [Online] Available from: http://www.kidney.org/professionals/KDOQI/guidelines_diabetesUp/diabetes-ckd-update-2012.pdf (Accessed: 1st July 2013).

[45] National Kidney Foundation. KDOQI Clinical Practice Guidelines on Hypertension and Antihypertensive Agents in Chronic Kidney Disease, 2004. [Online] Available from: http://www.kidney.org/professionals/kdoqi/guidelines_bp/ (Accessed: 1st July 2013).

[46] Chadban S, Howell M, Twigg S, Thomas M, Jerums G, Alan C, Campbell D, Nicholls K, Tong A, Mangos G, Stack A, McIsaac R, Girgis S, Colagiuri R, Colagiuri S, Craig J. National Evidence Based Guideline for Diagnosis, Prevention and Management of Chronic Kidney Disease in Type 2 Diabetes. Diabetes Australia and the NHMRC, Canberra 2009. CARI (2009): National Evidence Based Guideline for Diagnosis, Prevention and Management of Chronic Kidney Disease in Type 2 Diabetes. [Online] Available from: http://diabetesaustralia.com.au/PageFiles/763/Chronic%20Kidney%20Disease%20Guideline%20August%202009.pdf (Accessed 6th July 2013).

[47] Nigerian Association of Nephrology. Guidelines for the detection and management of CKD. Lagos: NAN, 2011.

[48] World Health Organization, International Society of Hypertension Writing Group. 2003 World Health Organization (WHO)/International Society of Hypertension (ISH) statement on management of hypertension. *J Hypertens*, 2003, 21:1983–1992.

[49] Nigerian Hypertension Society Guidelines Committee. Guideline for the manangement of hypertension in Nigeria. Onwubere, Kadiri ed. Enugu: NHS, 2005.

[50] U.S. Department of Health and Human Services. The Seventh Report of the Joint National Committee on Prevention, Detection, Evaluation, and Treatment of High Blood Pressure - Complete Report. [Online] August 2004. Available from: http://www.nhlbi.nih.gov/guidelines/hypertension/jnc7full.htm (Accessed: 1st July 2013).

[51] O'Riordan M New European hypertension guidelines released: Goal is less than 140 mm Hg for all. [Online] Available from: http://www.theheart.org/article/1552087.do (Accessed: 1st July 2013).

[52] Tigerstedt R, Bergman PG. Niere and Kreislauf. *Scand Arch Physiol* 1898; 8:223-71.

[53] Friedman B, Abramson DI, Marx W. Pressor substancein the cortex of the kidney. *Am J Physiol* 1938; 124:285-94.

[54] Page IH, Helmer OM. A crystalline pressor substance (angiotonin)resulting from the reaction between renin an and renin activator L *Exp Med* 1940; 71:29 – 42.

[55] Braun-Menendez E, Fasciolo J, Leloir LF, Munoz JM. The substance causing renal hypertension. *J. Physiol* 1940; 98: 283-98.

[56] Braun-Menendez E, Page IH. Suggested revision of nomenclature – Angiotensin. *Science* 1958; 127:242.

[57] Skeggs Jr LT. historical Overview of the Renin-Angiotensin System. In: Doyle AE, Bearn AG, editors. Hypertension and the Angiotensin System: Therapeutic Approaches. New York: Raven Press; 1983.

[58] Skidgel ra, Erdös EG. Novel activity of human angiotensin I converting enzyme: release of the NH2- and COOH-terminal tripeptides from the luteinizing hormone-releasing hormone. *Proc Natl Acad Sci U S A*. 1985 February; 82(4): 1025–1029.

[59] Donoghue M, Baronas E et al. A novel angiotensin converting enzyme-related carboxypeptidase (ACE2) converts angiotensin I to angiotensin 1-9. *Circ Res* 2000; 87: E1-9.

[60] Fyhrquist F, Saijonmaa O. Journal of Internal Medicine. doi: 10.1111/j.1365-2796.2008.01981.x

[61] Kramkowski K, Mogielnicki A, Leszcznska A, Buczko W. Angiotensin- (1-9), the product of angiotensin I conversion in platelets enhances arterial thrombosis in rats. *J Physiol Pharmacol* 2010; 61(3): 317-324.

[62] Paul M, Poyan Mehr A, Kreutz R. physiology of local angiotensin system. *Physiol Rev* 2006; 86:747-803

[63] Theodore L, Goodfriend MD. Angiotensins: actions and receptors. In:Izzo JL, Sica DA, black HR, editors. Hypertension Primer, chapter A17. Philadelphia:Lippincott Williams & Wilkins;2008.

[64] Baker KM, Chernin MI, Schreiber T et al. Evidence of a novel intracrine mechanism in angiotensin II-induced cardiac hypertrophy. *Regul Pept* 2004; 120:5-13

[65] Upadhyay A, Earley A, Haynes SM, Uhlig K. Systematic review: blood pressure target in chronic kidney disease and proteinuria as an effect modifier. *Ann Intern Med* 2011; 154:541.

[66] Materson BJ. Monotherapy of hypertension with angiotensin-converting enzyme inhibitors. *Am J Med.* 1984 Oct 5;77(4A):128-34.

[67] Tahiliani R, Khokhani RC, Damle VB, Dadkar VN, Jaguste VS, Patel K, Raghu CN, Oke VG. Comparative evaluation of captopril and methyldopa monotherapy for hypertension: double-blind study in Indians. *Clin Ther.* 1986;8(5):482-9.

[68] Fitscha P, Meisner W, Hitzenberger G. Antihypertensive effects of isradipine and captopril as monotherapy or in combination. *Am J Hypertens.* 1991 Feb;4(2 Pt 2):151S-153S

[69] Jamerson KA, Nwose O, Jean-Louis L, Schofield L, Purkayastha D, Baron M. Initial angiotensin-converting enzyme inhibitor/calcium channel blocker combination therapy achieves superior blood pressure control compared with calcium channel blocker monotherapy in patients with stage 2 hypertension. *Am J Hypertens.* 2004;17(6):495–501.

[70] Major outcomes in high-risk hypertensive patients randomized to angiotensin-converting enzyme inhibitor or calcium channel blocker vs diuretic: The Antihypertensive and Lipid-Lowering Treatment to Prevent Heart Attack Trial (ALLHAT). *JAMA.* 2002 Dec 18;288(23):2981-97.

[71] Heran BS, Wong MM, Heran IK, Wright JM. Blood pressure lowering efficacy of angiotensin converting enzyme (ACE) inhibitors for primary hypertension. *Cochrane*

Database Syst Rev. 2008 Oct 8;(4):CD003823. doi: 10.1002/14651858. CD003823.pub2.

[72] van Vark LC, Bertrand M, Akkerhuis KM, Brugts JJ, Fox K, Mourad JJ, Boersma E. Angiotensin-converting enzyme inhibitors reduce mortality in hypertension: a meta-analysis of randomized clinical trials of renin-angiotensin-aldosterone system inhibitors involving 158,998 patients. Eur Heart J. 2012 Aug;33(16):2088-97. doi: 10.1093/eurheartj/ehs075. Epub 2012 Apr 17.

[73] Mallareddy M, Parikh CR, Peixoto AJ. Effect of angiotensin-converting enzyme inhibitors on arterial stiffness in hypertension: systematic review and meta-analysis. *J Clin Hypertens* (Greenwich). 2006 Jun;8(6):398-403.

[74] Yousef Shahin, Junaid Alam Khan, Ian Chetter. Angiotensin converting enzyme inhibitors effect on arterial stiffness and wave reflections: A meta-analysis and meta-regression of randomised controlled trials. *Atherosclerosis*, Volume 221, Issue 1, March 2012, Pages 18–3

[75] *Veterans Administration Co-operative Study Group of Antihypertensive Agents. Racial differences in response to low-dose captopril are abolished by the addition of hydrochlorothiazide.* Br J Clin Pharmacol. 1982*;*14*:* 97S–*101S.*

[76] Creditor M, Loschky U. PRA in hypertension. *Am J Med.* 1967;43:371–382.

[77] Wisenbaugh PE, Garst JB, Hull C, Freedman RJ, Matthews DN, Haddy M. Renin, aldosterone, sodium and hypertension. *Am J Med.* 1972;52: 175–186.

[78] *Ku* Curtiss SC, Cohn JN, Vrobel T, Franciosa JA. Role of the renin-angiotensin system in the systemic vasoconstriction of chronic congestive heart failure. *Circulation.* 1978;58: 763–769.

[79] Gavras H, Faxon DP, Berkoben J, Brunner HR, Ryan TJ. Angiotensin converting enzyme inhibition in patients with congestive heart failure. *Circulation.* 1978;58:770 – 776.

[80] Turini GA, Brunner HR, Gribic M, Waeber B, Gavras H. Improvement of chronic congestive heart-failure by oral captopril. *Lancet.* 1979;1:1213–1215.

[81] Davis R, Ribner HS, Keung E, Sonnenblick EH, LeJemtel TH. Treatment of chronic congestive heart failure with captopril, an oral inhibitor of angiotensin converting enzyme. *N Engl J Med.* 1979;301:

[82] Vaughan DE, Pfeffer MA. Angiotensin converting enzyme inhibitors and cardiovascular remodelling. Cardiovasc Res. 1994;28:159–165.

[83] CONSENSUS Trial Study Group. Effects of enalapril on mortality in severe congestive heart failure: results of the Cooperative North Scandinavian Enalapril Survival Study (CONSENSUS). *N Engl J Med.* 1987;316:1429 –1435.

[84] The SOLVD Investigators. Effect of enalapril on survival in patients with reduced left ventricular ejection fractions and congestive heart failure. *N Engl J Med.* 1991;325:293–302.

[85] Cohn JN, Johnson G, Ziesche J, Frederick C, Francis G, Tristani F, Smith R, Dunkman WB, Loeb H, Wong M, Bhat G, Goldman S, Fletcher RD, Doherty J, Hughes CV, Carson P, Cintron G, Shabetai R, Haakenson C. A comparison of enalapril with hydralazine-isosorbide dinitrate in the treatment of chronic congestive heart failure. *N Engl J Med.* 1991;325:303–310].

[86] Swedberg K, Held P, Kjekshus J, Rasmussen K, Ryden L, Wedel H. Effects of the early administration of enalapril on mortality in patients with acute myocardial infarction:

results of the Cooperative New Scandinavian Enalapril Survival Study II (CONSENSUS II). *N Engl J Med.* 1992;327:678–684.

[87] ISIS Collaborative Group. ISIS-4: randomised study of oral captopril in over 50,000 patients with suspected acute myocardial infarction. *Circulation.*1993;88(suppl I):I-394.

[88] Ambrosioni E, Borghi C, Magnani B. The effect of the angiotensinconverting- enzyme inhibitor zofenopril on mortality and morbidity after anterior myocardial infarction. *N Engl J Med.* 1995;332:80–85.

[89] AIRE Study Investigators. Effect of Ramipril on mortality and morbidity of survivors of acute myocardial infarction with clinical evidence of heart failure. The Acute Infarction Ramipril Efficacy (AIRE) Study Investigators. *Lancet* 1993 Oct 2; 342(8875): 821 - 828

[90] Ravid M, Lang R, Rachmani R, Lishner M. Long-term renoprotective effect of angiotensin-converting enzyme inhibition in non-insulindependent diabetes mellitus: a 7-year follow-up study. *Arch Intern Med.*1996;156:286 –289.

[91] Lewis EJ, Hunsicker LG, Bain RP, Rohde RD. The effect of angiotensin- converting-enzyme inhibition on diabetic nephropathy. *N Engl J Med.* 1993;329:1456 –1462.

[92] Peterson JC, Adler S, Burkart JM *et al.* Blood pressure control, proteinuria, and the progression of renal disease: the Modification of Diet in Renal Disease Study. *Ann Intern Med*1995;123:754-62.

[93] De Zeeuw D, Remuzzi G, Parving HH *et al.* Proteinuria, a target for renoprotection in patients with type 2 diabetic nephropathy: lessons from RENAAL. *Kidney Int* 2004; 65: 2309 - 2320.

[94] Atkins RC, Briganti EM, Lewis JB *et al.* Proteinuria reduction and progression to renal failure in patients with type 2 diabetes mellitus and overt nephropathy. *Am J Kidney Dis* 2005; 45: 281-7.

[95] Remuzzi G, Benigni A, Remuzzi A. Mechanisms of progression and regression of renal lesions of chronic nephropathies and diabetes. *J Clin Invest* 2006; 116: 288-96

[96] Jackson T. Wright, Jr, George Bakris, Tom Greene, Larry Y. Agodoa, Lawrence J. Appel, Jeanne Charleston, et al. Effect of Blood Pressure Lowering and Antihypertensive Drug Class on Progression of Hypertensive Kidney Disease: Results From the AASK Trial. *JAMA*, 2002, 288 (19): 2421-2431.

[97] Maschio G, Alberti D, Janin G, Locatelli F, Mann JF, Motolese M, Ponticelli C, Ritz E, Zucchelli P. Effect of the angiotensin-converting-enzyme inhibitor benazepril on the progression of chronic renal insufficiency. The Angiotensin-Converting-Enzyme Inhibition in Progressive Renal Insufficiency Study Group. *N Engl J Med.* 1996 Apr 11; 334 (15): 939-45.

[98] Mann JF, Schmieder RE, McQueen M, Dyal L, Schumacher H, Pogue J, Wang X, Maggioni A, Budaj A, Chaithiraphan S, Dickstein K, Keltai M, Metsarinne K, Oto A, Parkhomenko A, Piegas LS, Svendsen TL, Teo KK, Yusuf S: Renal outcomes with telmisartan, ramipril, or both, in people at high vascular risk (the ONTARGET study): A multicentre, randomised, double-blind, controlled trial. *Lancet* 2008, 372: 547–553.

[99] Brown NJ and Vaughan DE. Angiotensin-Converting Enzyme Inhibitors *Circulation.* 1998;97: 1411-1420.

[100] Hodsman GP, Isles CG, Murray GD,Usherwood TP, Webb I, Robertson H. Factors related to first dose hypotensive effect of captopril; prediction and treatment *BMJ*, 1983;286:p832-834.

[101] Burnakis TG, Mioduch HJ,. Combined therapy with captopril and potassium supplementation: a potential for hyperkalemia. *Arch Int Med* 1984; 144: 2371-2372.
[102] Dzau VJ,. Renal effects of angiotensin-converting enzyme inhibition in cardiac failure. *Am J Kidney Dis*. 187; 10: 74 - 80.
[103] Quilley J, Duchin KL, Hudes EM, McGiff JC. The anti-hypertensive effect of captopril in essential hypertension: relationship to prostaglandins and the kalli-krein system *J Hypertens*. 1987; 5: 121-128.
[104] Erdos EG. The Angiotensin converting enzyme *Fed PROC*. 1977; 36:1760-1765.
[105] Nishizawa A. Angiotensin-Converting Enzyme Inhibitor induced cough among Asians. *UCLA Healthcare* 2000; 4: 35–38.
[106] Israili ZH, Hall WD. Cough and angioneurotic edema associated with angiotensin-converting enzyme inhibitor therapy. A review of the literature and pathophysiology. *Ann Intern Med*. 1992;177(3) : 234-242.
[107] Woo KS, Norris RM, Nicholls G. Racial difference in incidence of cough with angiotensin-converting enzyme inhibitors (a tale of two cities). *Am J Cardiol*. 1995; 75(14):967 – 968.
[108] Elliot WJ. Higher incidence of discontinuation of angiotensin converting enzyme inhibitors due to cough in black subjects. *Clin Pharmacol Ther*. 1996; 60 (5): 582 - 588.
[109] Tomaki M, Ichinose M, Miura M, et al. Angiotensin converting enzyme (ACE) inhibitor-induced cough and substance P. *Thorax*. 1996; 51(2):199-201.
[110] Gavras H, Gavras I. Angiotensin converting enzyme inhibitors. Properties and side effects. *Hypertension 11*, 1988;[Suppl II]: II-37 – II-41.
[111] 16Weber MA, Messerli FH. Angiotensin-converting enzyme inhibitor and angioedema. *Hypertension*. 2008;51: 1465-1467.
[112] 17Fennell; DJ, Nunan TO, O"Doherty MJ, Croft DN. Fatal Stevens-Johnson syndrome in a patient on captopril and allopurinol [Letter]. *Lancet* 1984;1:463
[113] Lisinopri lDrugs.com/Yahoo Medicine
[114] Bullo M, Tschumi S, Bucher BS, Bianchetti MG, Simonetti GD. Pregnancy outcome following exposure to angiotensin-converting enzyme inhibitors or angiotensin receptor antagonists. A systemic review. *Hypertension*. 2012;60:444-450.
[115] Sedman AB, Kershaw DB, Bunchman TE. Recognition and management of angiotensin converting enzyme inhibitor fetopathy. *Pediatr Nephrol*. 1995;9:382-385.
[116] Adigun AQ and Ajayi AA. Angiotensin converting enzyme inhibitor induced cough in Nigerians. *West Afr J Med*.2001 Jan-Mar;20910:46-47.

In: ACE Inhibitors. Volume 2
Editor: Macaulay Amechi Onuigbo
ISBN: 978-1-62948-422-8

Chapter 6

ACEIs as Antihypertensives in the Elderly (>65 Year Old): A South American Perspective

Carlos G. Musso, MD PhD* and Jose Alfie, MD
Hospital Italiano de Buenos Aires, Buenos Aires, Argentina

Abstract

Hypertension represents the most powerful risk factor for cardiovascular death in the elderly, and there is a significant reduction in stroke incidence, cardiovascular and global mortality in old people on antihypertensive treatment. Angiotensin converting enzyme inhibitors (ACEIs) are among the main antihypertensive drugs prescribed in this age group. Senescence induces changes in the renin-angiotensin-aldosterone system: a moderate decrease in circulating renin and aldosterone levels which is more pronounced in the up-right posture and with sodium-volume depletion. Additionally, angiotensin II represents a key molecule in the physiological and pathological mechanisms of heart, kidney, and brain, by promoting inflammation, cell growth, and reactive oxygen species generation at cellular and mitochondrial levels (oxidative stress). Studies in mice models have shown that disruption of angiotensin receptors promotes longevity. ACEIs should be handled with caution in the elderly, avoiding sudden reduction in blood pressure, hyperkalemia, hyponatremia, and syndrome of rapid-onset end-stage renal disease. In conclusion: ACEIs are useful drugs for treating hypertension in elderly population where they could even interfere with the ageing process beneficially.

Introduction

Hypertension represents the most powerful risk factor for cardiovascular death in the elderly, and there is a significant reduction in stroke incidence, cardiovascular and global mortality in old people on antihypertensive treatment [1]. The RENATA study updated the

* Corresponding author: Carlos G. Musso MD PhD. Email: carlos.musso@hospitalitaliano.org.ar

information about prevalence, awareness and treatment of hypertension in seven cities in Argentina (n: 4150 persons / 623 elderly) [2]. Systolic blood pressure increased with age in men and women, yet it was higher in men up to 54 years of age. Diastolic blood pressure showed a mild increase in men of up to 54 years of age and 64 in women. The prevalence of hypertension increased with age in both genders, from 11.1% in subjects < 35 years to 68.5% in ≥ 65 years, and was greater in men compared to women up to 54 years of age. Among those with hypertension 37.2% were unaware of their condition, while 6.6% knew they had hypertension but were not receiving treatment. Only 26.5% had their blood pressure well controlled. The following agents were most commonly used: angiotensin - converting enzyme inhibitors (ACEIs) (49.9%), beta blockers (29.9%), angiotensin II receptor blockers (22.4%), and calcium channel blockers (12.3%). The most common association was beta blockers + ACEI (34.7%) without significant differences between controlled vs. uncontrolled hypertension [2]. ACEIs, the main antihypertensive drugs prescribed in the elderly, are related with some phenomena particularly important in old people, such as renin-angiotensin-aldosterone senile serum levels, hypertension, longevity, Inflammation and fibrosis processes, dementia, and their adverse effect more prevalent in the elderly. Below we are going to describe each of them:

Senile Renin-Angiotensin –Aldosterone System

Senescence induces changes in the renin-angiotensin-aldosterone system which consists of a moderate decrease in circulating renin and aldosterone levels. These changes are more pronounced in the up-right posture and with sodium-volume depletion settings [3]. Angiotensin II represents a key molecule in physio-pathological mechanisms of the heart, kidney, and brain, by promoting inflammation, cell growth, and reactive oxygen species generation at cellular and mitochondrial levels (oxidative stress), all of them which could be positively influenced by ACEIs, with potentially blood-pressure lowering-independent beneficial effects [4].

Hypertension

It is known that the activation of the renal dopamine D1 (D1R) receptor and angiotensin II type 1 (AT1R) influences the activity of proximal tubular transporter NaKATPase and maintains sodium homeostasis and blood pressure. Studies performed on animal models (rats) have documented that a diminished D1R and exaggerated (AT1R) functions were associated with hypertension [5]. These findings could explain why clinical studies have documented significantly increased sodium proximal tubule reabsorption in old people; as well as the importance of ACEIs for treating hypertension in the elderly [1,6,7].

LONGEVITY

Angiotensin II regulates energy metabolism and affects the onset and the progression of cell senescence. Chronic activation of renin-angiotensin system promotes end-stage organ injury associated with ageing by increasing tissue and mitochondrial oxidative stress. Furthermore, a nicotinamide adenine dinucleotide positive protein (sirtuins) has been documented which is associated with mitochondrial and cell cycle regulation, apoptosis, DNA damage repair, and longevity, and it could be modulated by ARBs [8].

All the above mentioned facts could explain why ACEIs reduce age-associated cardiovascular, renal and brain damage, preserve mitochondria function, and consequently they could prolong life in humans. In the same sense, studies in mice models have shown that disruption of angiotensin- type 1 receptors promotes longevity, possibly through the attenuation of oxidative stress and over expression of pro-survival genes, such as Klotho gene [9,10].

INFLAMMATION AND FIBROSIS

Angiotensin II and related peptides are not exclusively involved in the regulation of systemic blood pressure and renal electrolyte balance but they are also a pro-inflammatory and pro-fibrotic agent. Increased generation of cellular reactive oxygen species and activation of redox-sensitive signaling cascades are critical events involved in angiotensin II actions. After binding to its AT1 receptors, angiotensin II triggers intracellular superoxide production. Under normal physiological conditions this pathway is closely regulated, but under conditions associated with renin-angiotensin system (RAS) over-activation, such as hypertension, diabetes, and normal ageing, angiotensin II – dependent oxidant generation becomes a significant contributor to cell oxidation and tissue damage. Due to the above espoused reasons, RAS blockade with ACEIs or ARBs, in the setting of hypertension, heart failure, and chronic renal failure, provided cardiac and renal benefits not limited to their antihypertensive effects alone [9,10].

DEMENTIA

Animal studies have suggested that angiotensin II promotes production of amyloid in brain, and they have also suggested ACEIs or ARBs may decrease amyloid-beta oligomerization. In a clinical study, Li et al. had documented that ARBs were associated with a significant reduction in the incidence and progression of Alzheimer´s disease and dementia, when compared with ACEs or other cardiovascular drugs in a predominantly male population [12]. Additionally, Hajjar et al. found that treatment with ARBs was associated with less Alzheimer disease-related pathology on autopsy evaluations [11-13]

Adverse Effects of ACEI in the Elderly

ACEIs should be handled with caution in the elderly since among the adverse effects secondary to these drugs the following are the main ones in this age group [14-19]:

Hypotension

Since healthy old people present a reduced water and sodium reabsorption capability, they are predisposed to hypovolemia. Besides, one third of elderly people suffer from orthostatism due to vascular dysautonomy. Consequently, all the above mentioned changes predispose old people to develop significant hypotension when they receive ACEIs.

Hyperkalemia

Despite renal potassium excretion capability being generally reduced in healthy old people, the serum potassium levels still are able to usually within the normal range in this group. However, old people easily develop hyperkalemia when they receive potassium sparing drugs, as is the case of ACEIs.

Hyponatremia

The combination of senile renal physiological changes (reduced free water clearance, and increased sodium loss) and concurrent ACEIs effects (sodium tubular loss, worsening renal perfusion during hypovolemic states) induces a trend to develop hyponatremia in this age group.

Syndrome of Rapid-Onset End-Stage Renal Disease (SORO-ESRD)

In 2010, Onuigbo described a new entity, the syndrome of rapid-onset end-stage renal disease (SORO-ESRD) in order to define an unpredictable, nonlinear, abrupt, and rapid progression to irreversible end-stage renal disease, often over a period of less than 2-4 weeks, following acute kidney injury resulting from medical and surgical events in chronic kidney disease patients with prior stable and non-progressive reduced levels of glomerular filtration rate (GFR), more so, in elderly patients on ACEIs/ARBs, and not explained by the presence of significant bilateral renal artery stenosis [19]. Probably, an interaction among the above mentioned factors with the senile renal physiological changes (vascular dysautonomy, reduced GFR and renal perfusion, tubule frailty) could explain the appearance of this syndrome, at least in some of the patients reported [19,20]. Indeed, one of us, working together with Onuigbo and a third researcher have contributed another chapter of this book which analyzes this newly described clinical syndrome of rapid onset ESRD further, together with an evaluation of the possible association of this syndrome with the ageing kidney and renal senescence [19,20].

Conclusion

ACEIs are useful drugs for treating hypertension in the older population where they could even proffer additional benefits by beneficially interfering with the ageing process, independent of simple blood-pressure lowering effects. Nevertheless, at the same time, ACEIs (and ARBs) in the elderly (>65 year old) must still be utilized with significant caution to avoid the compendium of sudden reductions in blood pressure, acutely worsening renal failure, hyperkalemia, hyponatremia, and the syndrome of rapid onset end stage renal disease (SORO-ESRD).

References

[1] Garcia-Donaire J, Rodicio-Diaz J, Ruilope M. Hypertension in the elderly. In Macías Núñez J, Cameron S, Oreopoulos D. (Eds). The aging kidney in health and disease. New York. Springer: 199-207

[2] Marin M, Fábregues G, Rodriguez P, Díaz M, Paez O, Alfie J, Caruso G, Pantalena P, Schiavi B, González M. National registry of hypertension. Awareness, treatment and control of hypertension. The RENATA study. *Revista Argentina de Cardiología*. 2012; 80(2): 121-128

[3] Weidmann P, De Myttenaere-Bursztein S, Maxwell M, De Lima J. Effect of aging on plasma renin and aldosterone in normal man. *Kidney International*. 1975; 8: 325-333

[4] Conti S, Cassi P, Benigni A. Aging and the renin-angiotensin system. *Hypertension*. 2012; 60:878-883

[5] Chung G, Lokhandwale M, Asghar M. Altered functioning of both renal dopamine D1 and angiotensin II type 1 receptors causes hypertension in old rats. *Hypertension*. 2012; 59(5):1029-36

[6] Arnold A, Gallagher P, Diz D. Brain renin-angiotensin system in the nexus of hypertension and aging. *Hypertension research*. 2013; 36: 5-13

[7] Musso C, Álvarez Gregori J, Jauregui J, Macías Núñez J. Creatinine, urea, uric acid, water and electrolytes renal handling in the healthy oldest old. *World Journal of Nephrology*. 2012; 1(5): 1-5

[8] Benigni A, Corna D, Zoja C, Sonzogni A, Latini R, Salio M, Conti S, Rottoli D, Longaretti L, Cassis P, Morigi M, Coffman T, Remuzzi G. Disruption of the angiotensin II type 1 receptor promotes longevity in mice. *The Journal of Clinical Investigation*. 2009; 119(3):524-30

[9] Inagami T. Mitochondrial angiotensin receptors and aging. *Circulation research*. 2011; 109:1323-1324

[10] Cavanagh E, Inserra F, Ferder L. Angiotensin II blockage: a strategy to slow ageing by protecting mitochondria? *Cardiovascular Research*. 2011; 89: 31-40

[11] Sink K, Leng X, Williamson J, Kritchevsky S, Yaffe K, Kuller L, Yasar S, Atkinson H, Robbins M, Psaty B, Goff D. Angiotensin converting enzyme inhibitors and cognitive decline in older adults with hypertension: Results from the cardiovascular health study. *Arch Intern Med.* 2009; 169(13): 1195-1202

[12] Li N, Lee A, Whitmer R, Kivipeito M, Lawler E, Kazis L, Wolozin B. Use of angiotensin receptor blockers and risk of dementia in a predominantly male population: prospective cohort analysis. *BMJ.* 2010; 340: 54-65

[13] Hajjar I, Brown L, Mack W, Chui H. Impact of angiotensin receptor blockers on Alzheimer disease neuropathology in a large brain autopsy series. *Arch Neurol.* 2012; 69(12):1632-8

[14] De Jong P. Angiotensin I converting enzyme inhibitors and angiotensin II receptor antagonists. In De Broe M, Porter G, Bennet W, Deray G (Eds.). Clinical nephrotoxins. Renal injury from drugs and chemicals. New York. Springer. 2008:481-494

[15] Musso CG, Liakopoulos V, et al. Correlation between creatinine clearance and transtubular potassium concentration gradient in old people and chronic renal disease patients. *Saudi Journal Kidney Dis Trasplant.* 2007; 18(4): 551-555

[16] Musso CG, de Miguel R, Algranati L, Farias E. Renal potassium excretion: comparison between chronic renal disease patients and old people. *Int Nephrol and Urol.* 2005; 37: 167-170

[17] Lacy C, Armstrong L, Goldman M, Lance L. *Drug Information Handbook.* Lexi-Comp. 2004: 526-529

[18] Musso CG, Alvarez Gregori J, Jauregui R, Macías Nuñez J. Creatinine, urea, uric acid, water and electrolytes reanl handling in the healthy oldest old. *World Journal of Nephrology.* 2011;6 (5):1-4

[19] Onuigbo M. Syndrome of rapid-onset end-stage renal disease: a new unrecognized pattern of CKD progression to ESRD. Renal failure. 2010; 32: 954-956.

[20] Onuigbo MA, Onuigbo NT. (2012). The Syndrome of Rapid Onset End-Stage Renal Disease (SOROESRD) – A New Mayo Clinic Dialysis Services Experience, January 2010-February 2011. In Di Iorio B, Heidland A, Onuigbo M, & Ronco C (Eds.), HEMODIALYSIS: When, How, Why. New York, NY. NOVA Publishers. p. 443-485.

In: ACE Inhibitors. Volume 2
Editor: Macaulay Amechi Onuigbo

ISBN: 978-1-62948-422-8

Chapter 7

THE IMPACT OF SALT RESTRICTION ON THE EFFECTIVENESS OF ANTIHYPERTENSIVE THERAPY

***Natale Gaspare De Santo, MD*[*1] *and Massimo Cirillo, MD*[2]**
[1]Department of Medicine, Second University of Naples, Naples, Italy
[2]Department of Medicine and Surgery, University of Salerno, Italy

ABSTRACT

"... if too much salt is added in foods the pulse hardens". This statement appearing in the *Yellow Emperor Textbook of Internal Medicine* (c2500 BC) indicates that a causal relation between sodium intake and blood pressure was already taken for granted in Ancient China some 4,500 years ago. Therefore our contemporary understanding that healthy diets are basically low in sodium has historical roots which finally attracted the interest of scientists of the twentieth century who provided controlled evidence that Kempner's rice diets reduced blood pressure because of their low sodium content. With that demonstration sodium restriction was identified as an effective treatment for hypertension to be controlled by continuous monitoring of urinary sodium over time. The list of papers on blood pressure profiles in people from low and high salt culture, going from populations with virtually no sodium intake to population with excessive sodium intake has widened the cultural horizons. This allowed Page to suggest in 1980 that "when all individuals of a population ingest small amounts of sodium, blood pressure does not increase with age and hypertension is virtually absent. When all members of the populations are ingesting large amount of sodium a high percentage develop hypertension. Between these extremes the relationship between blood pressure and sodium intake is difficult to perceive because of wide variation in genetic susceptibility and other type of "noise" introduced by other variables. The relationship, nevertheless, probably is present in all populations. A moderate reduction in sodium intake to 70 mmol/day would do no harm, and might do a great deal of good". Further advancement was achieved by learning that a small addition of sodium to the milk in feeding newborn babies significantly increased their blood pressure within short time. Finally clinical trials in the last decade have shown a reduction in blood pressure following a restriction in sodium intake in non-hypertensive persons ingesting typical American meals and have

[*] Corresponding author: Natale Gaspare De Santo MD; Email: nataleg.desanto@unina2.it

fixed at 65 mmol per day the ideal target of sodium intake. Although there are still reports and personal views not foreseeing benefits in blood pressure control by associating sodium restriction to antihypertensive drugs, there is good evidence of additive blood pressure lowering when sodium restriction is the associated with diuretics, ACE-inhibitors and beta-adrenergic blockers and Angiotensin II receptor blockers. However a reduction of sodium intake does not impact blood pressure readings in hypertensive patients receiving calcium-channel blockers.

INTRODUCTION

"... if too much salt is added in foods the pulse hardens". This statement in the *Yellow Emperor Textbook of Internal Medicine* (c2500 BC) indicates that a causal relation between sodium intake and blood pressure was already taken for granted in Ancient China some 4500 year ago. Therefore our present understanding that healthy diets are basically low in sodium has remote roots. This old concept finally attracted the interest of scientists of the twentieth century who provided controlled evidence that Kempner's rice diets reduced blood pressure because their low sodium content. The present chapter aims to show that low sodium diets are the prerequisite of any drug therapy. For the goal of this chapter proofs will be given that a low salt intake maximizes the effects of the pharmacological treatment of hypertensive persons as well as of hypertensive patients with renal disease. However, the association with calcium channel blockers is ineffective.

THE TASTE FOR SALT IN MAN: EVOLUTIONARY ASPECTS

During Miocene hominoids ate fruits (frugiverous) and leaves (foliverous). Their salt intake was around and 0.6 g of NaCl a day (10 mmol). Preagricultural humans of the Paleleolithic period–mainly hunter-gatherers–ate diets rich in potassium (up to 10,500 mg/day), no sodium chloride was added. Foods were not cooked, their net acid charge was not high. The Na to K ratio in urine was 0.13 as in it was seen in the second part of the last century in Yanomano, Xingo Amerindians and Asaro from New Guinea. The Paleolithic intake was that of chimpanzee, a species very close to humans [1,2].

The relation of sodium to blood pressure might go back to 12,000 years ago, to the times of the introduction of agriculture and the domestication of animals. Before that time, as Jeremiah Stamler [3], pointed out:

" ...man and his immediate predecessors—evolving in tropical and semitropical Africa as hunters and food gatherers—knew nothing of salt as a separate material to be added to foods. Man, the hunter, easily satisfied his small physiological needs for Na from approximately 30 to 35% of calories of animal origin. In fact he readily managed on less, even in a tropical climate, given his great ability, acquired in 70 million years of primate evolution, to minimize Na loss (via the kidney, skin and gut), and to conserve this electrolyte, vital for his homeostasis. In ancient times, based on the invention of agriculture, grain became the main source of food for the masses, i.e., most human beings became overwhelmingly vegetarian. A surplus of food became available. Salt began to be used as a preservative for some perishable foods and man developed a taste for sodium, perhaps aided and abetted by the paucity of Na in his high-grain diet". Thus the challenge of excreting a sizeable excess of salt, well above physiological need, almost every day from early childhood on is almost certainly relatively recent one for man, and a sizeable portion of the species seems not to possess the optimal genetic mechanisms to accomplish the task while maintaining low-normal optimal blood pressures, with no increase from late teens through middle age. Only a minority manage this optimal adaptation".

LESSONS FROM ANIMAL STUDIES

Chimpanzees (a species phylogenetically close to humans) were fed a fruit and vegetable diet (2-25 mmol/day of Na, that of a preliterate society where hypertension is the exception) whereas the treatment group were given increasing amounts of sodium chloride (5, 10 and 15 g a day corresponding to 85, 170 e 257 mmol of Na) for nearly 20 months. Salt caused a significant increase in systolic (SBP), diastolic (DBP) and mean blood pressure (MAP) which was completely abolished by a 6 month stopping of salt intake. The highest intake was associated with an increase of SBP, DBP and MBP of 33, 10 and 10 mm Hg respectively [4].

A more recent study in chimpanzees had an arm in Gabon (Africa) with 11 animals and the other arm was in Bastrop (USA) with 110 animals [5]. In Gabon, the baseline diet provided 75 mmol of Na per day, in Bastrop 250 mmol/day and was subsequently switched to 35 mmol/day, and to 120 mmol/day in Gabon and to 125 mmol/day in Bastorp. In both sites diets were rich in potassium and calcium.

The lower sodium intake was associated with a reduction in SBP, DBP and MAP. The adjusted fall for SBP was -12.7 mm Hg (95% CI -16.9 to -8.5 mm Hg) per 100 mmol/day lower sodium intake in Gabon and -5.7 mm Hg (95% CI -12.2 to -0.7 mm Hg) per 122 mmol/day reduction of Na intake in Bastorp.

The fall in DBP was -7.5 mm Hg (95% CI 5.10 to 10.0) in Gabon, and -4.4 mm Hg (-9.6 to -0.8 mm Hg) in Bastrop. MAP fell by – 9.9 mm Hg (95% CI -6.5 to -13.2 mm Hg) in Gabon and by -4.8 mm Hg (-10.2 to -0.7 mm Hg) in Bastrop.

The data obtained with a vegetarian diet rich in potassium in a species close to man disclose exciting perspectives for the use of sodium restriction to control blood pressure since they "are qualitatively and quantitatively consistent with result of human epidemiological studies and clinical trial data" thus they have "important policy implications for human populations" [3]. However, the animal model which disclosed the risk of high salt intake in man was not that of chimpanzee but rats, following a genial experiment of L.K. Dahl in 1961 [6]. Female rats fed diets containing sodium excess became hypertensive. Hypertension became self-sustaining; two/thirds of the animals did not reduce their blood pressure (BP) after withdrawal of sodium excess. The sober conclusion of the study, at a time when science was not vociferous, pointed out that "an etiologic relationship between Na intake and development of hypertension was not excluded" [6].

A Bit of History of Salt

Obtained from primordial elements (air water, earth and fire), salt has influenced human nutrition, health and our survival on earth. It has regulated politics, taxation systems, economy, freight, transport and commerce. The importance of salt is such that all human activities have been influenced by it, including religious beliefs, and practices, art, literature, and corpse preservation, in other words the whole gamut of history. Salt has associations with superstitions, has been used in exorcism and is a relevant symbol for psychoanalysis" [7]. "Il cristallise dans un réseau cubique, image de la perfection » [8]. "Salt is thus a product that can offer its attractions to the believer, to the surveyor, to the physician, to the chemist, and to the historian" [8]. The history of salt begins in ancient times and "is closely related to different aspects of human history" [9]. It has been an emblem for many cultures. It has been invested with many meanings. No sacral ceremony could take place in Rome without "*mola salsa*" /salty flour. Salt was used instead of money to compensate for work in Rome (salary, and salacious derive from salt) [9,10].

"It was regarded as the essence of living things and life, and as the very soul itself. Nothing could be eaten without salt and to be without salt was believed to lack an essential element and its name was used also to refer to mental pleasures (Plutarch, *Moralia VIII, Table Talk IV*). A civilized life was believed to be impossible without salt, and its name was also used to refer to mental pleasures as Pliny the Elder pointed out "*Sales appellantur omnisque vitae lepos et summa hilaritas laborumque requies non alio magis vocabulo constat*" (*Naturalis Historia*, Book XXXI, 54-98) (9). Other historical examples of the importance of salt may be found in the splendour of the maritime Republic of Venice, living on salt commerce, in the conquest of the Kingdom of Naples by the Anjou Family which began with a tax on salt, in the start of the French Revolution, and in the Indian Revolution started by Gandhi [9]. "The importance of finding salt is underlined by the fact that appetite for salt is innate and salt is a primary salt in vertebrates. Antropoids are vegetarians and man is similar to vegetarians both in dentition and in the gastrointestinal tract. Hominid evolution, initiated 30 million years ago mainly in tropical warm regions, was associated substantially with a vegetarian diet and some evidence supports the thesis that the diet of the feral man even in recent times was mainly vegetarian and characterized by a low salt intake. The hypothesis has been put forward that the practice of adding salt to food is typical of agricultural-vegetarian lifestyles, as there is no need to add salt when food contains a sufficiency of it" [9].

Many artists, among them Bellini, Brueghel, Hendricks, Poussin, Rafael, Romano, Titian, Tintoretto, and Veronese, have used the symbol of salt in both religious and profane works. By contrast only a few studies have examined the symbolism of salt as adopted in various works of arts [2-4]. If one might select some representative piece of arts to symbolize salt it would be difficult. Perhaps Botticelli (*Venus Saligena,* at the Uffizi in Florence), Leonardo (*The Last Supper,* at Santa Maria delle Grazie in Milan), Cellini (*The Salt Cellar,* Kunsthistorisches Museum in Vienna), and the "*The Enchanted Mountain*" a temporary piece of art, created by Mimmo Paladino in Plebiscito Square in Naples (December 1995-January 1996) might open the list [11-12].

SODIUM AND BLOOD PRESSURE: 1ST HALF OF THE TWENTIETH CENTURY

As thoroughly reviewed elsewhere, the first controversial data about sodium and blood pressure appeared in the 1st half of the 20th century [13]. The field was started by Ambard and Beaujard, and were written in French. Ambard and Beaujard reported on the effect on hypertension of chloride restriction, hence on an attendant restriction of sodium also [14,15]. They were heavily criticized and did not influence contemporary medical thinking. Subsequently Allen and his collaborators produced interesting data which were also not appreciated [16,17]. It was a Jewish physician [13], born in Germany but working in USA since 1934 at Duke University in North Carolina, who developed a diet based on rice (250-350 g) associated with fruit juice plus 100-500 g/day of sugar or dextrose to meet caloric requirements. It was poor in fat and the protein content averaged 20 g/day. The sodium intake was below 10 mmol/day [13]. Kempener showed that the diet was capable to reduce blood pressure in the majority of patients [18, 19]. Finally Corcoran, Taylor and Page, in a landmark paper extensively demonstrated the role of sodium intake in lowering BP [20]. Their paper can be considered either the first of modernity or the last of pre-modernity.

INITIAL CONTRIBUTIONS FROM EPIDEMIOLOGY

In the second half of the last century epidemiological studies disclosed a low sodium intake in low-blood pressure population (Table 1). This let Page to hypothesize that when *"all individuals in a population are habitually using very small amounts of sodium, blood pressure does not rise with age and hypertension is virtually absent. When all members of the population are ingesting a very large amount of sodium a high percentage, reflecting the maximum number of susceptible individuals (genetic noise), develop hypertension. Between the extremes the relationship between blood pressure and sodium is difficult to perceive because of the wide variation in genetic susceptibility and other type of noises. One can say that a moderate reduction in sodium intake to the range of 1,610 mg a day would not harm and might do a great deal of good"* [21].

Table 1. Sodium intake in low-blood pressure populations

Country	Populations	Na intake, mg/day
Brazil	Yanomano Indians	34.5
New Guinea	Tukisenda	34.5
Solomon Indians	Kwaio, Baegu, Aita	20-460
Uganda	Samburu	1150
Cook Islands	Pukapuka	1415
Solomon Islands	People of Ontong Java	1150-1610

Modified from ref.1.

LESSONS FROM STUDIES IN NEONATES AND CHILDREN

In 1980, 476 newborn infants participated in randomized double-blind trial on the six-month effects on blood pressure of low sodium intake and normal sodium intake (0.89±0.26 mmol) and (2.50±0.95 mmol) [22]. At the end of the study, systolic blood pressure was -2.1 mm Hg lower in the low sodium group than in the normal sodium group after appropriate adjustment for body weight, length at birth, and systolic blood pressure in the first week(90% CI -3.7 to -0.5, p<0.01) (22).

A subgroup of these children was re-evaluated fifteen years later to investigate whether this very early difference in sodium intake was still associated with blood pressure differences [23]. The study showed that at follow-up SBP was -3.6 mm Hg (95% CI -6.6 to -0.5) and DBP was -2.2 mm Hg lower (95% CI -4.5 to -0.2) in children who received a low sodium diet. The study showed that sodium restriction lasting six months after birth was associated with sizeable differences in blood pressure later in life [23].

THE INTERSALT STUDY

The Intersalt Study Group investigated on the relation with blood pressure of 24-hour urinary excretion of Na and K in more than 10,000 men and women aged 20-59 years (median age 40 years) from 52 centres all over the world [24, 25]. A significantly positive relation was found between daily urinary sodium excretion and systolic blood pressure in cross-sectional population analyses and at the individual level. Average sodium excretion of 52 populations associated with the slopes of systolic and diastolic blood pressure over age. The authors concluded that *"Estimates of the effect of median sodium excretion higher by 100 mmol/day over a 30 year period (age 55 minus age 25) were of 10-11 mm Hg in systolic blood pressure and 6 mm Hg in diastolic blood pressure"*. It was speculated that such an effect could affect the rates of cardiovascular diseases and mortality from all causes. Strong recommendations were made to reduce salt intake for *"prevention and control of adverse blood pressure levels and high blood pressure in populations"* [24, 25].

THE DASH TRIALS

The Dietary Approaches to Stop Hypertension (DASH) Trial was devised to test the blood pressure effects of a diet rich in fruits and vegetables but low in total and saturated fat in adults with SBP < 160 mm Hg and DBP 80-95 mm Hg [26]. A subsequent study examined the effects of the DASH Diet in association with three different levels of Na intake: High (150 mmol/day), Intermediate (100 mmol/day), and Low (50 mmol/day). Urinary sodium averaged 141 mmol, 106 mmol, and 67 mmol during high, intermediate, and low Na intake, respectively [27]. Baseline data of urinary sodium, SBP, and DBP were identical in control and DASH groups (Figure 1). After 8 weeks there were consistent differences in blood pressure between high and low sodium groups across all dietary regimens (Figure 1 and Figure 2).The differences tended to be larger in hypertensives, persons older than 45, African-Americans, and people abstaining from alcohol. Thus, *"the DASH diet associated to decreased sodium intake should be broadly recommended for preventing hypertension and its sequelae"* [28].

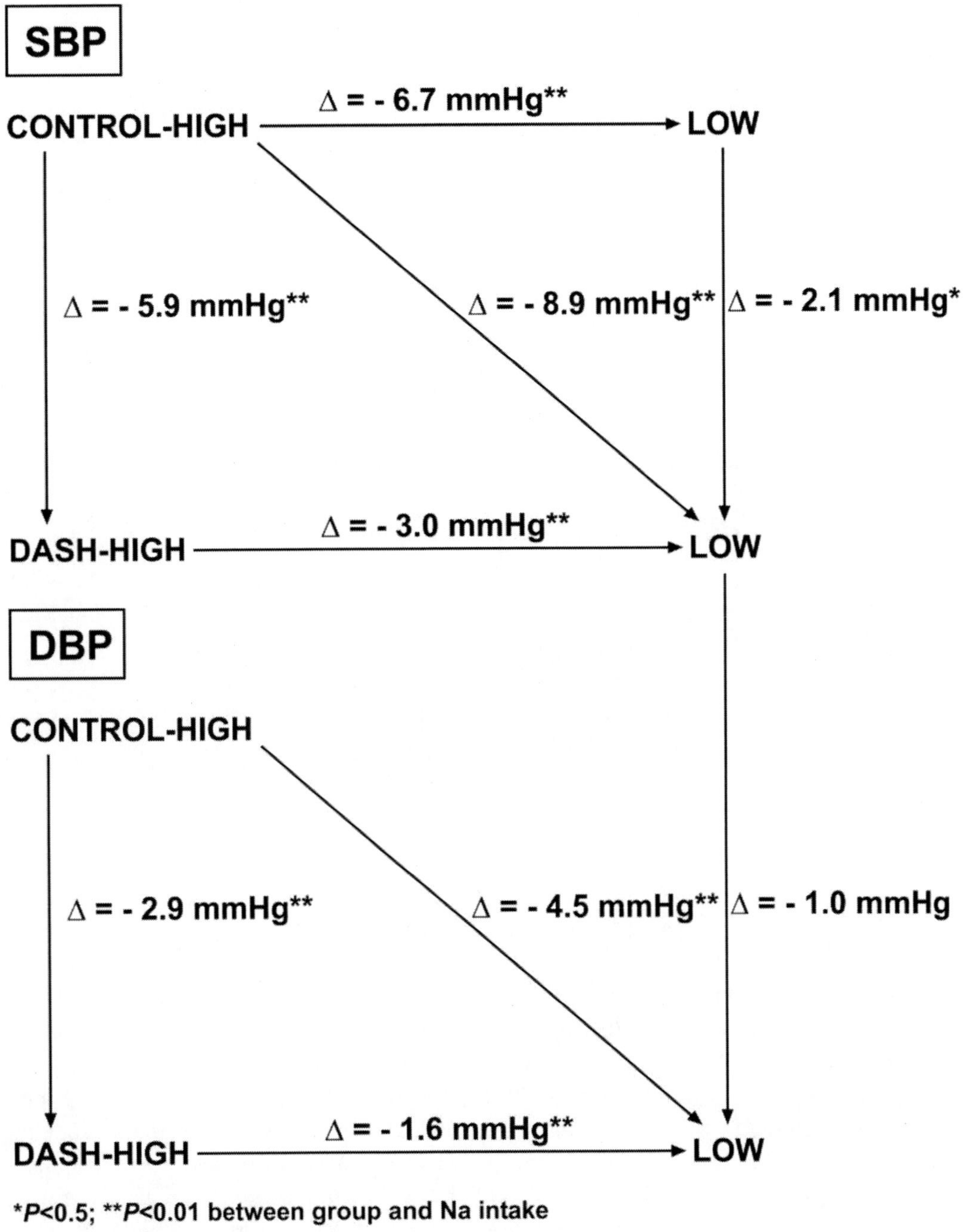

Figure 1. Systolic and Diastolic Blood Pressure according to sodium intake. Redrawn from data in reference no. 28.

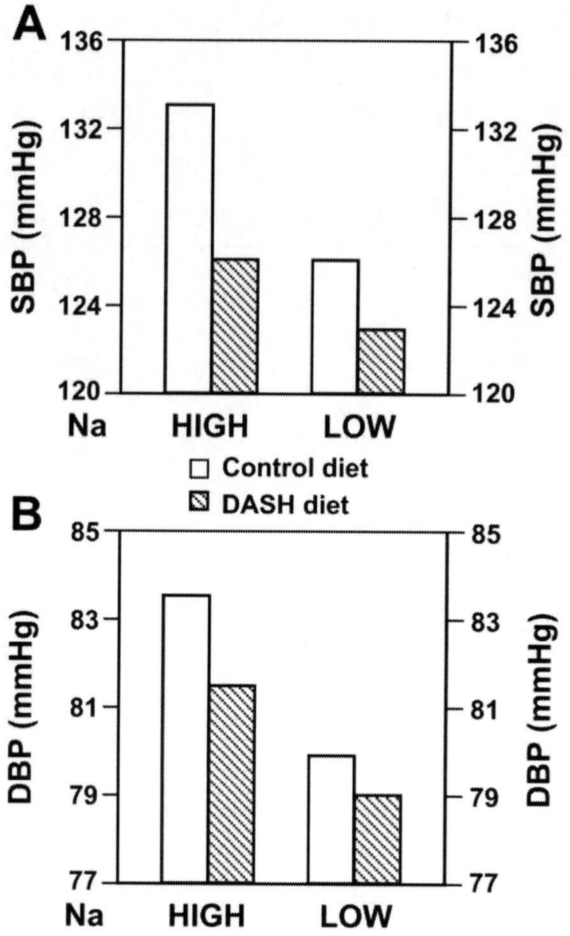

Figure 2. Systolic and Diastolic Blood Pressure according to sodium intake. Modified from data in reference no. 28.

META-ANALYSES AND STUDIES ON EVENTS

A recent paper analysed data of cohort studies and randomised controlled trials [29]. A total of 36 studies demonstrated that a reduction of sodium intake was associated with a reduction of SBP by -3.39 mm Hg (-2.46 to- 4.31 mm Hg) and of DBP by -1.54 mm Hg (-0.98 to -2.11 mm Hg). A difference of -3.47 mm Hg SBP (-0.76 to -6.16) and of -1.81 mm Hg DBP (-0.54 to -3.08) was found when sodium intake < 2 g/day was compared to sodium intake > 2 g/day. The results for SBP were obtained in studies lasting less than 3 months, regardless of sex, methods, and study design. *"Reductions in diastolic blood pressure was less pronounced but patterns in subgroups were similar to those for systolic blood pressure"* [29]. Another observation of the meta-analysis was that higher sodium intake increases the risk of stroke and fatal cardiovascular events whereas sodium restriction does not associate with significant adverse effects [29]. Another study based on 34 trials evaluated the long-term effects on blood pressure of modest differences in salt intake [30]. With a reduction in salt intake of -75 mmol/day SBP was reduced by -4.18 mm Hg (-5.18 to -3.18, p< 0.001) and

DBP by -2.06 mm Hg (-2.64 to -1.45, $p<0.001$). Age, blood pressure status (hypertensive and non-hypertensive), urinary sodium and ethnic group explained 68% of the variance between groups for SBP and 41% of the variance for DBP. Blood pressure effects tended to be larger in hypertensives than in normotensives. The reduction in salt intake was followed by a modest increase in plasma renin activity, aldosterone, and noradrenaline which did not associate with significant adverse events. The changes in serum total cholesterol, low and high density lipoprotein cholesterol and triglycerides were not significant.

These two meta-analyses contradicted the suspicions of possible harmful effects of salt restriction, and support the practice of salt intake reduction down to 5-6 g/day or lower levels [31-34].

Another meta-analysis focused on prospective studies published between 1996 and 2008 in 14 cohorts including 154,282 persons and 5,346 events [35]. The conclusion was that *"a higher salt intake of about 5 g (2,000 mg of sodium, 88 mmol/day) was associated with a risk of stroke of 1.23 (1.06 to 1.43, p<0.007) and a dose response of 6% increase in the risk of stroke for every 50 mmol(approximately 1,150 mg) sodium per day"*. A difference of 5 g in salt intake was also associated with a 17% increased risk for cardiovascular disease (1.02 to 1.32, P=0.07). Since 1 out 3 strokes and 1 out 5 cardiovascular disease are fatal such reduction in salt intake of 5 g/day might spare every year 1.25 million deaths for stroke and 3 million deaths for cardiovascular disease worldwide [35, 36].

The Northern Manhattan Study reported data collected in 2,657 participants aged 69±10 years during 10-year follow up. The study reported a large number of events with inclusion of 2202 ischemic strokes, 209 myocardial infarctions, and 371 vascular deaths [37]. The analysis of sodium intake as a continuous variable showed a 17% increase in stroke risk for each 500 mg/day increase in sodium consumption. The higher sodium intake was associated with a 14% increased risk of cardiovascular disease (p=0.07). The data are consistent with the meta-analysis of Strazzullo et al. [35], and support the importance of reducing sodium intake in the US population. During the last forty years there has been a continuous interest in the role of sodium intake in high blood pressure among children [22, 23, 38-44]. The meta-analysis of above showed that a restriction in sodium intake significantly reduces systolic and diastolic blood pressure in children also suggesting that low salt intake in childhood may be crucial to prevent the blood pressure increase with age [29]. This conclusion was based on data from 8 studies in childhood where a sodium intake restriction was associated with decreases in systolic and diastolic blood pressure [45-52]. Thus, sodium intake restriction in childhood is considered as an effective and powerful manoeuvre to prevent the increase of blood pressure with age.

Recommendations about Salt Intake in Adults and Children

In 2004 the Institute of Medicine of the American Academies established the requirements for sodium and other nutrient intake having recognized that "the effects of sodium and health have been reported often vociferous" [53]. The statement departed from the extreme amounts of sodium intake (10 mmol/day of Yanomano Indians of Brazil and 450 mmol/day in Northern Japan), and put emphasis on the minimal replacement quantity (180 mg/day, 8 mmol/day) which is a quantity that does not allow to formulate a diet with safe amounts of other nutrients. They therefore established the Adequate Intake (AI) and the tolerable Upper Limit (UL) for individuals living in US and Canada. AI was fixed at 1.5 g for young adults, 1.3 g for ages 50-70 years and 1.2 g for people≥ 71 years of age (corresponding to 65, 55, and 50 mmol/day).The UL was fixed at 2.3 g/day with a caveat for *"certain groups of individual who are most sensitive to the blood pressure effects of sodium intake, e.g. older persons, African Americans, and individuals with hypertension, diabetes, or chronic kidney disease for whom it may well be lower"*. UL may be greater for those with "*sodium sweat losses*" [30]. It was acknowledged that many individuals exceeded both the AI and UL allowances. The USDA 2010 Dietary Guidelines for American recommend *"sodium intakes of less than 2,300 mg daily for adolescents and adults 14 years of age or older, and no more than 1,500 mg daily for African Americans, individuals 51 years of age or older, and individuals with hypertension, diabetes or CKD"* [54]. In 2012, the World Health Organization (WHO) recommended *"a reduction of sodium intake to reduce blood pressure risk of cardiovascular disease, stroke and coronary heart disease in adults [≥ 16 years of age] to < 2g day sodium (5 g/day salt) [100 mmol]"*. In addition WHO recommended *"a reduction in sodium intake to control blood pressure in children [2-15 years of age]"* for whom *"the maximum level of sodium intake of 2 g/day in adults should be adjusted downwards based on the energy requirements of children relative to those of adults"*. Those recommendations apply to all individuals with or without hypertension [55].

Thus, animal studies, studies in low salt populations, migration studies, cohort studies, randomised controlled trials, limited controlled intervention studies, studies on surrogate markers of outcomes and WHO recommendations, unanimously support the benefits of a lower sodium intake [56].

Finally, the 2013 recommendations of the committee appointed by the Institute of Medicine of the National Academies *"found that data among pre-hypertensive participants from two related studies provided some evidence suggesting a continued benefit of lowering sodium intake in these patients down to 2,300 mg per day (and lower, although based on small numbers in the lower range) (57). In contrast, the committee found no evidence for benefit and some evidence suggesting risk of adverse health outcomes associated with sodium intake levels in ranges approximating 1,500 to 2,300 mg a day in other disease-specific population subgroups, specifically those with diabetes, chronic kidney disease (CKD) or pre-existing CVD. No relevant evidence was found on health outcomes for other population subgroup (i.e persons 51 years of age and older, and African Americans. In studies that explored interactions, race, age, or prevalence of hypertensions or diabetes did not change the effect of sodium on health outcomes"*.

Blood Pressure Effects of Sodium Restriction Associated with Antihypertensive Drugs in Hypertensive Persons

Inhibitors of Angiotensin-Converting Enzyme (ACE)

The effect of enalapril (10 mg BID) on blood pressure was studied under low (50 mmol/day) and high (200 mmol/day) sodium intake. During low sodium intake, mean arterial pressure (MAP) was significantly reduced from 110± 2 to 94±2 mm Hg. During high sodium intake, enalapril was associated with a significant fall of MAP from 109±2 to 98±2 mm Hg. The differences in MAP between high and low salt intake (- 4.0 mm Hg) was statistically significant (p<0.02). ACE-inhibition was associated with a more sustained effect on ERPF and GFR during salt restriction [58].

Table 3. Effects of ACE-inhibition on MAP during low and high sodium intake [58]

Sodium intake	Baseline MAP	MAP following ACEi
Low	110±2	94±2*
High	109±2	98±2*
		- 4.0 mm Hg**

Statistical significance *p<0.01; **p<0.02

ACE Inhibitors and Diuretics

In a double-blind, placebo-controlled, crossover study Singer et al studied the effects on blood pressure of a moderate salt restriction (104±11 mmol/day) in comparison with the usual salt intake (195±14 mmol/day) in patients receiving captopril and hydrochlorothiazide [59]. A reduction of 91 mmol/day in sodium intake caused significant changes in SBP both at 2 and 12 hours, and of DBP at 12 H. The decrease in blood pressure correlated with the reduction in sodium intake. Moderate sodium restriction had an additive effect on blood pressure when associated to a converting enzyme inhibitor and hydrochlorothiazide. Thus patients with hypertension uncontrolled by ACE-inhibitor and HCTZ will benefit of sodium restriction.

Table 4. Effects of sodium restriction on SBP, DBP and MAP in hypertensive patients receiving captopril and hydrochlorothiazie 2 and 12 hours after therapy [59]

Period	Na intake	SBP, mm Hg		DBP, mmHg		MAP, % fall	
	mmol/day	2H	12H	2H	12H	2H	12H
A	195±14	147±15	159±6	91±2	102±.2		
B	104±11	138±5*	148±5*	88±3	95±2**	5±2	7±2*

*p<0.01, **p<0.001 vs A

Indapamide or low sodium intake (96 mmol/day) independently reduced blood pressure in another study on patients with mild to moderate essential hypertension who were resistant to ACE inhibitor Perindopril while on sodium intake of 158 mmol/day [60]. The reduction was maximal when the low sodium intake and the diuretic were combined (Table 5).Thus, diuretics and low sodium intake can effectively reduce blood pressure of patients resistant to ACE inhibition. The effect is maximal when the low sodium intake and the diuretic are associated each other. This indicates that a sodium intake below 100 mmol/day is beneficial in essential hypertension and its effects may be further magnified by a small dose of a diuretic.

Table 5. Effects of a combination of Indapamide and low sodium intake on blood pressure of patients with essential hypertension resistant to Perindropril on high sodium intake [60]

	Perdindopril Na 158 mmol/day	Perindopril+Indapamide Na 96 mmol/day
SBP, mm Hg	160±2	144±2*
DBP, mm Hg	98±2	88±1*
MAP, mm Hg	121±4	110±1*

*statistical significant significant differences

Renin Inhibitors

Aliskiren is the first medication among the class of direct renin inhibitors and prevents the conversion of angiotensinogen to angiotensin I [61]. It was used at a dose of 300 mg a day in a randomised cross-over study in association with a low (84.8 mmol/day) and high sodium intake (207.6 mmol/day). Aliskiren was associated with ambulatory SBP of 124.2±10.4 mm Hg on low Na intake, and of 133.5±10.6 mm Hg on high sodium intake. The difference -9.4 mm Hg (95% CI -7.5 to -11.4) was statistically significant (p<0.001). Ambulatory DBP averaged 78.4±8.2 mm Hg on low Na intake and 84.1±8.6 mm Hg on high sodium intake. The difference between Na intakes was -5.7 mm Hg (95% CI -4.4to -6.9, p<0.001) (Figure 3).Furthermore 76.5% of patients on low sodium + aliskiren achieved either a successful BP response (SBP<130 mm Hg) or a reduction of baseline SBP≥20 mm Hg, whereas the proportion on the higher sodium intake was 42.6% (p<0.001). In addition when a different definition of BP response was used (SBP<135 mm Hg or a reduction ≥20 mm Hg from baseline the percentage of patients achieving the target raised up to 84.3% on low Na and to 54.7% on high intake [61].

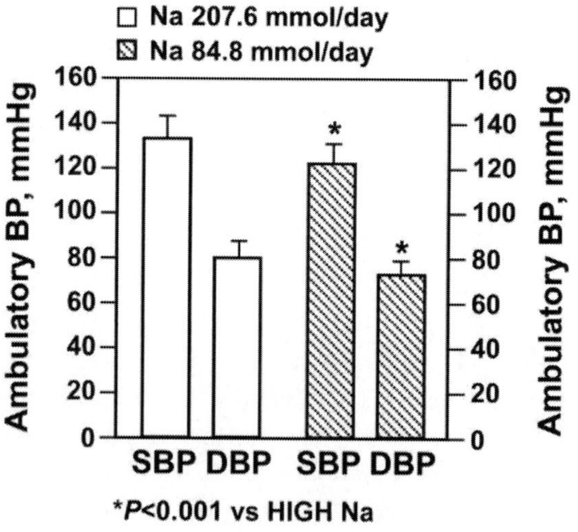

Figure 3. Effects of aliskiren, a direct renin inhibitor, on blood pressure of hypertensive subjects. Redrawn from data in reference no. 60.

β-blockers and Diuretics

Erweteman et al at the Department of Medicine of the University Centrum in Amsterdam studied hypertensive patients with normal plasma creatinine while on restricted sodium intake or normal sodium intake (70 and 130 mmol/day of Na) [62]. The patients were treated with placebo, chlorthalidone, metoprololo or a combination of chlorthalidone and metoprolol. The fall in blood pressure was maximal with the combination of the diuretic plus the β-blocker. Under restricted sodium intake the effects of treatment tended to be larger than on normal sodium intake. The data point out that a moderate sodium restriction increases the effectiveness of blood pressure reduction secondary to treatment with β-blockers (Table 6 and Table 7).

Table 6. Supine Systolic and Diastolic Blood Pressure (SDP, DBP) on restricted and normal sodium intake at screening and on placebo, diuretic, β-blocker or combination of diuretic and beta-blocker

	Sodium intake			
Treatment	**Restricted**	**Normal**	**Restricted**	**Normal**
	Systolic Blood Pressure		**Diastolic Blood Pressure**	
Screening	157.0±11.4	156.2±11.8	101.5±5.4	100.5±3.4
Placebo	141.0±15.4	142.9±16.4	92.9±10.4	94.4±12.0
Chlorthalidone	135.3±14.8	137.0±13.6	90.5±10.4	90.8±6.9
Metoprolol	128.5±16.3	134.6±15.9	83.7±8.6	87.6±9.1
Chlortalidone+Metoprolol	128.1±15.0	126.8±11.6	83.1±9.6	83.7±7.5

Data are in mm Hg (Mean ± SEM) [21].

Table 7. Changes of Systolic and Diastolic Blood Pressure (Δ) in comparison to the Screening period under restricted and normal sodium intake

	Sodium Intake			
Treatments	**Restricted**	**Normal**	**Restricted**	**Normal**
	Δ Systolic Blood Pressure		**Δ Diastolic Blood pressure**	
Placebo	- 16.0	- 13.3	- 8.6	- 6.1
Chorthalidon	- 21.7	- 20.3	- 11.5	- 9.7
Metoprolol	- 28.5	- 21.3	- 17.8	- 12.9
Chlorthalidone+Metoprolol	- 28.9	- 29.4	- 18.4	- 16.8

Data are given in mm Hg (Mean ± SEM) [62].

Calcium Channel Blockers

Salt-sensitive and non-salt sensitive patients with mild to moderate essential hypertension were studied in a single-blind crossover study, on low sodium intake (100±14 mmol/day) and high sodium intake (210±22 mmol/day) after the administration of the calcium antagonist Isradipine [63]. As reported in Table 8, similar levels of blood pressure are achieved in salt-sensitive and non-salt-sensitive persons on isradipine, irrespective of Na sodium intake, although slightly higher doses of Isradipne were used in salt-sensitive persons. Isradipine effects on the higher Na intake may be driven either by the high calciuric effect on high Na or by the effects of high Na on ionized Ca, PTH and 1,25$(OH)_2D_3$ or the natriuretic action.

Table 8. Effects of Isradipine on blood pressure during high and low salt intake [63]

Salt-Sensitive	No	Na intake	Basal BP	Final BP	ΔSBP	ΔDBP
				mm Hg		
+	5	High	157.2/102.9	138.5/83.3	-18.7	-19.6
+	5	Low	148.7/97.3	141.8/85.3	- 6.9	-12.0
				Δ = +3.3/+1.7 mm Hg		
-	16	High	155.0/98.6	142.7/91.0	-12.6	- 7.4
-	16	Low	141.8/91.7	141.8/91.7	-19.2	-10.9
				Δ=+0.9/+0.7 mm Hg		

Nicholson et al. demonstrated that verapamil reduces blood pressure more in persons on low Na intake than in persons on high Na intake (10 mmol/day and 200 mmol/day) (Figure 4) [64]. In another study, the same author proved that nitrendipine reduced blood pressure more in persons on a high Na intake (250 mmol/day) than in persons on a lower sodium intake (50 mmol/day) [65]. Similarly, the results of the study of Del Rio et al showed that nifedipine (40mg/day) caused a significant reduction of SBP (- 9.83%) and of DBP (-11.17%) which was not altered by the amount of salt in the diet during the experimental periods [67].Thus, sodium restriction may not be needed in patient on antihypertensive doses of calcium channel blockers which likely produce a modest but beneficial sodiuretic effect [68, 69].

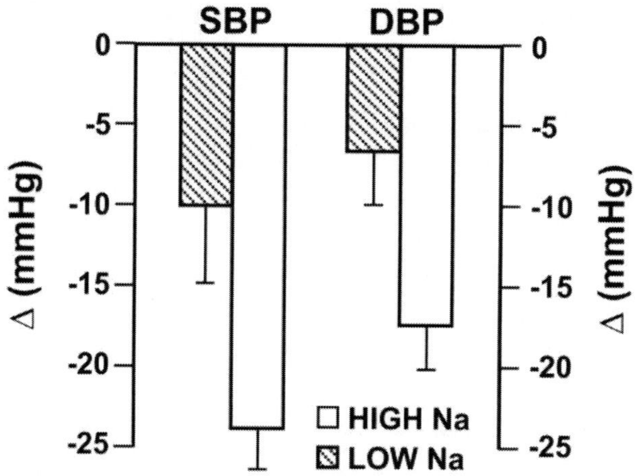

Figure 4. Verapamil effects on blood pressure during low and high Na intake. Modified from reference no. 64.

BLOOD PRESSURE EFFECTS OF SODIUM RESTRICTION ASSOCIATED WITH ANTIHYPERTENSIVE DRUGS IN CHRONIC KIDNEY DISEASE

ACE Inhibitors

Wapstra et al demonstrated that, in adramycin nephrosis, a course of 10 mg/kg a day of lisinopril significantly affected blood pressure and that the effect was greater under low sodium intake than in normal sodium intake (Table 9) [70].

Table 9. Effects of sodium intake on systolic blood pressure in experiment on adriamycin nephrosis treated with Lisinopril (10 mg/kg) for 8 weeks [70]

Sodium Intake	Systolic Blood Pressure, mm Hg	
	Basal	Lisinopril
Normal	121±5	89±2*
Low	119±4	77±3*†

* P<0.05 vs basal, †P<0.05 vs normal sodium + lisinopril

In patients with steroid-insensitive nephrotic syndrome J.E.Heeg et al studied the effects of the ACE inhibitor lisinopril and sodium intake on proteinuria and blood pressure in patients with baseline SBP of 134±13 mm Hg, a DBP of 83±13 mm Hg and MAP of 101±12 mm Hg [71].

Lisinopril reduced MAP in patients on low Na intake. The effect was reversed by high sodium intake and re-established by subsequent low Na intake. The effect was evident in patients with near- normal blood pressure (Table 10).

Table 10. Effects of lysinopril on Mean Arterial Pressure according to Na intake [70]

Period	Na intake	Lisinopril	MAP (mm Hg)
A	Low	-	101±11
B	Low	+	87±7*
C	High	+	89±8*†
D	Low	+	87±8*‡

Significant differences: * vs A, † vs B and ‡ vs C.

ACE-Inibitor and Diuretics

The blood pressure response of CKD patients with proteinuria (< 1 g/day) and creatinine clearance > 30 ml/min during treatment with ACE inhibitors (enalapril or lisinopril) was studied in three 4-week ambulatory periods: low sodium intake (100 mmol/day), high sodium intake (178 mmol/day) and high sodium + 50 mg of hydrochlorothiazide (HCTZ) [72]. As outlined in Table 11 high sodium intake was associated to an increased MAP as compared to the period on low Na intake (p<0.05). The addition of HCTZ to high sodium intake reduced MAP in comparison with high sodium alone (p<0.05), and MAP returned to levels seen with low Na intake. The study confirms that in CKD patients on chronic ACE inhibition the reduction of mean blood pressure is blunted or even lost during high sodium intake. Addition of HCTZ reduces MAP to level achieved with low Na intake [72].

Table 11. Restoration of the blood pressure effect of chronic ACE inhibition through hydrochlorothiaze during high sodium intake [72]

Period	Sodium intake	Drug	MAP, mm Hg.
A	Low	ACEi	89 (83-96)
B	High	ACEi	98 (91-104)*
C	High	ACEi+HCT	89(83-94)

p*<0.05 vs A and C

In diabetic patients, who have high sodium pool, impaired renal sodium excretion and hypertension, the antihypertensive blood pressure effect of Losartan (50 mg) was studied under low Na intake (85±14 mmol/day) and on regular Na intake (> 100 mmol/day).Under low Na intake SBP was reduced by - 9.7 mm Hg (95% CI -2.2 to - 17.2 mm Hg, p<0.002), DBP by - 5.5 mm Hg (95% CI - 2.6 to -8.4 mm Hg, p<0.002), MAP by -7.3 mm Hg (95% CI - 3.3 to -11.3 mm Hg, p<0.003). Comparable significant differences were also measured for proteinuria. In conclusion a low sodium intake potentiates the effectson blood pressure and proteinuria of losartan in type 2 diabetes [73].

Angiotensin II Receptor Antagonists and Diuretics

In patients with renal disease, uncontrolled hypertension, stable proteinuria (>2 g/day <10 g/day), eGFR > 30 ml/min but eGFR decline < 6 ml/year, a reduction in sodium intake from 196±9 to 92±8 mmol/day caused a significant reduction of systolic and diastolic blood pressure (Table 11) both on placebo, losartan and losartan+ HCT [49]. The low sodium intake was associated with statistical significant reduction of MAP on placebo, losaratan and losartan + hydrochlorothiazide. Sodium restriction maximized the effects of RAAS blockade with losartan, the Angiotensin II type 1 antagonist (AT1), and was additive with hydrochlorothiazide in a randomized, double-blinded, placebo-controlled, crossover study. The lower sodium intake maximized the reduction of proteinuria [74].

Table 12. Effects on blood pressure (mm Hg) of Losartan and Losartan +HCT on high and low sodium intake [74]

Parameter	Na intake	Placebo	Losartan	Losartan+ HCT
SBP	High	143±4‡	135±3*	125±3*†
	Low	137±3	128±3*H	121±2*†H
DBP	High	86±2‡	80±2	75±2*†
	Low	83±1	78±1*	74±1*†

Significant differences: * vs placebo, †vs Losartan, ‡ vs all periods, H vs High Na intake

RAASi and Non-RAASi Anthypertensive Therapy

In a recent study on 1177 patients participating in the RENAAL and IDNT studies (type 2 diabetic patients) ARB receptor blockade (Losartan and Irbersartan, RAASi-based therapy) was compared to non-RAASi –based therapy [75]. The analysis of data about urinary sodium gave interesting results. In the lowest tertile of sodium intake (152±76 mmol/day) RAASi was more protective on urinary albumin excretion and blood pressure in comparison with higher urinary sodium tertiles (179±82 mmol/day and 209±90 mmol/day). The reduction in systolic blood pressure was -5 mm Hg (-8.8 to -1.1 mm Hg) on the low sodium intake and -3.5 mm Hg (-7.4 to +0.4) with the high sodium intake ($p<0.05$ for trend). Also the urinary albumin/creatinine ratio (mg/g) was reduced more ($p<0.05$ for trend) with the low sodium intake (-44 mg/g (-55 to -30 mg/g) than with the high sodium intake -21 mg/g (-35 to - 2 mg/g). The protective effect of RAASi based therapy was lost when sodium intake was maximal. Estimated sodium intake in the lower tertile averaged 8.8 g/day. The favorable effects on urinary on albuminuria and blood pressure were associated with early eGFR reduction but with long-term smaller eGFR decline. The fact that in type 2 diabetic chronic nephropathy, the ARB effect is blunted by high sodium and is protective on low sodium intake suggests that a reduction of salt intake to 5-6 g a day might be more effective, and is a strong call for a policy of population based low sodium intake [75].

ACE Inhibition + Angiotensin II Receptor Antagonists

In non-diabetic CKD patients with proteinuria > 1 g/day, stable creatinine clearance > 30 ml/min, and blood pressure >125/75 on high (184±6 mmol/day) or low Na intake (106±5 mmol/day) the effects of ACE inhibition alone (lisinopril) or in combination with the Angiotensin II Receptor Antagonist (valsartan) were studied by Slagman et al in a randomized controlled study (Table 13) [76]. ACE inhibition alone or in combination with ARB (valsartan) did not affect SBP. On low sodium intake ACE inhibition significantly lowered SBP, an effect which was further increased by the addition of beta-blockade. On high sodium intake ACE inhibition alone did not reduce DBP which was reduced by the combination with ARB. A low sodium intake reduced significantly DBP below values on ACE inhibition and ACE inhibition associated with ARB. The association of low sodium intake with a ARB reduced DBP below values on high sodium intake receiving ACE inhibitor alone or in combination with ARB.

Table 13. Effects of ACE inhibition and ARB in renal patients on high and low sodium intake. Data are mean ± SEM [76]

Study Period	ACEi	ARB	Na intake	SBP (mm Hg)	DBP (mm Hg)
A	+	-	High	134±3	80±2
B	+	+	High	131±3	77±2†
C	+	-	Low	123±1*	73±2†‡
D	+	+	Low	121±2*	71±2†‡

Significant differences * vs A and B for DBP, † vs A, ‡ vs B for DBP.

Comment

The data points out that sodium restriction in combination with antihypertensive drugs significantly increase the anti-hypertensive effect in hypertensive patients and in CKD patients.

Conclusion

Sodium restriction reduced blood pressure in normotensive persons and in prehypertensive and hypertensive individuals including those aged 51 years of age or older. A restriction associated to other changes in lifestyle is a prerequisite to pharmacological treatment. Sodium restriction appears as an efficient and safe adjunct to all classes of antihypertensive drugs with the exception of calcium channel blockers, likely due to the mild sodiuretic effects of these drugs.

A small but significant reduction in resting SBP and DBP is seen in children following a reduction in sodium intake [14]. A small but not deleterious effect which over years may prevent BP increase with age and hypertension is observed. Salt restriction prevents stroke and cardiovascular mortality, reduces urinary calcium excretion and may be advantageous for calcium stone formers and osteoporosis, and increase the effect of ACE inhibitor in chronic kidney disease [77]. AHA and USDA strong recommendations for Na intake should be adopted extensively, having well in mind that the deleterious effects which have been hypothesized in patients on low salt intake are undemonstrated. Taken all together the data discussed herein generate a list of take home messages (Table 14) which may help in preventing the effects of high blood pressure in adults and children.

Table 14. Take home messages

1) Our hunter-gatherers progenitors lived on a low salt diet.
2) Our taste for salt in humans has been developed a few millennia ago, at the time agriculture and animal stabulation were developed, thus salt had to be used for food preservation.
3) With the advent of deep freeze and refrigerators, sodium is no longer needed to store foods however our taste is addicted and the food industry finds expensive to reduce sodium in processed foods.
4) Salt has been a companion for men and women during their history and has affected all human activities including arts and is a reason for the past splendor of Venice.
5) Animal studies (rat, dog, chicken, rabbits, baboon, chimpanzee), studies in low salt populations, migration studies, and intervention studies have shown a causal relation between usual salt intake and blood pressure.
6) The higher the sodium intake from food and beverages, the higher the prevalence of stroke and cardiovascular events.
7) The reduction in salt intake has important falls in hypertensive and normotensive persons irrespective of gender and ethnic group.

8) Population based intervention studies and meta-analysis of randomised controlled trial have shown that blood pressure may be significantly reduced by reducing salt intake.
9) Evidence on salt and blood pressure is consistent and persuasive (78).
10) Reducing of 5 g the habitual salt intake is associated with a 23% reduction in the rate of stroke and a 17% difference in cardiovascular diseases.
11) A reduction in NaCl intake of 5g/day might spare yearly 1250000 deaths from stroke, and some 3 million deaths cardiovascular disease worldwide.
12) The World Health Organization strongly recommended in 2012 "a reduction of sodium intake to reduce blood pressure risk of cardiovascular disease, stroke and coronary heart disease in adults [≥ 16 years of age] to < 2g day sodium (5 g/day salt) [100 mmol]". In addition WHO strongly recommended "a reduction in sodium intake to control blood pressure in children [2-15 years of age]" for whom "the maximum level of sodium intake of 2 g/day in adults should be adjusted downwards based on the energy requirements of children relative to those of adults". Those recommendations apply to all individuals with or without hypertension".
13) Sodium restriction is a prerequisite to prevent the consequences of high blood pressure.
14) Sodium restriction is preliminary to any pharmacological intervention in patients with high blood pressure.
15) A constant monitoring of salt intake should start in childhood since BP tracks.
16) In hypertensive patients a reduction of sodium intake < 100 mmol/day is a significant adjunct to the lowering BP effects of ACE inhibitors, ARB blockers alone or in combination, direct renin inhibitors, beta-blockers and diuretics.
17) In hypertensive and well as in patients with diabetic and non-diabetic renal disease the hypotensive effect of calcium channel blockers is not potentiated by sodium restriction.
18) Sodium restriction and/or diuretics should be not used to treat edema in patients on calcium channel blockers.
19) In diabetic and non-diabetic patients with renal disease, sodium restriction potentiates the lowering blood pressure effects of ACE inhibitors, angiotensin II receptor antagonists, diuretics, beta-blockers.
20) Na intake is a problem in countries with high, medium and low state economies.
21) Reducing sodium intake is a state problem.
22) Sodium restriction is feasible.
23) Industry should be supported in reducing the amount of salt in food processing.
24) The general population should be made aware of Na content in foods.
25) Labelling the sodium content of foods is of paramount importance.
26) The general public needs to be reminded regularly that reduction in salt intake prevents heart attacks and strokes. The media have this possibility and should consider it as a duty.

Abbreviations

BP	Blood Pressure
CKD	Chronic Kidnye Disease
DBP	Diastolic Blood Pressure
ERPF	Effective Renal Plasma Flow
GFR	Glomerular Filtration Rate
SBP	Systolic Blood Pressure
USDA	United States Department of Agriculture
WHO	World Health Organization

Acknowledgements

The chapter is dedicated to Carmelo Giordano, MD, Mario Mancini, MD, Jeremiah Stamler MD for their admirable mentoring and to the Second University of Naples, the University of Naples Federico II, and the Northwestern University in Chicago places for clinical scientists.

References

[1] Eaton SB, Eaton SB III, Konner MJ. Palelithic nutrition revisited: A twelve-year retrospective on its nature and implications. *Eur J Clin Nutr* 1997; 51: 207-216.

[2] Konner M, Eaton SB. Paleolithic nutrition, twenty-five years after. *Nutrition in Clinical Practice* 2010; 25: 594-602.

[3] Stamler J. Improved Life Styles: their Potential for the Prevention of Atherosclerosis and Hypertension in Childhood". In Lauer M and Shekelle RR Eds, Childhood Prevention of Atherosclerosis ans Hypertension. New York, Raven Press, 1980¸291.op.cit., 1980; pp.3-36.

[4] Denton D, Weisinger R, Mundy NI, Wicking EJ, Dixon A, Moisson P, Pingard AM, Shade R, Carey D, Ardaillou R, Paillard F, Chapman J, Thillet J, Michel JB. The effect of increased salt intake on blood pressure in cimpanzees. *Nature Medicine* 1995; 1: 1009-1016.

[5] Elliott P, Walker LL, Little MP, Blair-West JR, Shade RE, Lee R, Rouquet P, Leroy E, Jeunemaitre X, Ardaillou R, Paillard F, Meneron P, Denton DA. Change in Salt Intake Affects Blood Presure of Chimpanzees. Implications for Human Population. *Circulation* 2007; 116: 1563-1568.

[6] Dahl LK. Effects of chronic excess salt loading. Induction of self-sustaining hypertension in rats. *J Exp Med* 1961; 114: 231-6

[7] De Santo NG, Bisaccia C, Cirillo M, De Santo RM, De Santo LS, De Santo D, Papalia T, Capasso G, and De Napoli N. A contribution to history of common salt. *Kidney Int* 1997; 51, Suppl. 59, S127S134

[8] Hocquet J-C. Le Sel de la Terre. Paris, Du May, 1989, p.44.

[9] Cirillo M, Capasso G, Di Leo VA, De Santo NG. A history of salt. *Am J Nephrol* 1994; 14:

[10] De Santo NG, Capasso G, Giordano DR, Aulisio L, Anastasio P, Annunziata F, Armanini B, Coppola S, Musacchio R. Nephrology in the Natural History of Pliny the Elder. *Am J Nephrol* 1989; 9: 252-260.

[11 Bisaccia C, De Santo RM, De Santo LS, De Santo D, Bellini L, De Santo NG. The Symbolism of Salt in Paintings. *Am J Nephrol* 1997; 17: 318-329.

[12] De Santo NG, Bisaccia C, De Santo RM, De Santo LS, Gallo L, Petrelli L, Cirillo M, Capasso G. Common salt: nutrition, symbolism and iconology. In *Contributions for the history of nutrition*, De Santo NG and Marotta P, Eds, Naples, Citta del Sole, 1996; pp. 135-199.

[13] Cirillo M, Del Giudice L, Bilancio G, Franzese MD, De Santo NG. Low salt diet and treatment of hypertension. *J Nephrol* 2009; 22(S14):S136-S138.

[14] Ambard L, Beaujard E. Causes de l'hypertension arterielle. *Arch Gen Med* 1904; 1: 520-533.

[15] Ambard L, Beaujard E. La retention clorurée sèche. Semaine Med 1905;25 :133-136.

[16] Allen FM. Arterial Hypertension. *JAMA* 1920;74:652-655.

[17] Allen FM, Sherrill JW. The treatment of essential hypertension. *J Metab Res* 1922;2:429-545.

[18] Kempner W. Treatment of kidney disease and of hypertensive vascular disease with rice diet. *North Carolina Med J* 1944;5:125-133.

[19] Kempner W. Treatment of hypertensive vascular disease with rice diet. *Am J Med* 1948;4:545-

[20] Corcoran AC, Taylor RD, Page IH. Controlled observations on the effect of low sodium dietotherapy in essential hypertension. *Circulation* 195; 3:1-16.

[21] Page LB. Dietary sodium and blood pressure: Evidence from human studies. In Lauer M and Shekelle RR, Eds, *Childhood prevention of Atherosclerosis and Hypertension*. New York, Raven Press 1980; pp. 261.

[22] Hofman A, Hazebroek A, Valkenburg HA. A randomized trial of sodium intake and blood pressure in newborn infants. *JAMA*. 1983;250:370-373

[23] Geleijnse J, Hofman A, Witteman CM, Hazebroek AAJM, Valkenburg HA, Grobbee DE. Long term effects of neonatal Sodium Restriction on Blood Pressure, *Hypertension* 1997; 29: 913-917.

[24] Intersalt: an international study of electrolyte excretion and blood pressure. Results from 24 hour urinary sodium and potassium excretion. *BMJ* 1988; 297: 319-328.

[25] Elliot P, Stamler J, Nichols R, Dyer AR, Stamler R, Kestelot H, Marmot M for the Intersalt Cooperative Research Group. *BMJ*, 1996; 312: 1249-1253.

[26] Appel LJ, Moore TJ, Obarzenek E, Vollmer WM, Svetkey LP, Sacks FM, Bray GA, Vogt TM, Cutler JA, Windhauser MM, Lin P-H, and Karanja N for the DASH Collaborative research Group. A clinical trial of the effects of dietary patterns on blood pressure. *N Engl J Med* 1997; 336: 1117-24.

[27] Sacks FM, Svetkey LP, Vollmer WM, Appel LJ, Bray GA, Harsha D, Obarzanek E, Conlin PR, Miller II ER, Simons-Morton DG, Karanja N, and Lin P-H, for the DASH-Sodium Collaborative Research Group. *N Engl J Med* 2001; 344: 3-10.

[28] Vollmer WM, Sacks FM, Appel LJ, Bray GA, Simons-Marton DG, Conlin PR, Svetkey LP, Erlinger TP, Moore TJ, and Karanja N, for the DASH-Sodium Trial Collaborative

research Group. Effects of Diet and Sodium Intake on Blood Pressure: Subgroup Analysis of the Dash-Sodium Trial. *Ann Intern Med* 2001; 135: 1019-1028.

[29] Aburto NJ, Ziolkovska A Hooper L, Elliot P, Cappuccio FP, Meerpohl JJ. Effects of lower sodium intake on health: systematic review and meta-analyses. BMJ 2013; 346: f1326.

[30] He FJ, Li J, MacGregor G. Effect of longer term modest salt reduction on blood pressure: Cochrane systematic review and meta-analysis of randomized trials. *BMJ* 2013; 346: f1325.

[31] Stolarz-Skrzypek K, Kuznetsova T, Thijs L, Tikhonoff V, Seidlerova J, Richart T et al. Fatal and non fatal outcomes, incidence of hypertension, and blood pressure changes in relation to urinary sodium excretion. *JAMA* 2011; 305: 1777-85.

[32] O'Donnel MJ, Yusuf S, Mente A, Gao P, Man JF, Teo K, et al. Urinary sodium and portassium excretion and risk of cardiovascular events. *JAMA* 2011; 306: 2229-38

[33] Taylor RS, Ashton KE, Moxham T, Hooper L, Ebrahim S. Reduced dietary salt for the prevention of cardiovascular disease: a meta-analysis of randomized controlled trails (Cochrane Review). *Am J Hpertens* 2011, 24: 843-53.

[34] Paterna S, Gaspare P, Fasullo S, Sarullo FM, Di Pasquale P. Normal-sodium diet compared with low-sodium diet in compensated congestive heart failure: is sodium an old enemy or a new friend? *Clin Sci (London)* 2008; 114. 221-30.

[35] Strazzullo P, D'Elia L, Kandala NB, Cappuccio FP. Salt intale, stroke, and cardiovascular disease: meta-analysis of prospective studies. *BMJ* 2009; 339:b4567.

[36] Cappuccio F, Chen Ji. Less salt and less risk of stroke. Further support to action. *Stroke* 2012; 43: 1195-96.

[37] Gardner H, Rundek T, Wright CB, Elkind MSV, Sacco RL. Dietary sodium and stroke in Northern Manhattan Study. *Stroke* 2012; 43: 1200-1205.

[38] Clarke WR,. Schrott HG, Leaverton PE, Connor WE, and Lauer RM. Tracking of blood lipids and blood pressures in school age children.the Muscatine Study. *Circulation* 1978; 58: 626-634.

[39] Lauer RM, Clarke WR, Beaglehole R. level, trend and variability of blood pressure during chidlhood: The Muscatine Study. *Circulation* 1984; 69: 242-249.

[40] Amnest JL, Sing CF, Biron P, Mongeau JG. Familial aggregation of blood pressure and weight in adoptive families.II. Estimation of the relative contributions of genetic and common environmental factors to blood pressure correlations between family members. *Am J Epidemiol1987*; Suppl.3, 110: 479-491.

[41] Report of the Second Task Force on Bood Pressure Control in Children-1987. *Pediatrics* 1987; 70:1-25.

[42] De Santo NG, Trevisan M, Capasso G. Hypertension in childhood, *Semin Nephrol* 1989; 9:207-303.

[43] Alon U and De Santo NG. Pediatric Hypertension. *Child Nephrol Urol* 1992 ; 12 : 69-175.

[44] Cirillo M, Laurenzi M, Stamler J. Factors Related to Blood Pressure in a Sample of Italian Children Age 5 to 14: The Gubbio Population Study. *Semin Nephrol* 1989; 267-271.

[45] Ellison RC, Capper AL, Stephenson WP, Goldberg RJ, Hosmer DW Jr, Humphrey KF, et al. Effects on blood pressure of a decrease in sodium use in institutional food preparation: The Exeter-Andover Project. *J Clin Epidemiol*1989;42:201-8.

[46] Howe PR, Jureidini KF, Smith RM. Sodium and blood pressure in children—a short-term dietary intervention study. *Proc Nutr Soc Austr* 1985;10:121-4.

[47] Miller JZ, Weinberger MH, Daugerty SA, Fineberg NS, Christian JC, Grim, CE. Blood pressure response to dietary sodium restriction in healthy normotensive children. *Am J Clin Nutr1988*;47:113-9.

[48] Palacios C, Wigertz K, Martin BR, Jackman L, Pratt JH, Peacock M, et al. Sodium retention in black and white female adolescents in response to salt intake. *J Clin Endocrinol Metab*2004;89:1858-63.

[49] Trevisan M, Cooper R, Ostrow D, Miller W, Sparks S, Leonas Y, et al. Dietary sodium, erythrocyte sodium concentration, sodium-stimulated lithium efflux and blood pressure. *Clin Sci (Lond)* 1981;61(Suppl 7):29-32.

[50] Calabrese EJ, Tuthill RW. The Massachusetts blood pressure study, part 3. Experimental reduction of sodium in drinking water: effects on blood pressure. *Toxicol Ind Health* 1985;19-34.

[51] Gillum RF, Elmer PJ, Prineas RJ. Changing sodium intake in children. The Minneapolis Children's Blood Pressure Study. *Hypertension* 1981;3:698-703.

[52] Sinaiko AR, Gomez-Marin O, Prineas RJ. Effect of low sodium diet or potassium sup plementation on adolescent blood pressure. Hypertension1993;21(6 Pt2):989-94.

[53] IOM. Dietary Reference Intakes for Water, Potassium, Sodium, Chloride, and Sulfate. Washington, D.C, National Academies Press, 2004-424.

[54] HHS and USDA (U.S. Department of Health and Human Services and U.S. Department of Agriculture). The report of Dietary Guidelines Advisory Committee on Dietary Guidelines for Americans, 2010, to the Secretary of Agriculture and the Secretary of Health and Human Services, Washington DC; 2010, USDA/ARS

[55] WHO. Guidelines: Sodium intake for adult and children. Geneva, World Health Organization (WHO), 2012, p.18

[56] Campbell NRC, Cappuccio FP, and Tobe SW. Unnecessary controversy regarding dietary sodium: A lot about a little. *Can J Cardiol* 2011; 27: 404-406.

[57] IOM (Institute of Medicine). Sodium intake in Populations. Assessment of Evidence. Washington DC, The National Academic Press, 2013.

[58] Navis G, De Jong PE, Donker ABJM, Van Der Hem GK, and Dick de Zeeuw. Moderate sodium restriction in hypertensive subjects: Renal effects of ACE-inhibition. *Kidney Int* 1987; 31: 815-819

[59] Singer DRJ, Markandu ND, Sugden AL, Miller MA, and MacGregor GA. Sodium Restriction in Hypertensive Patients Treated With a Converting Enzyme Inhibitor and a Thiazide. *Hypertension* 1991; 17: 798-803.

[60] Wing LMH, Arnolda LF, Harvey PJ, Uptom J, Molloy D, Gabb GM, Bune AJC, and Chalmers JP. Low-dose diuretic and/or dietary sodium restriction when blood pressure is resistant to ACE inhibitors. *Blood Pressure* 1998; 7: 299-307

[61] Weir MR, Yadao AM, Prkhayastha D, and Charney AN. Effects of High- and Low-Sodium Diets on Ambulatory Blood Pressure in Patients with Hypertension Receiving Aliskiren. *J Cardiovascular Pharmacol* 2010; 15: 356-363

[62] Erweteman TM, Nagelkerke N, Kubsen J, Koster M, Dunning AJ. βBlockade, diuretic, and salt restriction for the management of mild hypertension: a randomised double blind trial. *BMJ* 1984; 289: 406-409.

[63] Weir MR, Hall PS, Behrens MT, Flack JM. Salt and Blood Pressure Response to Calcium Antagonism in Hypertensive Patients. Hypertension 1997: 30: 422-427.

[64] Nicholson JP Pickering TG, Resnick LM, Laragh JH. The hypotensive effects of calcium channel blockade with verapamil is enhanced by increased sodium intake. (Abstract). *Clin Res* 1084; 32: 245A.

[65] Nicholson JP, Resnick LM, James JD, Jennis R. Sodium restriction and the antiproteinuric effect of nitrendipine (abstract). *Clin Res* 1986; 34: 404A.

[66 Nicholson JPW, Resnick LM, Laragh JH. The antihypertensive effect of Verapamil a extreme of dietary salt intake. *Ann Intern Med* 1987; 107: 329-334.

[67] Del Rio A, Rodriguez-Villamil JL, López-Campos JM, Carrera F. Effect of moderate salt restriction on the antihypertensive action of nifedipine: a double blind study. *Rev Clin Esp* 1990; 186: 5-10.

[68] Luft FC, Weinberger MH. Review of salt restriction and the response to antihypertensive drugs. Satellite symposium on calcium antagonists. *Hypertension* 1988; 11: I-229-I231.

[69] Sica DA. Calcium Channel Blocker-Related Peripheral Edema: Can It Be Resolved? *J Clin Hypertension* 2003; 5: 291-295.

[70] Wapstra FH, van Goor H, Navis G, de Jong PE, de Zeeuw D. Antiproteinuric effect predicts renal protection by angiotensin-converting enzyme inhibition in rats with established adryamicin nephrosis. *Clin Sci (Lond)* 1996; 90: 393-401.

[71] Heeg JE, de Jong PE, Van Der Hem GK, de Zeeuw D. Efficacy and variability of the antiproteinuric effect of ACE inhibition by Lisinopril. *Kidney Int* 1989; 36: 272-279.

[72] Buter H, Hemmelder MH, Navis G, de Jong PE, de Zeeuw D. The bluntiung of the antiproteinuric efficacy of ACE inhibition by high sodium intake can be reversed by hydrochlorothiazide. *Nephrol Dial transplant* 1998; 13: 1682-1685.

[73] Houlihan C, Allen TJ, Baxter AL, Panagiotopoulos S, Casley DJ, Cooper ME, Jerums G. A low sodium diet potentiates the effects of losartan in type 2 diabetes. *Diabetes Care* 2002; 25: 663-671.

[74] Vogt L, Waanders F, Broomsa F, dee Zeeuw D, and Navis G. Effects of Dietary Sodium and Hydrochlorothiazide on the Antiproteinuric efficacy of Losartan. *J Am Soc Nephrol* 2008; 19: 999-2007.

[75] Lambers Heerspink HJ, Holtkamp FA. Parving H-H, Navis G, Lewis JB, Ritz E, de Graeff PA, and de Zeeuw D. Moderation of dietary sodium potentiates the renal and cardiovascular protective effects of angiotensin receptor blockers. *Kidney In.* 2012; 82. 330-7]

[76] Slagman MCJ, Waanders F, Hemmelder MH, Janssen WMT, Lambers HJ, Navus G, Laverman GD. Moderate dietary sodium restriction added to angiotensin converting enzyme inhibition compared with dual blockade in lowering proteinuria and blood pressure: randomised controlled trial. *BMJ* 2011;343: d4366.

[77] Kaplan N. Salt intake, salt restriction, and essential hypertension. *UpToDate* 2013; 2013.

[78] Elliott P, Stamler J. Commentary: Evidence on salt and blood pressure is consistent and persuasive. *Int J Epidemiol* 2002; 34: 316-319.

SECTION 2. ACE INHIBITORS AND ANGIOTENSIN RECEPTOR BLOCKERS IN SPECIAL PATIENT POPULATIONS

In: ACE Inhibitors. Volume 2
Editor: Macaulay Amechi Onuigbo
ISBN: 978-1-62948-422-8

Chapter 8

ARE ARBS THE PREFERRED AGENTS TO TREAT HYPERTENSION IN PATIENTS WITH HIV-NEPHROPATHY WITH ALBUMINURIA?

Biagio Di Iorio, MD,[1,*] Antonio Bellasi, MD[2] and Giovanni Guaraldi, MD[3]
[1]Department of Nephrology and Dialysis, PO "A Landolfi" – Solofra (AV), Italy
[2]Department of Nephrology and Dialysis, Azienda Ospedaliera Sant'Anna-Como, Como, Italy
[3]Department of Medical and Surgical Sciences for Adults and Children, Clinic of Infectious Diseases, University of Modena and Reggio Emilia, Italy

ABSTRACT

Numerous signs of renal dysfunction such as proteinuria, crystalluria and microhematuria as well as a variety of other renal syndromes may characterize the course of HIV infection and lead to renal failure. It is estimated that approximately 1% to 2% of patients starting dialysis suffer from HIV-associated renal disease.

HIV-associated nephropathy (HIVAN) occurs in about 10% of HIV-infected subjects with a distinct predilection for Blacks and Hispanic individuals. This nephropathy is characterized by glomerular basement membrane thickening, wrinkling and folding, segmental or global collapse of the glomerular tufts, increase in the Bowman space, and podocytes abnormalities. Large podocytes filled with protein droplets often accumulate in layers around the collapsed areas forming the pseudocrescents. Tubular atrophy, interstitial inflammation and different degree of fibrosis are generally associated with the glomerular damage.

Until antiretroviral therapy (ART) became available, HIVAN was characterized by a rapid renal function decline and progression to end-stage renal disease. Aside from the HIV direct injury to the nephron, numerous experimental observations lend support to the notion that Angiotensin II contributes to podocytes damage and treatment with angiotensin-converting enzyme inhibitors (ACE-Is) as well as angiotensin receptor

* E-mail: br.diiorio@gmail.com.

blockers (ARBs) may attenuate renal function decline in HIVAN. However, clinical data on the impact of these antihypertensive agents in HIV infected individuals are still scanty and uncertainties still remain to be properly addressed. We herein analyze the studies that investigated the use of ACE-Is and ARBs in the treatment of hypertension in patients with HIV-nephropathy (HIVAN) and albuminuria.

RENAL DYSFUNCTION AND FAILURE IN HIV

The prevalence of kidney disease among HIV infected individuals is higher in people with long standing HIV infection [1]. Both acute renal failure and chronic kidney disease (CKD) occurring in HIV infection maybe due to theincreasing age and comorbidities such as diabetes mellitus and hypertension or exposures tonephrotoxic drugs such as antibiotics and antifungals, tobacco, hepatitis C and other chronic infections that are among the strongest risk factors for renal dysfunction. A recent survey from the EUROSIDA Cohort analyzed predictors of advanced CKD, end-stage renal disease and renal death among 9044 HIV-positive individuals in Europe [2]. According to this survey, the incidence rate of CKD/ESRD/renal death was 1.32/1000 person-years of follow-up and the independent predictors of the endpoint included any cardiovascular event, lower eGFR and CD4 count [2]. Other studies investigating the prevalence of CKD among HIV infected subjects (defined as the presence proteinuria and/or glomerular filtration rate (GFR) lover than 60 ml/min) report on 3.5-4.7% in Europe, Argentina and Israel [3], 11 % in USA [4], 33 to 38 % in Zambia [5] and Nigeria [6], and 48.5% in Uganda [7], respectively. In our experience, in a sample of 1151 subjects with HIV infection followed at the University of Modena and Reggio Emilia, a normal renal function (defined as an estimated GFR greater than 90 ml/min/1.73 m^2 without evidence of proteinuria or hematuria) was found in only about 50% subjects (Table 1). All other patients had different degrees of renal impairment or dysfunction (Figure 1). The peak incidence of HIVAN requiring dialysis occurred in the 1990's and remained stable after thanks to early detection of HIV and the wide spread of HAART [8,9]. Nonetheless, it is estimated that about 10% of HIV-1–infected individuals suffer from HIVAN, a condition characterized by severe podocyte abnormalities, heavy proteinuria, and rapid progression to end-stage renal failure (ESRD). Of interest, the marked racial predilection for Black and Hispanic people observed in many studies suggests a genetic predisposition to HIVAN [10].

Table 1. Renal function and urinary abnormalities in 1151 subjects followed at University of Modena and Reggio Emilia

	N of patients	% of patients
Total patients	1151	
Normal Renal function*	560	48.6
GFR decline no urinary abnormalities	299	25.9
Proteinuria (detected via urinary dipstick)	154	13.4
Ematuria (detected via urinary dipstick)	175	15.2
Proteinuria+Ematuria (detected via urinary dipstick)	37	3.2

*defined as an estimated GFR greater tha 90 ml/min/1.73 m^2 without evidence of proteinuria or ematuria detected via urinary dipstick.

eGFR estimated via CKD-EPI formula

	>90		89-60		<60	
	No proteinuria	Proteinuria	No proteinuria	Proteinuria	No Proteinuria	Proteinuria
No Ematuria	77.9	6.9	71.8	13.6	45.2	33.3
Ematuria	12.5	2.6	11.8	2.8	4.8	16.7

	>90	89-60	<60
Overall prevalence of ematuria	15.1	14.6	21.4
Overall prevalence of proteinuria	9.6	16.4	50.0
Overall prevalence of ematuria and proteinuria	2.6	2.8	16.6

Figure 1. Renal function (%) and urinary abnormalities (%) in 1151 subjects followed at University of Modena and Reggio Emilia.

Furthermore, HIVAN incidence varies depending on the geographic distribution of HIV infection though the lack of consensus on the diagnostic criteria adopted to define HIVAN may partly account for some of the reported variability. The term HIVAN should be used if the typical histologic lesions such as focal segmental glomerular sclerosis (FSGS) with glomerular capillary collapse, glomerular basement membrane retractation and podocyte hypertrophy and hyperplasia as well as tubulointerstitial changes are detected [11-19]. Another histological pattern of renal lesions characterized by immune-complex deposition has also been described prevalently in African-American HIV infected individuals (HIVICK, HIV immune-complex kidney disease). Though the pathophysiology of this pattern is far from being elucidated, this form of nephropathy seems less likely to result in ESRD when compared to HIVAN [20].

Irrespective of the histological pattern, the Infectious Disease Society of America suggests Black race, male sex, CD4 count less than 200 cell/mm3, HIV RNA levels greater than 4000 copies/ml as risk factors for proteinuria and CKD [21-22].

In 1994, Burns and coworkers first reported a significant reduction in proteinuria and renal function decline in a subject with biopsy-proven HIVAN treated with fosinopril suggesting the clinical relevance of the Renin-Angiotensin-Aldosterone-System (RAAS) inhibition in HIVAN [23].

This as well as subsequent reports and experimental evidence corroborate the notion that RAAS inhibition with a combination of agents may be beneficial and preserve the renal function beyond the antihypertensive action of these agents [26-27]. Indeed,
angiotensin II-associated glomerular damage may share common features with the hemodynamic as well as the histopathologic changes observed in HIVAN. Though we currently lack randomized controlled trials (RCTs) in HIV subjects, it is widely accepted that in patients treated with ACE inhibitors or ARBs, the reduction in 24-hour urinary protein excretion as well as serum creatinine stabilization are strictly dependent on the attenuation of the glomerular hemodynamic and fibrotic actions of angiotensin II. It is plausible that

inhibition of the RAAS may potentially slow the renal function decline in HIV subjects with proteinuria especially in the era of HAART that allows for an efficient HIV infection control, and has undoubtedly increased life expectancy in HIV infected individuals [8, 9].

Though not specifically meant for HIVAN, the American Society of Nephrology in 1997 made a strong recommendation in favor of the use of ACE-Is in non-diabetic renal disease, particularly in high-risk groups with rapidly declining glomerular filtration rate or increased proteinuria [28], such as HIVAN patients [29].

RAAS Attenuation in HIV: Evidence from Experimental Studies

Animal models such as transgenic mice expressing the envelope, regulatory, and accessory genes of HIV-I may develop renal disease that resemble HIVAN and provide the scientific community an experimental model to test the efficacy of different drugs. Bird and coworkers studied the effect of captopril in 25 mice with HIVAN [30]. At study completion, renal function, glomerular and interstitial changes, as well as survival were all improved among treated animals [30]. Other studies suggest that Angiotensin II mediated part of the renal damage seen in HIVAN. Ideura and coworkers demonstrated in a transgenic mice model that Angiotensin II infusion was associated with an accelerated podocyte injury similar to what was seen after a nephrectomy [31]. These lesions were prevented by RAAS inhibition [31]. These authors hypothesized that agiotensin II may induce or accelerate the podocyte injury by increasing the intraglomerular capillary pressure and/or via a direct toxic effect on podocytes [32-37]. In a transgenic mice model (podocin/Vpr) expressing vpr (one of the HIV-1 accessory genes) selectively in podocytes, the same group of investigators demonstrated that treatment with doxycycline for 8 to 12 week induced renal injuries similar to HIVAN [38]. However, the concomitant administration of olmesartan (Angiotensin II type 1 receptor blocker) exerted a renoprotective effect by reducing proteinuria and preventing glomerulosclerosis independent of systemic blood pressure reduction [38]. All taken together, these data suggest that as renal function declines, the reduction in nephron mass amplifies the podocyte injury and subsequent glomerulosclerosis, possibly worsening glomerular hypertension. Nevertheless, Angiotensin II receptor blocker administration can ameliorate glomerular hypertension, podocyte injury and attenuate renal function loss [38].

Kumar and coworkers reached similar conclusions [39]. They evaluated the effect of aliskiren, an inhibitor of the renin activity, on the progression of renal lesions in two different mouse models (Vpr and Tg26) of HIVAN. At study completion, Aliskiren administration resulted in significant reductios in renal lesions progression, proteinuria and blood urea levels ($p<0.01$) [39]. Although treated mice also experienced a significant blood pressure drop, these findings further corroborate the notion that RAAS modulation may slow down the progression of HIVAN [39].

To evaluate the contribution of Angiotensin II in HIVAN, Shimizu generated two transgenic mice models carrying either the HIV-1 gene (control/HIV-1) or both HIV-1 gene and podocyte-selectively nullified AT1 gene (AT1KO/HIV-1) [40]. Both models developed HIVAN at 8 months of age. Indeed, urinary albumin/creatinine ratio (median 2.5 versus 9.1 mg/mg), glomerulosclerosis (median 0.63 versus 0.45 on 0–4 scale) and down-regulation of nephrin (median 6.90 versus 7.02 on 0–8 scale) were statistically identical in AT1KO/HIV-1 as well as control/HIV-1 mice [40]. Nevertheless, after AT1 blocker treatment, a significant reduction in proteinuria and glomerulosclerosis was noted in control/HIV-1 but not AT1KO/HIV-1 mice, suggesting that the protective effect of ARB therapy was mediated through its receptors on cells other than podocytes, such as efferent arteriolar smooth muscle cells [40].

Finally, using a different experimental approach, Zhong and coworkers concluded that the combination of an ACE-I with a histone deacetylase inhibitor (HDACI) could reverse the maximal number of genes altered in mice models of HIVAN suggesting that ACEI may interfere with HIV genes expression at the kidney level [41].

In summary, experimental evidence suggests that RAAS inhibition may represent a valid clinical target to attenuate HIVAN; however whether the use of ACE-I or ARB should be preferred is yet to be clarified.

RAAS Attenuation in HIV: Evidence from Clinical Studies

Though no RCTs have ever formally tested the impact of RAAS inhibition on HIVAN, various clinical reports suggest that the use of ACE-Is and ARBs is safe and can be beneficial in HIVAN. Burns and coworkers documented in 7/11 and 5/9 HIV infected subjects with non-nephrosic and nephrosic proteinuria, respectively, that treatment with fosinopril (10 mg/day for 12 to 24 weeks) was associated with renal function stabilization and a significant reduction in proteinuria [42]. In another case series of 18 patients, Kimmel et al reported on a significant increase in renal survival among patients treated with captopril when compared to patients not treated with ACE-Is (mean renal survival 156 vs 37 days, respectively), in addition to HAART [43].Though blood pressure control was not reported, multivariable adjustments for CD4 count, age, serum creatinine and urine protein/creatinine ratio did not significantly affect these results [43].

In another observational study of 44 HIV infected subjects with biopsy-proven HIVAN, Wei and coworkers reported significant renal progression attenuation associated with ACEI use [44]. All recruited subjects had a serum creatinine less 2 mg/dl at study inception whereas 24 (54.5 %) and 20 (45.5%) presented a non-nephrotic or nephrotic proteinuria, respectively. Sixteen of the 16 (100%) patients that did not receive treatment with ACE-I as compared to only 1 of the 28 (4%) patients treated with fosinopril (10 mg/day) progressed to ESRD [44]. Of interest, treated patients were followed up for 180 to 1890 days (median 479 days; of note 10 subjects had a followup longer than 1000 days) as compared to 33 to 360 days of the untreated patients (median 140 days) [44]. The greater renal survival was also coupled with a better overall survival (6 v.s. 14 deathsin the fosinopril and control group, respectively) [44]. Though encouraging, the effect of fosinopril on blood pressure was not analyzed in this as in previous studies.

In another retrospective study, Szczech and collaborators observed that the use of ACE-Is or ARBswas associated with a significant risk reduction of ESRD (Hazard Ratio: 0.41; 95% Confidence Interval: 0.15-0.96; p<0.04) in a cohort of 87 HIVAN patients followed at the Indiana University School of Medicine, Mount Sinai School of Medicine, Wake Forest University, Emory University, MetroHealth Medical Center (Cleveland), and Duke

University Medical Center between January 1, 1995 and January 1, 2001. Similar to previous reports, these authors did not analyze the impact of blood pressure on the risk of CKD progression [45].

In a small double blinded, randomized clinical trial aimed at testing the safety of the use of lisinopril in combination with pravastatin in HIV–infected subjects, Baker and coworkers randomized 34 subjects to 4 different treatment regimens (Lisinopril 10 mg/day + placebo; lisinopril 10 mg/day + pravastatin 20 mg/day; placebo + pravastatin 20 mg/day; placebo + placebo) for 4 months [46]. At study completion, the combination of lisinopril and pravastatin was well tolerated and associated with a significant reduction of markers of inflammation (high sensitivity C-reactive protein, interleukin-6 and tumor necrosis factor-alpha) and blood pressure, suggesting an anti-inflammatory effect of the combined treatment that may potentially contribute to reduced CKD progression [46].

Bigé and coworkers in another retrospective study that recruited 57 patients with HIVAN treated with highly active antiretroviral therapy between 2000 and 2009 described a significant renal survival benefit associated with RAAS blockade [47]. In this cohort of relatively young (median age 41, range 18-58) individuals prevalently of African origin (87%) with severe renal dysfunction (mean eGFR 20 mL/min/1.73m^2), high-grade proteinuria (4.1 g/day; range 0.6–16.8 g/day), high proportion of sclerotic glomeruli (mean 31.5%), and low CD4 count (mean 127/mm^3), treatment with RAAS-blockers was associated with a significantly greater life expectancy (Hazard Ratio: 5.23; 95%Confidence Interval: 1.19-23.0; p=0.028) [47]. Of interest, systolic blood pressure (Hazard Ratio: 3.97; 95% Confidence Interval: 0.88-17.98; p=0.07) and diastolic blood pressure (Hazard Ratio: 0.98; 95% Confidence Interval: 0.33-2.93; p=0.97) were not associated with evolution to ESRD during follow-up [47].

Though the results of these observational studies are promising, [42-47], they were not confirmed by a very recent systematic review published in 2013 that searched the medical literature for RCTs and quasi-RCTs of any therapy used in the treatment of HIVAN [48]. The authors of this systematic review could only identify 4 different RCTs of which 3 are still unpublished and one, registered in 2004 (NCT 00089518), was terminated before study conclusion without any specific reasons being provided [48]. This was a phase III study aimed at comparing the impact of valsartan (ARB) in association with HAART vs HAART alone, on physical examination, medication assessment and blood pressure readings. This Cochrane group of investigators concluded that there is not currently any RCT to base recommendations on treatment of HIVAN and that only data from observational studies are available to support the use of steroids and RAAS blockage in patients with HIVAN [48].

CONCLUSION

In summary, current use of ACE-Is or ARBs in HIVAN relies upon experimental and observational data. Though there is a strong rationale and encouraging preliminary data, the role of RAAS blockage in HIVAN remains to be confirmed in any RCT studies. However, in consideration of the new highly effective anti-viral regimens, which have significantly improved survival of HIV-infected individuals, a larger number of patients may experience renal dysfunction during the course of HIV infection [8,9].While future RCT studies aiming at shedding further light on this cogent question are awaited, the use of compounds to block the RAAS seems safe and effective, particularly in high-risk groups with rapidly declining glomerular filtration rate or increased proteinuria,[28], such as HIVAN patients [29].

References

[1] Mocroft A., Kirk O., Reiss P., de Wit S., Sedlacek D., Beniowski M., et al. Estimated glomerular filtration rate, chronic kidney disease and antiretroviral drug use in HIV-positive patients. *AIDS*, 2010; 24: 1667–1678.

[2] Ryom L., Kirk O., Lundgren J. D., Reiss P., Pedersen C., De Wit S., Buzunova S., Gasiorowski J., Gatell J. M., Mocroft A. EuroSIDA in EuroCoord. Advanced chronic kidney disease, end-stage renal disease and renal death among HIV-positive individuals in Europe. *HIV Med.,* 2013 Apr 16. doi: 10.1111/hiv.12038. [Epub ahead of print].

[3] Mocroft A., Kirk O., Gatell J., Reiss P., Gargalianos P., Zilmer K. et al. Chronic renal failure among HIV-1-infected patients. *AIDS.*, 2007; 21: 1119-1127.

[4] Wyatt C. M., Winston J. A., Malvestutto C. et al. Chronic kidney disease in HIV infection: an urban epidemic. *AIDS.,* 2007; 21: 2101-2103.

[5] Mulenga L. B., Kruse G., Lakhi S., Cantrell R. A., Reid S. E., Zulu I. et al. Baseline renal insufficiency and risk of death among HIV-infected adults on antiretroviral therapy in Lusaka, Zambia. *AIDS.,* 2008; 22: 1821-1827.

[6] Emem C. P., Arogundade F., Sanusi A., Adelusola K., Wokoma F., Akinsola A. Renal disease in HIV-seropositive patients in Nigeria: an assessment of prevalence, clinical features and risk factors. *Nephrol. Dial. Transplant.*, 2008; 23: 741-746.

[7] Peters P. J., Moore D. M., Mermin J., Brooks J. T., Downing R., Were W. et al. Antiretroviral therapy improves renal function among HIV-infected Ugandans. *Kidney Int.*, 2008; 74: 925-929.

[8] Ross M. J., Klotman P. E. Recent progress in HIV-associated nephropathy. *J. Am. Soc. Nephrol.*, 2002; 13:2997–3004.

[9] Lucas G. M., Eustace J. A., Sozio S. Highly active antiretroviral therapy and the incidence of HIV-1-associated nephropathy: a 12-year cohort study. *AIDS.,* 2004; 18: 541–546.

[10] Gupta S. K., Mamlin B. W., Johnson C. S., Dollins M. D., Topf J. M., Dubé M. P. Prevalence of proteinuria and the development of chronic kidney disease in HIV-infected patients. *Clin. Nephrol.*, 2004;61:1-6.

[11] D'Agati V., Suh J. I., Carbone L., Cheng I. T., Appel G.: The pathology of HIV nephropathy: A detailed morphologic and comparative study. *Kidney Int.,* 1989;35: 1358-1370.

[12] Rao T. K., Filippone E. J., Nicastri A. D., Landesman S. H., Frean E., Chen C. K., Friedman E. A.: Associated focal and segmental glomerubosclerosis in the acquired immunodeficiency syndrome. *N. Engl. J. Med.,* 1984;310: 669-673.

[13] Rao T. K. S., Nicastri A. D., Friedman E. A.: Natural history of heroin associated nephropathy. *N. Engl. J. Med.,* 1974; 290: 19-23.

[14] Rao T. K., Friedman E. A., Nicastri A. D.: The types of renal disease in the acquired immunodeficiency syndrome. *N. Engl. J. Med.,* 1987; 316:1062-1068.

[15] Carbone L., D'Agati V., Cheng I. T., Appel G. B.: The course and prognosis of human immunodeficiency virus-associated nephropathy. *Am. J. Med.,* 1989;87: 389-395.

[16] Barisoni L., Bruggeman L. A., Mundel P., D'Agati V. D., Klotman P. E. HIV-1 induces renal epithelial dedifferentiation in a transgenic model of HIV-associated nephropathy. *Kidney Int.,* 2000;58: 173–181.

[17] Barisoni L., Kriz W., Mundel P., D'Agati V. The dysregulatedpodocyte phenotype: a novel concept in the pathogenesis of collapsing idiopathic focal segmental glomerulosclerosis and HIV-associated nephropathy. *J. Am. Soc. Nephrol.,* 1999;10: 51–61.

[18] Kopp J. B., Winkler C. HIV-associated nephropathy in African Americans. *Kidney Int. Suppl.,*: 2003;S43–S49.

[19] Kriz W., LeHir M. Pathways to nephron loss starting from glomerular diseases-insights from animal models. *Kidney Int.,* 67: 404–419, 2005.

[20] Foy M. C., Estrella M. M., Lucas G. M., Tahir F., Fine D. M., Moore R. D., Atta M. G. Comparison of Risk Factors and Outcomes in HIV Immune Complex Kidney Disease and HIV-Associated Nephropathy. *Clin. J. Am. Soc. Nephrol.,* 2013 in press.

[21] Naicker S., Fabian J. Risk factors for the development of chronic kidney disease with HIV/AIDS. *Cli. Nephr.,* 2010;74 (S1):51-56.

[22] D'Agati V., Appel G. B. HIV infection and the kidney. *J. Am. Soc. Nephrol.,* 1997; 8:138-152.

[23] Burns G. C., Matute R., Onyema D., Davis I., Toth I. Response to inhibition of angiotensin-converting enzyme in human immunodeficiency virus-associated nephropathy: a case report. *Am. J. Kidney Dis.,* 1994;23:441-3.

[24] Klotman P. E. Early treatment *Am. J. Kidney Dis.,* 1998 Apr; 31(4):719-20.

[25] Wyatt C. M., Meliambro K., Klotman P. E. Recent progress in HIV*Annu Rev Med.,* 2012;63:147-59.

[26] Wolf G., Ritz E. Combination therapyblockers to halt progression of chronic renal disease: pathophysiology*international,* 2005 ;67:799-812.

[27] Komine N., Khang S., Wead L. M. et al. Effect of combining an ACE inhibitorangiotensin II*journal of kidney diseases;*39*:*159-64.

[28] American Society of Nephrology 30th Annual Meeting and Scientific Exposition. Short Course Syllabus, 1997, p 305-309.

[29] Rao T. K. S.: Clinical features of human immunodeficiency virus-associated nephropathy. *Kidney Int.,* 1991;40:35,s-13-18.

[30] Bird J. E., Durham S. K.,Giancarli M. R., Gitlitz P. H., Pandya D. G., Dambach D. M., Mozes M. M., Kopp J. B. Captopril prevents nephropathy in HIV-transgenic mice. *J. Am. Soc. Nephrol.,* 1998;9:1441-7.

[31] Ideura H., Hiromura K., Hiramatsu N., Shigehara T., Takeuchi S., Tomioka M., Sakairi T., Yamashita S., Maeshima A., Kaneko Y., Kuroiwa T., Kopp J. B., Nojima Y. Angiotensin I *Am. J. Physiol. Renal Physiol.,* 2007 Oct; 293(4):F1214-21.

[32] Denton K. M., Fennessy P. A., Alcorn D., Anderson W. P. Morphometric analysis of the actions of angiotensin II on renal arterioles and glomeruli. *Am. J. Physiol. Renal Fluid Electrolyte Physiol.,* 1992;262: F367–F372.

[33] Brinkkoetter P. T., Holtgrefe S., van der Woude F. J., Yard B. A. Angiotensin II type 1-receptor mediated changes in heparan sulfate proteoglycans in human SV40 transformed podocytes. *J. Am. Soc. Nephrol.*, 2004;15: 33–40.

[34] Gloy J., Henger A., Fischer K. G., Nitschke R., Mundel P., Bleich M., Schollmeyer P., Greger R., Pavenstadt H. Angiotensin II depolarizes podocytes in the intact glomerulus of the Rat. *J. Clin. Invest.,* 1997;99: 2772–2781.

[35] Doublier S., Salvidio G., Lupia E., Ruotsalainen V., Verzola D., Deferrari G., Camussi G. Nephrin expression is reduced in human diabetic nephropathy: evidence for a distinct role for glycated albumin and angiotensin II. *Diabetes,* 2003;52: 1023–1030, 2003.

[36] Macconi D., Abbate M., Morigi M., Angioletti S., Mister M., Buelli S., Bonomelli M., Mundel P., Endlich K., Remuzzi A., Remuzzi G. Permselective dysfunction of podocyte-podocyte contact upon angiotensin II unravels the molecular target for renoprotective intervention. *Am. J. Pathol.*, 2006;168: 1073–1085.

[37] Chen S., Lee J. S., Iglesias-de la Cruz M. C., Wang A., Izquierdo-Lahuerta A., Gandhi N. K., Danesh F. R., Wolf G., Ziyadeh F. N. Angiotensin II stimulates alpha3(IV) collagen production in mouse podocytes via TGFbeta and VEGF signalling: implications for diabetic glomerulopathy. *Nephrol. Dial. Transplant.*, 20: 1320–1328, 2005.

[38] Hiramatsu N., Hiromura K., Shigehara T., Kuroiwa T., Ideura H., Sakurai N., Takeuchi S., Tomioka M., Ikeuchi H., Kaneko Y., Ueki K., Kopp J. B., Nojima Y. Angiotensin I *J. Am. Soc. Nephrol.*, 2007;18:515-27.

[39] Kumar D., Plagov A., Yadav I., Torri D. D., Sayeneni S., Sagar., Rai P., Adabala M., Lederman R., Chandel N., Ding G., Malhotra A., Singhal P. C. Inhibition of renin activity slows down the progression of HIV-associated nephropathy. *Am. J. Physiol. Renal Physiol.*, 2012;303:F711-20.

[40] Shimizu A., Zhong J., Miyazaki Y., Hosoya T., Ichikawa I., Matsusaka T. ARB protects podocytes from HIV *Nephrol. Dial. Transplant.,* 2012;27:3169-75.

[41] Zhong Y., Chen E. Y., Liu R., Chuang P. Y., Mallipattu S. K., Tan C. M., Clark N. R., Deng Y., Klotman P. E., Ma'ayan A., He J. C. Renoprotective *J. Am. Soc. Nephrol.,* 2013;24:801-11.

[42] Burns G. C., Paul S. K., Toth I. R., Sivak S. L. Effect of angiotensin-converting enzyme *J. Am. Soc. Nephrol.,* 1997 ;8:1140-6).

[43] Kimmel P. L., Mishkin G. J., Umana W. O. Captopril *Am. J. Kidney Dis.,* 1996;28:202-8.

[44] Wei A., Burns G. C.,. Williams B. A., Mohammed N. B., Visintainer P., Sivak S. L. Long-term renal survival in HIV-associated nephropathy with angiotensin-converting enzyme inhibition. *Kidney International*, 2003;64:1462–1471.

[45] Szczech L. A., Gupta S. K., Habash R., Guasch A., Kalayjian R., Appel R., Fields T. A., Svetkey L. P., Flanagan K. H., Klotman P. E., Winston J. A. The clinical epidemiology *Kidney Int.,* 2004;66:1145-52.

[46] Baker J. V., Huppler Hullsiek K., Prosser R., Duprez D., Grimm R., Tracy R. P., Rhame F., Henry K., Neaton J. D. Angiotensin converting enzyme *PLoS One.* 2012;7(10):e46894. doi: 10.1371/ journal.pone.0046894.

[47] Bigé N., Lanternier F.,Viard J. P., Kamgang P., Daugas E., Elie C., Jidar K., Walker-Combrouze F., Peraldi M. N., Isnard-Bagnis C., Servais A., Lortholary O., Noël L. H.,

Bollée G. Presentation of HIV-associated nephropathy and outcome in HAART-treated patients. *Nephrol. Dial. Transplant.*, 2012;27:1114-21.

[48] Yahaya I., Uthman O. A., Uthman M. M. Interventions for HIV-associated nephropathy.*Cochrane Database Syst. Rev.*, 013 Jan 31;1:CD007183. doi: 10.1002/ 14651858.CD007183.pub3.

In: ACE Inhibitors. Volume 2
Editor: Macaulay Amechi Onuigbo
ISBN: 978-1-62948-422-8

Chapter 9

The Use of ACEIs and ARBs in ESRD Patients on Maintenance Hemodialysis and Peritoneal Dialysis

Donald A. Molony**, *MD
Professor of Medicine, Division of Renal Diseases and Hypertension and Center for Clinical Research and Evidence-based Medicine, University of Texas HSC Houston Medical School, Houston, TX, US

Abstract

Angiotensin Converting Enzyme inhibitors (ACEI) and angiotensin receptor blockers (ARB) are widely prescribed to individuals receiving dialysis for the treatment of ESRD. These medications are used to treat hypertension especially if the patient has other comorbid conditions such as congestive heart failure (CHF), left ventricular hypertrophy, proteinuria, or diabetes mellitus. Based largely on evidence from non-ESRD patient populations, thought leaders in nephrology have advocated the use of ACEIs/ARBs for the treatment of hypertension and CHF in ESRD patients undergoing dialysis. In this chapter, we shall briefly discuss the rationale for use of ACEIs/ARBs in ESRD and we shall review in detail the most robust evidence that either supports or questions the view that these agents confer particular benefits or potential harms in this unique population. Potential benefits include ACEI/ARB therapy-related regression of left ventricular hypertrophy and preservation of residual renal function. Each of these outcomes is supported by some RCT evidence. We shall review the potential role of ACEI/ARB in preserving modality in patients treated with peritoneal dialysis. The more fundamental question of whether improvements in these intermediate outcomes translate into real improvements in morbidity or mortality is less well supported by the epidemiologic and experimental evidence. There is limited RCT evidence comparing ACEI/ARB treatment to standard of care. Systematic reviews with meta-analysis of this evidence fail to support a survival advantage with the use of ACEI/ARB compared to other antihypertensive medications. The RCT evidence might provide a distorted or biased reflection of the truth and we shall review some of the potential sources of this

* E-mail: donald.a.molony@uth.tmc.edu.

bias. If there is a survival advantage for ESRD patients, it is likely that this benefit is either subpopulation/comorbid disease state specific or that the overall advantage is smaller than predicted form the experience in non-ESRD populations and may require more rigorous, larger, long-term clinical trials to prove and characterize.

INTRODUCTION

Up to 80% of patients on maintenance dialysis have hypertension and a significant portion of these patients have developed ESRD in part or entirely due to antecedent hypertension [1-3]. Most patients on dialysis when treated for hypertension require multiple medications for the successful management, on average more than 3 medications [4]. Additionally, the majority of dialysis patients have multiple comorbid conditions including diabetes with proteinuria, cardiovascular disease, and congestive heart failure [3-6]. Efforts have been directed importantly toward the control of cardiovascular (CV) risk factors since cardiovascular events are the most commonly identified cause for mortality in the ESRD population. Thus, significant efforts have been directed towards control of blood pressure and reduction of other CV risk factors. In the absence of specific evidence from randomized controlled trials (RCTs) in ESRD populations, much of the management of cardiovascular risk factors and the treatment of hypertension in patients on dialysis have been extrapolated from experience in non-CKD populations [7]. Despite the high percentage of patients initiating dialysis care with hypertension, congestive heart failure, diabetes, or atherosclerotic vascular disease, fewer than 40% of these patients are typically treated with agents that block the renin angiotensin system [5]. Thus, the use of antihypertensive agents that block the renin-angiotensin aldosterone system, the angiotensin converting enzyme inhibitors (ACEIs) and the angiotensin I receptor blockers/antagonists (ARBs) has been advocated by some as potentially beneficial in the ESRD population and thought likely to reduce further morbidity and mortality. The low number of patients treated with ACEI/ARB is seen as an opportunity missed for improved care and hence, a potential quality issue [7-9]. However, recent clinical trials' evidence highlights the risk of extrapolating experience in non-CKD populations to ESRD populations or in relying too heavily on observational data [10-13]. Indeed, recent epidemiologic evidence suggests that the definition of hypertension and optimal targets for BP management in ESRD patients may differ from those for the general population.

In this chapter we will review the evidence from RCTs, from systematic reviews of the RCT evidence, and from well-designed cohort studies that inform this question. We will discuss the evidence regarding the effect of ACEI/ARB or their combination on mortality in hemodialysis and peritoneal dialysis patients. We will not consider the RCT evidence informing care of patients with severe CKD but not yet on dialysis. We will discuss evidence evaluating some proposed benefits of ACEI/ARB therapy in ESRD patients on morbidities including improvements in left ventricular hypertrophy (LVH/LVMI), slowing of cognitive decline, and preservation of residual renal function in both hemodialysis and peritoneal dialysis patients. We will also review the evidence on potential adverse side effects including hemodialysis membrane reactions and hyperkalemia. The core patient-centered question with regards to the use of ACEI/ARB medications is whether their use in patients on dialysis is safe when compared to other antihypertensive strategies, and whether their use will result specifically in a reduction in mortality/morbidity beyond that expected or achieved from simply controlling the blood pressure. It is important to consider principally those trials that achieve equivalent BP control given the known effect of BP control in ESRD patients on mortality and morbidity. Furthermore, surrogate or intermediate outcomes may not translate into patient-centered outcomes but are cited as the rationale supporting the current recommendations for the use of ACEI/ARB in certain populations of ESRD patients. Potentially beneficial effects of ACEI /ARB on reducing cardiac fibrosis and LVH/LVM, on vascular stiffness and PWV, on preservation of residual renal function and reduction of proteinuria, on the inflammatory state and insulin sensitivity, may each be predicted to translate into beneficial effects on morbidity and mortality in ESRD patients. We shall examine these intermediate outcomes first. These are listed in table 1.

Table 1. Benefits from the Use of ACEI/ARB that May Result in Improved Survival

		RCT evidence in General Population (Yes / No)	Epidemiologic Evidence in the General Population	RCT Evidence in ESRD population	Epi evidence in ESRD
Cardiovascular	Reduced risk of stroke	Y	Y	N	N
	Improvements in LVH	Y	Y	Y	Y
	Improvements in Inflammation and oxidative stress	Y	Y	Y	Y
	Improved outcomes with A Fib	Y	Y	N	Y
	Preservation of vascular access			N	Y
Non-cardiovascular	Preservation of residual renal function			Y	Y
	Reduction in proteinuria			N	Y
	Preservation of peritoneal membrane integrity of PD			Y	Y
	Avoidance of Dialyzer reactions			N	Y
	Slowing of cognitive decline in dementia	N	Y	N	N

RAAS Blockade and Left-Ventricular Hypertrophy (LVH)

Shortly after the introduction of ACEIs for the treatment of hypertension and the subsequent recognition of the impact of ACEI therapy on congestive heart failure, London and coworkers interrogated the impact of two antihypertensive treatment regimens on a small group of established hemodialysis patients with left-ventricular hypertrophy [14]. In this small RCT, BP control was achieved with either an ACEI (perindopril, n = 14) or a calcium channel blocker (nitrendipine, n = 10). After one year of treatment, they observed a significant improvement in measures of LVH and left ventricular mass (LVM) in the patients assigned to ACEI therapy compared to the group that achieved comparable BP control with the calcium channel blocker. They subsequently reported in a long-term prospective hemodialysis cohort an association between reductions in LVH achieved through dual control of BP and anemia with improvements in survival [15]. London et al argued that the effect of ACEI on LVM in their patients is independent of its antihypertensive effect. Others have proposed that ACEI impact LVM via beneficial effects on the neurotransmitters levels, in particular, on sympathetic hyperactivity [16].

The association between reductions in LVH and improved survival has been observed by others [17]. Cannella and coworkers studied 18 prevalent hemodialysis patients using a non-randomized design and reported a reduction in LVM in patients treated with a small dose of lisinopril compared to concurrent patients with LVH who did not receive an ACEI [18]. However, neither London nor subsequent investigators have demonstrated with epidemiologic studies that a reduction in LVH or LVM in association specifically with ACEI/ARB therapy has resulted in improved survival in HD patients. More recently, Tai and colleagues conducted a meta-analysis of RCT evaluating ACEI or ARB therapy in patients on HD (See Table 2) [19]. Their conclusions were limited by the small size of the clinical trials identified for inclusion in their systematic review. For the surrogate outcome of LVH/LVMI, treatment with ACEI/ARB resulted in reductions in LVH (151 patients, 82 ACEI/ARB, 69 control). Improvements in all-cause or cardiovascular mortality did not reach statistical significance (3 studies with 837 prevalent HD patients). Yang and coworkers performed a systematic review with meta-analysis to re-examine the question of whether ARB treatment in patients with ESRD resulted in improvements in LVH and LVMI where such improvements might translate into improvements in cardiovascular and overall mortality [20]. They included 6 studies in their meta-analysis with a total of 107 patients receiving an ARB compared to alternate therapy or placebo in 100 patients. No trial was larger than 40 subjects. Yang concluded that ARB treatment resulted in superior reduction in LVH when compared to other non-RAAS related anti-hypertensive therapies or placebo. They were unable to determine if outcomes with ARB therapy differed from those achieved with ACEI. They did not examine mortality.

Table 2. Meta-analyses that Included an Evaluation of Surrogate Outcomes

Trial	Yr	PD/HD	Metaanalysis Question	Main Finding
Yang	2013	HD	LVH	+
Tai	2010	HD	Mortality and CV Mortality / LVH	- / +
Akbari	2009	PD	Mortality / residual renal function	- / +

ACEI/ARB THERAPY AND THE INFLAMMATORY STATE

A number of possible mechanisms have been proposed (see table 1) for the observed increases in cardiovascular and all-cause mortality in dialysis patients that are resistant to conventional CV risk factor management. Increased oxidative stress and an intense pro-inflammatory state as seen, in particular, in patients treated with hemodialysis, may be an important or even key risk factor for CV mortality and morbidity in this population. Oxidative stress and increased inflammation as possible mediators of increased fibrosis and cardiovascular risk in ESRD patients have recently been supported by a number of different lines of complementary evidence. This evidence has been summarized in a recent review by Himmelfarb [21]. Relevant to this question are the observations that inflammatory markers and mediators are increased in dialysis patients and in particular increased during the dialysis procedure. These changes in inflammatory markers have been associated with an observed increase in mortality [22].

If inhibition of the RAAS cascade reduces inflammation in experimental models, it is possible that ACEIs and ARBs will have important, potentially exploitable therapeutic effects on inflammatory mediators and their dysregulation in ESRD patients on hemodialysis. Gambao and coworkers hypothesized that the impact of ACEI and ARB on markers of inflammation and on endothelial dysfunction might differ because their impact on bradykinnin levels differ [23]. To test this hypothesis, they performed a randomized controlled cross-over study on 15 established stable dialysis patients evaluating the effects of 1 week each of ramipril (5 mg/day), valsartan (160 mg/day), or placebo on markers of inflammation and endothelial function [23]. They found, in the absence of any impact on intradialytic BP, that during a standard hemodialysis session that the ACEI ramipril increased IL-1b concentrations ($P=0.02$) and decreased IL-10 concentrations ($P=0.04$) when compared to placebo. Valsartan increased F2-isoprostane levels, whereas both valsartan and ramipril lowered IL-6 levels ($P = 0.01$). With regards to markers of endothelial dysfunction both valsartan and ramipril lowered D-dimer levels ($P = 0.01$), but only ramipril blocked an increase in von Willibrandt factor levels ($P=0.04$). Thus, during a conventional hemodialysis treatment, Gambao and colleagues observed that valsartan appeared to produce a greater anti-inflammatory effect when compared with ramipril, and ramipril appeared to be superior to valsartan in preventing hemodialysis-related endothelial dysfunction.

RCT evidence demonstrating the effectiveness of interventions that improve oxidative stress and endothelial function during dialysis resulting in improving cardiovascular or all-cause mortality and CV morbidity are in progress. However, no definitive results demonstrating a mortality-benefit from the effects of ACEI/ARB interventions on markers of inflammation are yet available [24-26].

Miscellaneous Potential CV Benefits from Use of ACEI/ ARB in Dialysis Patients

Longstanding hypertension, dysregulation of mineral metabolism, dyslipidemias, and an increased inflammatory state all potentially contribute to the increased vascular stiffness observed in ESRD patients. As demonstrated by Guerin and colleagues, this increased vascular stiffness and resultant increased pulse-wave velocity (PWV) is associated with increased CV events and mortality [27]. In a small RCT ($n = 24$) described above, London and his colleagues observed a favorable effect of ACEI compared to a CCB on measures of aortic stiffness concurrent with their observations on LVH [16]. Subsequently, Ichihara el al conducted a RCT on a small number of prevalent HD patients to examine the effects of an ACEI, an ARB, or placebo on PVW over one year [28]. Sixty four patients were randomly assigned to receive low dose ACEI (trandolapril), low dose ARB (losartan) or placebo. They observed that PWV increased in patients assigned to placebo, but decreased significantly and equivalently in the losartan and trandolapril groups. They observed no group specific changes in blood pressure, hematocrit, erythropoietin dose, ankle-brachial index, serum lipid levels, serum 8-isoprostane levels, or serum C-reactive protein levels during the 12-month study period. These results have not been confirmed in a larger study nor did Ichihara report on the impact of improvements in PWV measurements from treatment with ACEI/ARB on mortality.

Extrapolating from experience in the non-CKD population, use of ACEIs/ARBs has been advocated in dialysis patients with atrial fibrillation. Genovesi and colleagues followed a large Italian cohort of hemodialysis patients and demonstrated increased risks of mortality and hospitalization for patients with atrial fibrillation [29]. They also observed a reduced risk of new onset atrial fibrillation associated with ACEI use. These findings have not yet been confirmed in an RCT.

ACEI/ARB Therapy and Preservation of Renal Function; Special Consideration with Peritoneal Dialysis

Preservation of renal function in both hemodialysis (HD) and peritoneal dialysis (PD) patients is associated through epidemiologic surveillance and observational cohort studies with improved survival and reduced cardiovascular events and possibly reduced risk of serious infections and hospitalizations[30-35]. Upon further examination of the epidemiologic data, the observational studies support the hypothesis that the preservation of residual renal function is not simply a surrogate marker for better overall health status which would result in the observed association with improved health outcomes, but rather that residual renal function might have direct beneficial effects on the inflammatory state, on mineral bone metabolism, and on vascular endothelial function, each of which might independently result in improved mortality and morbidity [31, 32]. Additionally, in ESRD patients treated with peritoneal dialysis, the preservation of residual renal function is often central to maintaining adequate total clearance and preservation of PD as a treatment modality. For the latter reason, it is reasonable to implement strategies that will preserve residual renal function and the integrity of peritoneal membrane function. It is therefore important for both HD and PD patients to know whether ACEI/ARB therapy will preserve renal function and, for PD patients, will improve peritoneal membrane efficacy [36]. It is biologically plausible that a mortality benefit associated with PD compared to HD might be dependent on preservation of peritoneal membrane integrity.

Animal/experimental models demonstrate a reduction in peritoneal membrane fibrotic change in models of PD with ACEI and ARB treatment. To determine whether such protective effects of ACEI/ARB therapy might also occur in patients undergoing PD, Kolesnyk and colleagues have investigated the effects of ACEI/ARB on the peritoneal membrane transport characteristics in a stable cohort of 66 established peritoneal dialysis patients followed for more than 2 years [37, 38]. Patients who had received ACEI/ARB therapy as part of their routine care were more likely to demonstrate a decrease in small solute transport and an improvement in the mass transfer coefficient for creatinine with increasing vintage of PD. The authors argued that these findings support a possible protective effect of ACEI/ARB on peritoneal membrane kinetics.

A larger body of evidence from human trials addresses the potential role of ACEI/ARB therapy for the preservation of residual renal function (RRF) in both PD and HD patients. Two large observational studies first raised the question of whether ACEI/ARB therapy might result in improved preservation of RRF. Moist and coworkers evaluated a large prospective sample of patients initiating PD and HD in the US and followed prospectively [39]. They observed in this sample that RRF was better preserved in patients who initiated PD versus HD and that the overall preservation of RRF was better in patients who were treated with either ACEI or calcium channel blockers. These observational data support the hypothesis that BP control and not specific antihypertensive agents might be mediating the beneficial effect on RRF. Similarly, Johnson et al observed in a prospective cohort of incident PD patients that a number of treatment factors were associated with RRF perseveration but that antihypertensive medications including ACEI were not [40].

Most of the randomized clinical trials relevant to the current question of whether ACEI/ARB treatment helps preserve RRF have compared the rate of decline in RRF after initiation of either PD or HD in patients treated with either an ACEI or an ARB versus conventional therapy. These trials have been small and almost entirely conducted in Japanese dialysis patients. Li and coworkers performed a randomized trial in 60 established PD patients with an average RRF of 3.55 and 3.74 ml/min/1.73 m^2 for the ACEI and control patient groups and followed patients randomized to receive either 5 mg of ramipril or control anti-hypertensives to achieve a target BP [41]. Li et al demonstrate a 0.9-mL/min (95% confidence interval, 0.1 to 1.8) slower rate of decrease in RRF at 1 year in the PD patients treated with ramipril compared with controls. The benefit of improved preservation of RRF was observed only after 6 months of follow-up. Indeed, Li el al observed an increased risk of anuria in ramipril-treated patients prior to 6 months. The authors performed post-hoc adjustment to the groups due to an imbalance in the prognostic factors at allocation despite randomization. This problem highlights the instability in the results inherent in RCTs of very small size and introduces a degree of uncertainty into these findings.

Subsequently, Suzuki and coworkers conducted a small RCT trial to evaluate the effects of an ARB (valsartan) versus placebo on preservation of RRF [42]. They examined 34 CAPD patients who had been on CAPD for >3 months but less than 2 years and followed them after random allocation to valsartan or customary anti-hypertensive medications for 24 months with similar control of their blood pressure. These patients, on average at the start of the trial produced more than 900 ml of urine daily. Those treated with valsartan demonstrated a small increase in RRF compared to a decline in those allocated to conventional therapy. The valsartan treated CAPD patient also demonstrated a substantial (nearly doubling) increase in peritoneal creatinine clearance. It is quite possible that the preservation of RRF in the valsartan group was due, in part, to better maintenance of volume homeostasis as a result of an effect of ARBs on peritoneal membrane transport kinetics. Additionally, similarly to the study by Li, the small size of the Suzuki study increases substantially the uncertainty of their findings.

Recently, Akbari and colleagues, conducted a systematic review of RCTs in PD patients to determine if ACEI/ARB therapy improved either survival or preservation of RRF [43]. (See Table 2). One would predict that if RRF is improved, that this would translate into a survival benefit. They identified 5 studies that meet the grade and only two that addressed

RRF [41, 42]. With regards to RRF, they reported a weighted mean difference of 0.91 mL/minute/1.73 m^2 (95% CI 0.14 – 1.68) per year favoring ACEI or ARB therapy when compared to conventional therapy. At the same time, because of the small number of patients studied and the scarcity of events, they were unable to demonstrate a reduction in mortality. This appearance of a contradiction supports that notion that the magnitude of benefit from use of ACEIs/ARBs in PD patients if present must be modest at best. There are currently 2 additional RCTs in progress to evaluate the effects of RAAS blockade on RRF and on survival in PD patients. An up-dated systematic review for the Cochrane library is pending [44].

ACEI/ARB and Cognitive Decline

Multiple observational studies have noted a progressive decline in cognitive and executive function in a large proportion of dialysis patients [45]. Mild to moderate degrees of dementia are commonly noted in ESRD patients where the prevalence of dementia amongst dialysis patients is higher than amongst age-matched controls. The dementias seen in elderly ESRD patients have been attributed to multiple causes. Most observational studies demonstrate an increase in prevalence of vascular dementias. Alzheimer's dementia may be common albeit it is less certain whether the prevalence of Alzheimer's is uniquely increased in ESRD patients. Blood pressure control and ACEI/ARB use in the non-CKD population has been associated with improved outcomes for individuals with vascular dementia and most recently, it has been demonstrated that use of ACEIs that are known to cross the blood brain barrier is associated with a slowing of the decline of cognitive function in a cohort of patients with Alzheimer's [46]. A similar benefit from this subclass of ACEI in ESRD patients has yet to be demonstrated.

ACEI/ARB Therapy and Survival, Observational Evidence

Early observational studies implied that treatment with ACEIs and ARBs might affect cardiovascular health and hence mortality in ESRD patients. This notion has been largely supported by assumptions arising from an extrapolation of evidence from RCT conducted in non-CKD populations and from an argument of the biological plausibility of the benefit of ACEI/ARB therapy; the latter, supported by the observed effects of ACEI/ARB therapies on intermediate outcomes such as levels of biomarkers of inflammation, degree of proteinuria, renal function preservation, and regression of LVH. Indeed, it has been advocated by a number of nephrology thought leaders and reflected in guidelines that ACEIs/ARBs should be considered as first line therapy for patients with comorbid conditions such as congestive heart failure, coronary artery disease, and diabetes [47, 48].

Clearly from these assumptions arises a critical, clinically important, core question, namely, beyond the effects attributable to improvement in BP, do ACEIs or ARBs confer some unique additional benefits for some or all patients with ESRD on dialysis? Are there any circumstances in which the use of ACEIs/ARBs could cause harm? As noted below, recent observational studies call into question the view that ACEIs/ARBs confer the benefit predicted from an extrapolation from the experience in non-CKD populations. Additionally, two meta-analysis of RCT evidence in dialysis populations failed to demonstrate any additional benefit from ACEI/ARB usage compared to other anti-hypertensive regimens achieving similar BP goals. In these early meta-analyses, any findings regarding mortality were considered inconclusive due to the small number of studies evaluating the different treatment strategies side by side.

Evidence supports the view that pharmacologic control of hypertension results in improved survival and other important outcomes for patients on dialysis. Two recent systematic reviews have summarized this body of evidence [49, 50]. Both of the systematic reviews were motivated by the seeming paradox of an observed increase risk of mortality and adverse CV outcomes in patients with ESRD demonstrating lower BP with antihypertensive treatment and the proven benefits of hypertension treatment in classes of patients with hypertension including patients with CKD but without ESRD. This is particularly problematic given the prevalence of hypertension and the frequency of cardiovascular events and premature deaths in ESRD patients. Lambers-Heerspink et al performed a systematic review of the published literature indexed in Medline, Embase, or the Cochrane library registry of randomized trials from 1950 to 2008, investigating the evidence of the effects of BP treatment in patients on dialysis on cardiovascular outcomes [49]. They identified 8 trials with 1679 patients and 495 cardiovascular events. With active therapy, blood pressures were lowered on average by 4.5 mmHg systolic and 2.3 mmHg diastolic and active antihypertensive therapy compared to placebo was associated with a relative risks for CV events, all-cause mortality, and CV mortality of 0·71 (95% CI 0·55–0·92), 0·80 (0·66–0·96), and 0·71 (0·50–0·99), respectively. Lambers-Heerspink et al did not observe any differences in outcomes with the different classes of medications but the data were too sparse to make meaningful comparisons of one class of antihypertensive agents with the others. Indeed, they noted that for two of the trials where ACEI/ARB were used, a clear benefit of BP treatment was not demonstrated.

Agarwal et al performed a systematic review to address a very similar question [50]. They evaluated the RCT evidence informing the management of long-term dialysis patients with antihypertensive agents. Most of these patients were treated for hypertension but some may have received antihypertensive agents for other indications. They identified 5 RCTs with 1202 subjects. The hazard ratios for cardiovascular events with active treatment compared to control were 0.69 (95% CI: 0.56 to 0.84) using a fixed-effects model and 0.62 (95% CI: 0.45 to 0.86) using a random-effects model for all patients and fell to 0.49 (95% CI: 0.35 to0.67) when only hypertensive patients were included in the analysis. These results are limited by a significant degree of statistical heterogeneity when the mixed populations of ESRD patients with and without hypertension are included in the analysis and by evidence of a publication bias. The latter might magnify the appearance of benefit of treating dialysis patients with antihypertensive agents. Similarly to Lambers-Heerspink, Agarwal and coworkers did not demonstrate a class specific benefit with agents from any antihypertensive agent class compared to agents from the other classes.

Thus, these two recent systematic reviews both support a probable benefit from lowering BP in hypertensive patients on dialysis although a degree of uncertainty remains. Both sets of investigators have noted that the literature they evaluated was too sparse to evaluate the different classes of antihypertensive therapy for their comparative effectiveness. Recent RCT evidence may allow for more definitive conclusions. We will review the RCT evidence examining the effects of ACEI/ARB therapy on mortality in ESRD patients compared to active customary care. The relevant studies examining the impact of ACEI/ARB agents on mortality in dialysis patients are listed in table 3.

Table 3. Mortality Trials

Trial	year	PD/HD	RCT Yes/No	Benefit + /-
Randomized Clinical Trials				
Zannad - FOSIDIAL	2002	HD	Y	- (+)
Takhashi	2006	HD	Y	+
Suzuki	2008	HD	Y	-
Cice et al	2010	HD	Y	+ with combination therapy
Iseki - OCTUPUS	2013	HD	Y	-
Peters	2013	HD	Y	??
ARCADIA trial	2014	HD	Y	??
Cohort or Cross-sectional studies				
Efrati	2002	HD	N	+
Kestenbaum	2002	HD	N	-
Fang	2008	PD	N	+
Lopes AA, et al	2009	HD	N	+
Chang (HEMO study cohort)	2011	HD	N - cohort	-
Chan (Fresenius database)	2011	HD	N-observational	+ ?

Initial considerations of ACEIs for treatment of hypertension in patients with CKD evolved out of the clinical trials evidence examining small relatively short-term RCTs and the possible benefits of ACEI treatment for patients with uncomplicated hypertension, or hypertension complicated by diabetes with or without nephropathy or congestive heart failure. The effectiveness of ACEIs and their kinetics in patients on HD were reported in the late 1980's early 1990's [51, 52]. Widespread use of the ACEI/ARB agents in patients with advanced CKD or ESRD, however was constrained because of concerns regarding the loss of residual renal function especially for patients with advanced CKD not yet on dialysis, the risks of hyperkalemia, and any consequent increased risk of sudden death. Some of the early epidemiologic observations seemed to validate some of these theoretical concerns.

The observational study by Efrati and coworkers provided some of the first support, albeit weak, for the view that ACEI therapy in dialysis patients might save lives [53]. This study was a retrospective analysis of a small convenient sample of patients followed in a single dialysis practice during a 6 year time period in which patients were treated at the discretion of their physicians with various antihypertensive agents. The authors reported a 52% reduction in mortality in the entire cohort and a 79% reduction in patients <65 years of age for the 60 patients treated with an ACEI compared to 66 patients managed without an ACEI (73% with a calcium channel blocker). These authors did not adjust for potassium levels, residual renal function, or vintage of dialysis. This study is problematic because the risk of bias/confounding is substantial and the population studied is quite small. Nonetheless, this study has been widely cited as evidence supporting the benefits of ACEI treatment in HD patients. Concurrent with the Efrati study, Kestenbaum and colleagues interrogated data from a large prospective longitudinal cohort of US incident ESRD patients (WAVE II) and asked whether treatment with a calcium channel blocker (CCB) was associated with an observed improvement in survival in the 3716 patient included in their analysis [54]. They noted a substantial improvement in survival associated with use of a CCB. Fifty-one percent of patients in this cohort were treated with a CCB and 46.3 % were treated with an ACEI. Kestenbaum et al did not observe any associated reduction in risk for all-cause or CV mortality amongst patients treated with ACEIs. The observations arising from the WAVE II prospective dialysis cohort would support the view that if the ACEIs were conferring a unique survival advantage on dialysis patients compared to the other antihypertensive agents, it is likely that this advantage was relatively modest at best. Equally plausible is the hypothesis that any effect of ACEIs in dialysis patient is likely complex and modified importantly by comorbidities, duration of dialysis, and complex interactions with other medications. A third observational study in HD patients from the DOPPS cohort demonstrated an association between ACEI/ARB prescriptions and a modest reduction in CV mortality that is similar in magnitude to a reduction in mortality observed in the same study associated with beta-blocker prescriptions and that parallels the temporal increase in prescriptions for these two medications [4]. The possibility that confounding or a temporal bias might be responsible for this association is significant. A fourth retrospective analysis in a cohort of PD patients demonstrated by Cox proportional hazard analysis a 62% reduction (HR 0.382, 95% CI 0.232–0.631) in the risk of death in association with ACEI/ARB use [55]. In this retrospective analysis, the BP goals achieved were not equivalent in the two groups. Additionally, opportunities for confounding and bias remain a real issue in this study. These four studies however, provided an evidentiary basis for advocating use of ACEI/ ARB in dialysis patients.

Two larger prospective cohort studies have recently been published that call into question the findings reported in the prior observational studies [56, 57]. These observational studies largely differ from many of the previously published studies discussed above in that they were performed on large datasets. Chang and colleagues conducted a secondary analysis of the HEMO study, a well-characterized cohort of maintenance HD patients, to evaluate the impact of ACEI use on all-cause mortality and CV/heart failure hospitalizations and composite of all-cause mortality and either CV or CHF hospitalizations [56]. Using proportional hazards regression and a propensity scoring, they were unable to demonstrate any significant associations between ACEI use and mortality, CV hospitalizations or the composite outcomes. Their hazard ratio from the multivariable-adjusted analyses for all-cause mortality was 0.97 (95% CI 0.82-1.14). Importantly, however, in the multivariable-adjusted analysis, ACEI use was associated with a higher risk of heart failure hospitalization with a hazard ratio of 1.41 (95% CI 1.11-1.80). In the propensity score–matched cohort, ACEI use was not significantly associated with any of the adverse outcomes evaluated. While the authors concluded that the observed higher risk of CHF hospitalization associated with ACEI use may be the result of residual confounding, a true effect cannot be excluded, thus, highlighting the risk inherent in simply applying evidence from the general population to patients with ESRD. These results are particularly of interest since the potential benefits of targeted treatment of CHF with ACEI/ARB is cited as one of the principal rationales for using ACEIs in the dialysis population.

Chan and colleagues provided additional support to this cautionary note [57]. Chan and colleagues conducted an observational analysis of all patients initiated on ACEI or ARB therapy undergoing chronic hemodialysis at a large dialysis provider (Fresenius) over a 6 year period. Kaplan–Meier and Cox regression were used to determine mortality hazard ratios (HRs) and outcomes were compared using propensity score matching. Out of a population of 291,607 HD patients, 22,800 were newly initiated on an ACEI and 5828 on an ARB. Patients were followed for an average of 1.26 years. After adjustment, Chan and colleagues observed no significant difference in the risk of cardiovascular, all-cause, or cerebrovascular mortality in patients initiated on an ARB compared with an ACEI (HR of 0.96). However, amongst the majority of patients that required addition of another antihypertensive agent, Chan et al demonstrated that the 701 patients initiated on combined ACEI and ARB therapy (HR of 1.45) or the 6866 patients on ACEI and non-ARB antihypertensive agent (HR of 1.27) were at increased risk of cardiovascular death compared with 1758 patients initiated on an ARB and non-ACEI antihypertensive therapy. As an observational study, it remains possible, despite propensity score matching, that the results may be confounded by indication or location of practice.

The observational studies thus provide a mixed picture, with the larger studies, after adjustment, demonstrating no unique advantage to ACEI/ARB use when compared to other patients on HD treated either for hypertension or CHF with non ACEI/ARB regimens. Thus, despite multiple epidemiologic studies, robustly conducted RCTs of sufficient size and duration and reflecting the complexities of practice are required to best understand the "true" efficacy of ACEI/ARB therapy in ESRD patients where the risks of confounding and bias are minimized.

Randomized Trials Examining the Impact of ACEI/ARB Therapies on Mortality in Dialysis Patients

A number of small RCTs have been and are being conducted to test the hypothesis that treatment with the ACEIs/ARBs confers a survival benefit on patients with ESRD [58-60]. Zannad et al conducted a large RCT comparing HD patients treated with an ACEI (fosinopril 5 mg titrated to 20 mg to control BP, n=196) to patients treated with placebo plus conventional non-ACEI antihypertensive therapy (n = 201) for 24 months (> 90% follow-up) [58]. The primary end point was combined fatal and nonfatal first major CV events. Zannad and colleagues found no statistically significant benefit with fosinopril therapy in either the intention to treat analysis without adjustment and after adjusting for independent predictors of CV events, with the latter resulting in a relative risk of 0.93 (95% confidence interval (CI) 0.68–1.26). In the patients who were hypertensive at baseline, systolic and diastolic blood pressures were significantly better controlled in the fosinopril group compared to placebo and in the as treated analysis, this group demonstrated a trend towards benefit. The possible small benefit demonstrated in the patients who were hypertensive at baseline could not be attributed specifically to the ACEI but rather might be due to a general effect of better BP control.

The study by Zannad was followed by a smaller study by Takahashi et al in a Japanese prevalent HD population [59]. In this small study, 80 chronic hemodialysis patients without pre-existing clinical evidence of cardiac disease were randomly assigned either to candesartan

4–8 mg/day (n = 43) or no additional medications (control group; n =37), and followed for an average of close to 20 months and monitored for fatal/non-fatal CV events. A total of 24 CV events were observed (7 in the ARB group and 17 in the control). The authors reported that CV events and mortality rates were significantly (P<0.01) reduced with ARB therapy. These results are however, uncertain since in a study of this small size, randomization could not insure that both measured and unmeasured baseline prognostic factors were truly equivalent in both groups. Suzuki and colleagues conducted an open-label RCT to study the effects of treatment with an ARB (valsartan, candesartan or losartan) on CV events [60]. Three hundred and sixty prevalent adult hemodialysis patients were randomized after stratification by sex, age, diabetes status and BP and followed for the occurrence of a fatal or non-fatal CV event. There were 34 events in the ARB group and 39 in the non-ARB group. Despite stratification at randomization, the authors further adjusted for age, sex, diabetes, systolic BP and center and reported that assignment to the ARB treatment arm was associated with a reduction in fatal and nonfatal CV events with a hazard ratio of 0.51 (95% CI, 0.33 to 0.79). In the adjusted analysis, they reported 63 deaths; 25 in the ARB and 38 in the non-ARB groups. Even after adjustment, all-cause mortality did not differ between the 2 groups with a hazard ratio of 0.64; (95% CI of 0.39 to 1.06). The study results may be further biased by the open-label design and the use of 3 different ARBs. Thus, neither the study by Takahashi nor Suzuki definitively addresses the issue of ACEI/ARB therapy in HD patients and mortality. Similarly the study by Cice and colleagues which have been included in systematic reviews published to date, does not permit a direct evaluation of the potential benefits of RAAS blockade per say [61]. Cice and colleagues investigated the effects of the addition of the ARB telmisartan on all-cause and cardiovascular mortality and morbidity in hemodialysis patients with chronic heart failure (CHF) where the ARB was added to standard therapy with an ACEI. They randomized 332 patients to telmisartan 80 mg plus an ACEI (n = 165) or placebo plus and ACEI (n=167) and followed the study subjects for a mean of 36 months to determine the occurrence of all-cause mortality, CV mortality, or CHF hospitalization. They reported that telmisartan when added to ACEI therapy significantly reduced all-cause (35.1% vs. 54.4%) and CV mortality (30.3% vs. 43.7%;), and CHF hospitalizations (33.9% vs. 55.1%). They concluded that addition of telmisartan to standard therapies with an ACEI significantly reduced all-cause and CV mortality, and CHF hospitalizations. The study by Cice and colleagues does not specifically address the core question of RAAS blockade and the findings are counter to the findings from much larger RCTs in the general population where combination ACEI and ARB therapies result in poorer outcomes. All of the RCTs on the effects of ACEI/ARB treatments on mortality in ESRD patients summarized above, however, have been included in the systematic reviews published to date.

A recent study by Iseki and colleagues has not been included in the systematic reviews published to date [62]. This study is distinguished from the earlier studies by its larger size and longer follow-up and active treatment control arm with equivalent BP control achieved in both arms of the study. Iseki and colleagues conducted a multicenter open-label RCT with masked allocation and masked adjudication of outcomes. Hypertensive prevalent HD were assigned to receive the angiotensin receptor blockade (ARB) olmesartan (10–40 mg daily; n = 235) or another antihypertensive regimen that excluded either ACEIs or ARBs (n = 234) and study subjects were followed for a mean of 3.5 years for the primary outcomes of either a composite of death, nonfatal stroke, nonfatal myocardial infarction and coronary revascularization or all-cause mortality. Sixty-eight patients (28.9%) in the olmesartan group and 67 patients (28.6%) in the control group had either of the primary outcomes for a hazard ratio of 1.00, (95% CI 0.71–1.40). Death from any cause occurred in 38 patients (16.2%) in the olmesartan group and 39 (16.7%) in the control group for a HR of 0.97 (95% CI, 0.62–1.52). Thus, in this multi-centered RCT, ARB treatment of hypertension did not significantly reduce the absolute risk for mortality or for a major CV event in prevalent HD patients.

Two additional RCTs are currently in progress [63, 64]. The first by Peters and colleagues, the SAFIR study, has been completed as of January 2013, but the results of this study have not been published. This is a RCT including 82 prevalent HD patients with significant residual renal function randomized to an ARB or customary care [63]. The second study, the ARCADIA study, is an Italian multi-centered RCT that is currently recruiting patients with an intended enrollment of 266 patients assigned to either receive customary care or low dose ramipril and followed on treatment for 2 years; to be completed in March of 2015 [64].

The last comprehensive systematic review with meta-analysis evaluating the effects of ACEI or ARB therapy in dialysis patient on mortality included studies through March of 2008 [19]. The study by Iseki has not been included. Additionally, a number of long-term RCTs have evaluated the impact of ACEI/ARB on LVH but the published results from these studies have not reported any mortality data. Clearly an updated systematic review of the published evidence and any additional patient-level data on mortality in RCTs evaluating other patient outcomes such as LVH or preservation of RRF, would be informative. We are then left with the summary of the data by Tai and coworkers through 2008 in which they were unable to demonstrate a statistically significant benefit of ACEI/ARB treatment on mortality in dialysis-dependent patients. The evidence from the study by Iseki and colleagues should further strengthen this conclusion, namely that ACEI/ARB treatment in dialysis-dependent patients does not provide a unique benefit to these patients. Larger, long-term RCTs will be required to be sufficiently powered to interrogate the possibility of rare harms caused by use of ACEI/ARB to treat hypertension in the ESRD population when compared to treatment with other anti-hypertensive agents. The question of potential for harm is raised by the findings from the observational studies.

The uncertainty in the results of the systematic reviews/meta-analyses, and the contradictions between the findings from the observational studies and individual RCTS, however, illustrate some of the potentially important sources of gaps in the evidence on the question of the use of ACEI/ARB in ESRD patients. First, the experience with observational studies on surrogate or intermediate outcomes (i.e. LVH regression, preservation of RRF) suggesting benefit and subsequent lack of effect on mortality illustrates the principle that epidemiologic observations may not be confirmed when interrogated with an RCT; second, that small RCT's may provide a biased answer or an answer that has limited generalizability; and third, that achieving desired changes with a therapy in surrogate outcomes does not always translate into improvements in patient centered outcomes. Additionally, the meta-analyses examining the relationship between ACEI/ARB therapy and mortality in dialysis patients exhibit a significant degree of statistical heterogeneity. This heterogeneity could arise from fundamental differences in the interventions, outcomes, or populations studied. Given the small size of many of the studies examining this question, it is likely that some of the heterogeneity (or variance in the measured effect size) arises from the inherent uncertainty/ instability of the observed treatment-effect differences in small RCTs where random allocation might not insure equivalence of the groups' prognostic factors at baseline. Finally, as expressed by Onuigbo and Onuigbo, the benefit of any intervention in ESRD patients, including any potential benefit from ACEI/ARB therapy, will be modified by concurrent therapies and will vary from patient to patient as determined by their unique baseline risk profile and their unique constellation of comorbid conditions [65].

CONCLUSION

The core questions (Table 4) regarding the use of ACEI/ARB in patients with ESRD center on whether observed changes in intermediate outcomes such as changed in inflammatory markers, LVH, or preservation of residual renal function will translate into improvements in important patient-centered outcomes such as survival, cardiovascular events, hospitalizations and quality of life. The RCT evidence does provide some support for the conclusion that ACEIs/ARBs do result in regression in LVH and in preservation of residual renal function. However, the evidence from the larger observational studies and from the more robust RCT's do not support the likelihood that ACEI/ARB therapy in ESRD patients results in significant patient-centered benefits beyond those likely to be achieved with the proper control of BP. Given the small size of most of the studies that comprise most of the evidence published to date, a fair degree of uncertainty persists with regards to the role of ACEIs/ARBs in the treatment of hypertension in ESRD. There remains a real possibility that ACEI/ARB therapy in ESRD patients could produce important benefits for patients. However, the interrogation of the question of whether such therapy might result in actual harm is even less well served by the small, relatively short-term RCT studies that dominant the scope of published studies and the possibility that ACEI/ARBs cause some measure of harm cannot be excluded. The evidence obtained from studies in ESRD patients does not justify a recommendation that ACEIs/ARBs be considered as first line therapy in ESRD patients.

Table 4.

The core questions regarding the use of ACEI / ARB in patients with ESRD
1. Are ACEIs / ARBs safe in HD patients?
2. Will ACEI / ARB therapy result in improvements in LVH in ESRD patients?
3. Does ACEI / ARB therapy improve preservation of residual renal function?
4. Does ACEI / ARB therapy improve peritoneal dialysis effectiveness?
5. Do ACEIs/ARBs improve outcomes with CHF in ESRD patients?
6. Do ACEIs / ARBs improve survival in ESRD patients, in particular patients with DM, CAD, or CHF?

REFERENCES

[1] Inrig JK: Antihypertensive Agents in hemodialysis patients: A current perspective. *Semin Dialysis* 2010; 23: 290 – 297.

[2] Toto RD: Improving outcomes in hemodialysis patients: The need for well-designed clinical trials. *Am J Kidney Dis.* 2008; 52: 400-02.

[3] Renal Data System, USRDS 2012 Annual Data Report: Atlas of Chronic Kidney Disease and End-Stage Renal Disease in the United States, National Institutes of Health, National Institute of Diabetes and Digestive and Kidney Diseases, Bethesda, MD, 2012.

[4] Lopes AA, Bragg-Gresham JL, Ramirez SP, Andreucci VE, Akiba T, Saito A, Jacobsen SH, Robinson BM, Port FK, Mason NA, Young EW. Prescription of antihypertensive agents to haemodialysis patients: time trends and associations with patient characteristics, country and survival in the DOPPS. *Nephrol Dial Transplant* 2009; 24(9): 2809-16.

[5] Stack AG, Bloembergen WE. A Cross-sectional study of the prevalence and clinical correlates of congestive heart failure among incident US dialysis patients *Am J Kidney Dis* 2001; 38: 992-1000.

[6] Brown JH, Hunt LP, Vites NP, Short CD, Gokal R, Mallick NP. Comparative mortality from cardiovascular disease in patients with chronic renal failure. *Nephrol Dial Transplant* 1994; 9: 1136-1142.

[7] Cravedi P, Remuzzi G, Ruggenenti P. Targeting the renin angiotensin system in dialysis patients. *Semin Dialysis* 2011; 24: 2990 – 297.

[8] Marrs JC. Optimizing outcomes in patients with cardiovascular disease and chronic kidney disease. *Am J Manag Care.* 2011; 17 Suppl 15: S403-11.

[9] Sica DA, Gehr TW, Fernandez A: Risk-benefit ratio of angiotensin antagonists versus ACE inhibitors in endstage renal disease. *Drug Saf* 2000; 22: 350-360.

[10] Winkelmayer WC, Heinze G. Assessments of causal effects--theoretically sound, practically unattainable, and clinically not so relevant. *Clin J Am Soc Nephrol.* 2013; 8: 520-2

[11] Winkelmayer WC, Charytan DM, Levin R, Avorn J. Poor short-term survival and low use of cardiovascular medications in elderly dialysis patients after acute myocardial infarction. *Am J Kidney Dis* 2006; 47: 301-8.

[12] Horl WH. ACE inhibitors in hemodialysis patients: Does survival improve? *Am J Kidney Dis* 2002; 40: 1100 – 02.

[13] Sipahi I, Fang JC. Treating heart failure on dialysis. Finally Getting Some Evidence* *JACC* 2010; 56: 1709-11.

[14] London GM, Pannier B, Guerin AP, Marchais SJ, Safar ME, Cuche JL. Cardiac hypertrophy, aortic compliance, peripheral resistance, and wave reflection in end-stage renal disease. Comparative effects of ACE inhibition and calcium channel blockade. *Circulation* 1994; 90:2786–96.

[15] London GM, Pannier B, Guerin AP, Blacher J, Marchais SJ, Darne B, Metivier F, Adda H, Safar ME. Alterations of left ventricular hypertrophy in and survival of patients receiving hemodialysis: Follow-up of an interventional study. *J Am Soc Nephrol* 2001; 12: 2759–67.

[16] Lichtenberg G, Blankestijn PJ, Oey L, Klein IHH, Dijkhorst L-T, Boomsma F, Wieneke GH, van Huffelen AC, Koomans HA. Reduction of sympathetic hyperactivity by enalapril in patients with chronic renal failure. *N Engl J Med* 1999; 340: 1321-8.

[17] Lopez-Gomez JM, Verde E, Perez-Garcia R. Blood pressure, left ventricular hypertrophy and long-term prognosis in hemodialysis patients. *Kidney Int Suppl* 1998; 68: S92-S98.
[18] Cannella G, Paoletti E, Delfino R, Peloso G, Rolla D, Molinari S. Prolonged therapy with ACE inhibitors induces a regression of left ventricular hypertrophy of dialyzed uremic patients independently from hypotensive effects. *Am J Kidney Dis* 1997; 30:659–64.
[19] Tai DJ, Lim TW, James MT, Manns BJ, Tonelli M, Hemmelgarn BR; Alberta Kidney Disease Network. Cardiovascular effects of angiotensin converting enzyme inhibition or angiotensin receptor blockade in hemodialysis: a meta-analysis. *Clin J Am Soc Nephrol.* 2010; 5: 623-30.
[20] Yang LY, Ge X, Wang YL, Ma KL, Liu H, Zhang XL, Liu BC. Angiotensin receptor blockers reduce left ventricular hypertrophy in dialysis patients: a meta-analysis. *Am J Med Sci.* 2013; 345: 1-9
[21] Himmelfarb J: Uremic toxicity, oxidative stress, and hemodialysis as renal replacement therapy. *Semin Dial* 2009;22: 636–643
[22] Kimmel PL, Phillips TM, Simmens SJ, Peterson RA, Weihs KL, Alleyne S, Cruz I, Yanovski JA, Veis JH: Immunologic function and survival in hemodialysis patients. *Kidney Int* 1998;54: 236–244
[23] Gambao JL, Pretorius M, Todd-Tzanetos DR, Luther JM, Yu C, Ikizler TA, Brown NJ. Comparative effects of angiotensin-converting enzyme inhibition and angiotensin-receptor blockade on inflammation during hemodialysis. *J Am Soc Nephrol* 2012; 23: 334–342
[24] de Cavanagh EM, Ferder L, Carrasquedo F, Scrivo D, Wassermann A, Fraga CG, Inserra F. Higher levels of antioxidant defenses in enalapril-treated versus non-enalapril-treated hemodialysis patients. *Am J Kidney Dis.* 1999; 34: 445-55.
[25] Morena M, Delbosc S, Dupuy AM, Canaud B, Cristol JP: Overproduction of reactive oxygen species in end-stage renal disease patients: A potential component of hemodialysis-associated inflammation. *Hemodial Int* 2005; 9: 37–46
[26] Caglar K, Peng Y, Pupim LB, Flakoll PJ, Levenhagen D, Hakim RM, Ikizler TA: Inflammatory signals associated with hemodialysis. *Kidney Int* 2002; 62: 1408–1416
[27] Guerin AP, Blacher J, Pannier B, Marchais SJ, Safar ME, London GM. Impact of aortic stiffness attenuation on survival of patients in end-stage renal failure. *Circulation.* 2001;103:987-992.
[28] Ichihara A, Hayashi M, Kaneshiro Y, Takemitsu T, Homma K, Kanno Y, Yshizawa M, Furukawa T, Takenaka T, Saruta T. Low doses of losartan and trandolapril improve arterial stiffness in hemodialysis patients. *Am J Kidney Dis* 2005; 45: 866-874.
[29] Genovesi S, Vincenti A, Rossi E, Pogliani D, Acquistapace I, Stella A, Valsecchi MG. Atrial fibrillation and morbidity and mortality in a cohort of long-term hemodialysis patients. *Am J Kidney Dis.* 2008; 51: 255-62.
[30] Bargman JM, Thorpe KE, Churchill DN. Relative contribution of residual renal function and peritoneal clearance to adequacy of dialysis: a reanalysis of the CANUSA study. *J Am Soc Nephrol* 2001; 12:2158–62.
[31] Rocco MV, Frankenfield DL, Prowant B. Risk factors for early mortality in US peritoneal dialysis patients: impact of residual renal function. *Perit Dial Int* 2002; 22:371–9.

[32] Termorshuizen F, Korevaar JC, Dekker FW, Boeschoten EW, Krediet RT. The relative importance of residual renal function compared with peritoneal clearance for patient survival and quality of life: an analysis of the Netherlands Cooperative Study on the Adequacy of Dialysis (NECOSAD-2). *Am J Kidney Dis* 2003; 41:1293–302.

[33] Wang AY, Woo J, Wang M. Important differentiation of factors that predict outcome in peritoneal dialysis patients with different degrees of residual renal function. *Nephrol Dial Transplant* 2005; 20:396–403.

[34] Konings CJAM, Kooman JP, Schonck M. Fluid status in CAPD patients is related to peritoneal transport and residual renal function: evidence from a longitudinal study. *Nephrol Dial Transplant* 2003; 18:797–803.

[35] Wang AY, Sea MM, Ip R. Independent effects of residual renal function and dialysis adequacy on actual dietary protein, calorie and other nutrient intake in patients on continuous ambulatory peritoneal dialysis. *J Am Soc Nephrol 2001*; 12:2450–7

[36] Kolesnyk I, Dekker FW, Boeschoten EW, Krediet RT. Time-dependent reasons for peritoneal dialysis technique failure and mortality. *Perit Dial Int. 2010*; 30: 170-7

[37] Kolesnyk I, Dekker FW, Noordzij M, le Cessie S, Struijk DG, Krediet RT. Impact of ACE inhibitors and AII receptor blockers on peritoneal membrane transport characteristics in long-term peritoneal dialysis patients. *Perit Dial Int. 2007*; 27: 446–453.

[38] Kolesnyk I, Noordzij M, Dekker FW, Boeschoten EW, Krediet RT. Treatment with angiotensin II inhibitors and residual renal function in peritoneal dialysis patients. *Perit Dial Int.* 2011; 31: 53-9.

[39] Moist LM, Port FK, Orzol SM, Young EW, Ostbye T. Predictors of loss of residual renal function among new dialysis patients. *J Am Soc Nephrol* 2000; 11:556–64.

[40] Johnson DW, Mudge DW, Sturtevant JM, Hawley CM. Predictors of decline of residual renal function in new peritoneal dialysis patients. *Perit Dial Int* 2003; 23:276–83.

[41] Li PK, Chow KM, Wong TY, Leung CB, Szeto CC. Effects of an angiotensin-converting enzyme inhibitor on residual renal function in patients receiving peritoneal dialysis. A randomized, controlled study. *Ann Intern Med* 2003; 139: 105–12.

[42] Suzuki H, Kanno Y, Sugahara S, Okada H, Nakamoto H. Effects of an angiotensin-II receptor blocker, valsartan, on residual renal function in patients on CAPD. *Am J Kidney Dis* 2004; 43:1056–64.

[43] Akbari A, Knoll G, Ferguson D, McCormick B, Davis A, Biyani M. Angiotensin-converting enzyme inhibitors and angiotensin receptor blockers in peritoneal dialysis: systematic review and meta-analysis of randomized controlled trials. *Perit Dial Int.* 2009; 29: 554-61.

[44] Zhang L, Zeng X, Fu P, Wu HM. Angiotensin converting enzyme inhibitors and angiotensin II receptor blockers for preserving residual kidney function in peritoneal dialysis patients. *Cochrane Database of Systematic Reviews* 2011, Issue 5. Art. No.: CD009120. DOI: 10.1002/14651858.CD009120.

[45] Tamura MK, Yaffe K. Dementia and cognitive impairment in ESRD: diagnostic and therapeutic strategies. *Kidney Int.* 2011; 79: 14–22.

[46] Gao Y, O'Caoimh R, Healy L, Kerins DM, Eustace J, Guyatt G, Sammon D, Molloy DW. Effects of centrally acting ACE inhibitors on the rate of cognitive decline in dementia. *BMJ Open* 2013; 3:e002881.

[47] K/DOQI Clinical practice guidelines on hypertension and antihypertensive agents in chronic kidney disease. *Am J Kidney Dis* 2004; 43:1–290.

[48] Taler SJ, Agarwal R, Bakris GL, Flynn JT, Nilsson PM, Rahman M, Sanders PW, Textor SC, Weir MR, Townsend RR. KDOQI US commentary on the 2012 KDIGO Clinical Practice Guideline for management of blood pressure in CKD. *Am J Kidney Dis* 2013; 62: 201-13.

[49] Lambers Heerspink HJ, Ninomiya T, Zoungas S, de Zeeuw D, Grobbee DE, Jardine MJ, Gallagher M, Roberts MA, Cass A, Neal B, Perkovic V. Effect of lowering blood pressure on cardiovascular events and mortality in patients on dialysis: a systematic review and meta-analysis of randomised controlled trials. *Lancet* 2009; 373: 1009–15.

[50] Agarwal R, Sinha AD. Cardiovascular protection with antihypertensive drugs in dialysis patients: Systematic review and meta-analysis. *Hypertension.* 2009; 53: 860-866.

[51] Kelly JG, Doyle GD, Carmody M, Glover DR, Cooper WD: Phamacokinetics of lisinopril, enalapril, and enalaprilat in renal failure: Effect of hemodialysis. *Br J Clin Pharmacol* 1988; 26:781-786.

[52] Fillastre JP, Baguet JC, Dubois D, Vauquier J, Gordin M, Legallicier B, Luus HG, de la Rey N, Carcone N, Genthon R: Kinetics, safety, and efficacy of ramipril after long-term administration in hemodialyzed patients. *J Cardiovasc Pharmacol* 1996; 27: 269-274.

[53] Efrati S, Zaidenstein R, Dishy V, Beberashvili I, Sharist M, et al. ACE inhibitors and survival of hemodialysis patients. *Am J Kidney Dis* 2002; 40: 1023-9.

[54] Kestenbaum B, Gillen DL, Sherrard DJ, Seliger S, Ball A, Stehman-Breen C. Calcium channel blocker use and mortality among patients with end-stage renal disease. *Kidney Int* 2002; 61: 2157–2164.

[55] Fang W, Oreopoulos DG, Bargman JM. Use of ACE inhibitors or angiotensin receptor blockers and survival in patients on peritoneal dialysis. *Nephrol Dial Transplant* 2008; 23(11): 3704-10.

[56] Chang TI, Shilane D, Brunelli SM, Cheung AK, Chertow GM, Winkelmayer WC. Angiotensin-converting enzyme inhibitors and cardiovascular outcomes in patients on maintenance hemodialysis. *Am Heart J.* 2011; 162: 324-30.

[57] Chan KE, Ikizler TA, Gamboa JL, Yu C, Hakim RM, Brown NJ. Combined angiotensin-converting enzyme inhibition and receptor blockade associate with increased risk of cardiovascular death in hemodialysis patients. *Kidney Int.* 2011; 80: 978-85.

[58] Zannad F, Kessler M, Lehert P, Grunfeld JP, Thuilliez C, Leizorovicz A, Lechat P: Prevention of cardiovascular events in end-stage renal disease: Results of a randomized trial of fosinopril and implications for future studies. *Kidney Int* 2006; 70: 1318–24.

[59] Takahashi A, Takase H, Toriyama T, Sugiura T, Kurita Y, Ueda R, Dohi Y: Candesartan, an angiotensin II type-1 receptor blocker, reduces cardiovascular events in patients on chronic haemodialysis—A randomized study. *Nephrol Dial Transplant* 2006; 21: 2507–2512.

[60] Suzuki H, Kanno Y, Sugahara S, Ikeda N, Shoda J, Takenaka T, Inoue T, Araki R: Effect of angiotensin receptor blockers on cardiovascular events in patients undergoing hemodialysis: An open-label randomized controlled trial. *Am J Kidney Dis 2008;* 52: 501-506.

[61] Cice G, Di Benedetto A, D'Isa S, D'Andrea A, Marcelli D, Gatti E, Calabrò R. Effects of telmisartan added to angiotensin-converting enzyme inhibitors on mortality and morbidity in hemodialysis patients with chronic heart failure. A double-blind, placebo-controlled trial. *J Am Coll Cardiol* 2010; 56: 1701-8.

[62] Iseki K, Arima H, Kohagura K, Komiya I, Ueda S, Tokuyama K, Shiohira Y, Uehara H, Toma S; Olmesartan Clinical Trial in Okinawan Patients Under OKIDS (OCTOPUS) Group. Effects of angiotensin receptor blockade (ARB) on mortality and cardiovascular outcomes in patients with long-term haemodialysis: a randomized controlled trial. *Nephrol Dial Transplant.* 2013; 28: 1579-89.

[63] Peters CD, Kjærgaard KD, Jespersen B, Christensen KL, Jensen JD. Renal and cardiovascular effects of irbesartan in dialysis patients--a randomized controlled trial protocol (SAFIR study). *Dan Med J.* 2013; 60: A4602.

[64] Ruggenenti P. ARCADIA trial; ClinicalTrials.gov identifier: NCT00985322.

[65] Onuigbo MAC, Onuigbo NTC. Is combined angiotensin-converting enzyme inhibition and angiotensin receptor blockade associated with increased risk of cardiovascular death in hemodialysis patients? *Current Hypertension Rev* 2012; 8: 256-66.

In: ACE Inhibitors. Volume 2
Editor: Macaulay Amechi Onuigbo
ISBN: 978-1-62948-422-8

Chapter 10

The Use of Angiotensin-Converting Enzyme Inhibitors in the Renal Transplant Recipient

Matthew R. Weir, MD* and Manju Mavanur, MD
Division of Nephrology, University of Maryland School of Medicine Medical Center, Baltimore, MD, US

Abstract

Renin angiotensin system (RAS) inhibition has proven to be helpful in reducing cardiovascular (CV) and kidney disease progression in the general population; whether kidney transplant patients would derive similar benefits is unknown. RAS inhibition also reduces post-transplantation erythrocytosis (PTE) in kidney transplant recipients, but its effect on hemoglobin levels in patients without PTE is unclear. RAS in inhibition can also cause changes in serum creatinine which can be of concern to clinicians. In this chapter, we will review the available evidence supporting the use of these drugs in kidney transplant recipients and discuss their therapeutic index.

Keywords: ACE inhibitor, hypertension, renal transplantation

Introduction

Hypertension (defined as blood pressure greater than 140/90 mm Hg) after kidney transplantation is common with most studies reporting incident rates between 60% and 80% [1-3]. Post-transplant hypertension is associated with reduced graft and patient survival [4-8]. Inadequate blood pressure control can lead to a 20% to 40% higher risk of graft loss from chronic allograft dysfunction or death from cardiovascular disease [6,9-11]. The pathogenesis is multifactorial and optimal treatment strategies and goals have yet to be clearly defined. The use of renin angiotensin system blocking drugs raises concern about safety in a patient with a

* Corresponding Author: Matthew R. Weir, MD, Division of Nephrology, University of Maryland School of Medicine Medical Center, Baltimore, MD, USA. Email: mweir@medicine.umaryland.edu

single kidney if there is renal artery stenosis. Yet there is evidence that these medications in patients with certain types of renal disease or heart disease reduce kidney and cardiovascular events by approximately 20% [12, 13]. This chapter will review clinical aspects of hypertension in kidney transplant recipients and discuss the pros and cons of blocking the renin angiotensin system with an ACE inhibitor.

Blood Pressure Targets

Blood pressure levels vary widely depending upon time of the day, methods of measurement, and study conditions [14]. Ambulatory blood pressure monitoring (ABPM) is considered the gold standard for assessing BP, particularly in the diagnosis of white coat and masked hypertension. In the kidney transplant population, white coat hypertension is common [15, 16]. On the other hand, patients may have masked hypertension (Table 1). It is defined as a condition for which office blood pressure (BP) measurements indicate adequately controlled BP, but BP outside the clinic is elevated. Hypertension has been associated with accelerated kidney function loss and increased cardiovascular deaths in studies of general and chronic kidney disease populations including transplant recipients [17, 18]. Disturbances in circadian blood pressure rhythm are common following kidney transplantation. Loss of nocturnal systolic BP fall is associated with higher left ventricular mass index, increased cardiovascular events, reduced allograft function and increased risk of renal graft failure (Figure 1) [19-22]. When ABPM is not readily available, self-measured BP is a reasonable alternative. Home BP readings better correlate with ABPM values than BP obtained in office settings [23].

Table 1. Thresholds of hypertension diagnosis using different methods of measurement

Method of Measurement	Threshold (mmHg)
Office or clinic	140/90
Overall ABPM average	125-130/80
ABPM-daytime	130-135/85
ABPM-nighttime	120/70
Home	130-135/85

ABPM: ambulatory blood pressure monitoring.
KDIGO guidelines.

There are no prospective randomized controlled trials to evaluate optimal blood pressure in kidney transplant patients. We only have epidemiological information to examine. This is not surprising as there are only three prospective randomized controlled trials in people with native kidney disease that examine blood pressure targets and there are no prospective studies in people with diabetes and kidney disease to examine optimal levels of blood pressure to delay either progression of kidney disease or the development of cardiovascular events. Thus, most of the guidelines are based on expert opinion. The KDIGO Clinical Practice Guidelines encourage a blood pressure below 130/80 mmHg in transplant patients [24]. In patients with proteinuria, a blood pressure goal of less than 125/75 mm Hg is desirable based on data from the chronic kidney disease population and as published in the European best practice guidelines [25].

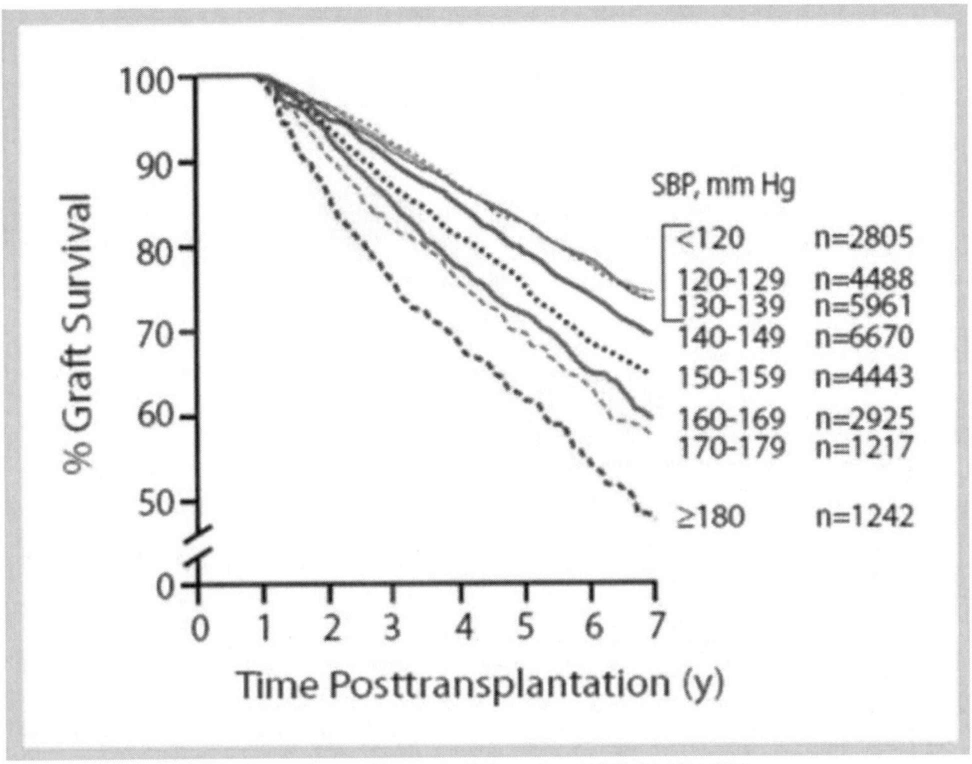

Adapted with permissision from Opetz, G., et al. *Kidney Int*. 1998;53:217-222.

Figure 1. Association of Systolic Blood Pressure (SBP) with Decreased Graft Survival.

PATHOGENESIS OF HYPERTENSION IN TRANSPLANT PATIENTS

Multiple factors increase the likelihood of hypertension post-transplantation including pre-existing hypertension, excessive weight gain, male gender, African-American ethnicity, recipients of kidneys from older donors, cyclosporine, tacrolimus, steroid therapy, renal artery stenosis and impaired graft function (Table 2). Impaired graft function associated with hypertension can be both from acute or chronic rejection as well as recurrent or de novo glomerular disease. In the immediate post-transplant period, especially in patients with delayed graft function, hypertension is often mediated by salt and water retention.

One also has to consider that many patients with chronic kidney disease or end-stage renal disease have developed structural alterations in vascular beds leading to increased stiffness and calcification. In fact, some investigators have demonstrated that aortic stiffness directly correlates with blood pressure at three and twelve months post-transplantation [26]. Interestingly, it is also affected by donor age, with younger donors having less stiff aortae whereas older donors have stiffer aortae. Diabetes is also an important factor that can lead to vascular changes whether pre-transplant or such development post-transplant.

Table 2. Factors that increase the likelihood of post-renal transplantation hypertension

Donor Factors
Old age
Pre-existing hypertension or diabetes mellitus
Nephron under dosing (female to male donor or donor-recipient BMI mismatch)
Subclinical kidney disease
Genetic factors (ABCB1 polymorphisms, MYH9 risk alleles)

Recipient Factors
Pre-transplant
Arteriosclerosis associated with CKD, DM, HTN, old age
Obesity
Male gender
Black race
Post-transplant (early <1 month)
Delayed graft function
High dose steroids
Volume overload
Post-transplant (late)
Immunosuppression medications
Calcineurin inhibitors
Corticosteroids
Transplant renal artery stenosis
Poor allograft function
Presence of native kidneys
Excessive weight gain

The mechanisms of calcineurin inhibitor-induced vasoconstriction are complex (Figure 2). This class of drugs activates both the sympathetic nervous system and the renin angiotensin system [26]. Cyclosporine also augments the vasoconstrictive effect of angiotensin II [27]. Calcineurin inhibitors alter the balance between vasodilator and vasoconstrictor prostaglandins in favor of greater vasoconstriction [28]. These drugs affect glomerular hemodynamics largely through pre-glomerular constriction and a reduction in GFR. The by-product of these effects is an increase in renal tubular reabsorption leading to the development of a salt sensitive form of hypertension. Recent experimental evidence indicates that calcineurin inhibitors can directly activate the renal sodium chloride cotransporter, an effect that can importantly be reversed by administering thiazide diuretics

[29, 30]. Of the two calcineurin inhibitors used in immunosuppression, tacrolimus has less pronounced effects on blood pressure compared to cyclosporine [31, 32].

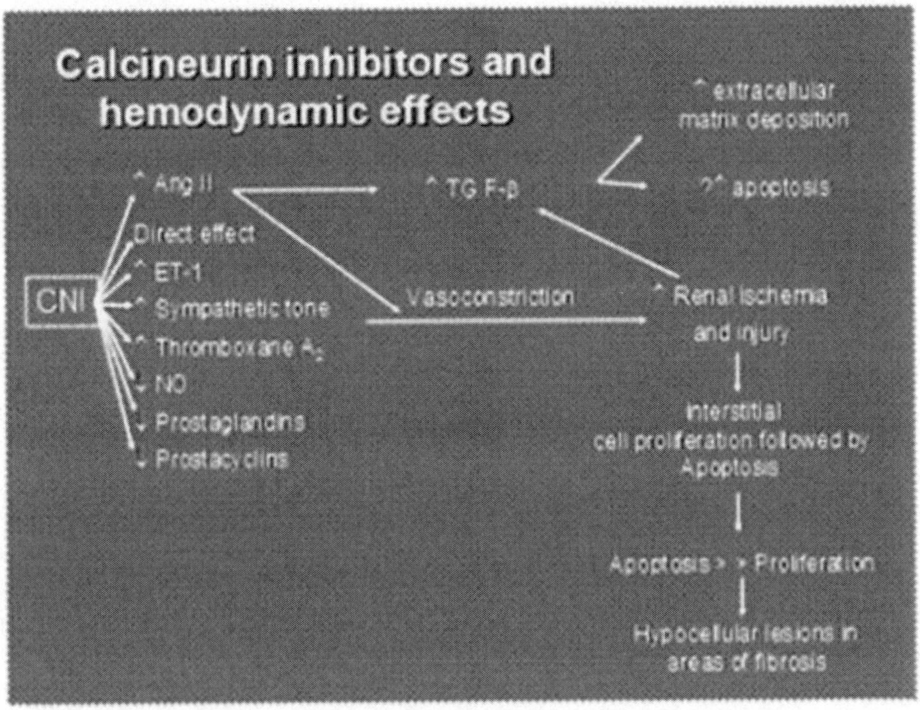

Figure 2. Calcineurin inhibitors and hemodynamic effects.

Corticosteroids especially when dosed in large amounts can have a substantial mineralocorticoid effect [33]. This leads to sodium and water retention and salt sensitive form of hypertension which may require some diuretic support. There is also evidence that glucocorticoid-receptor mediated activation of the vascular smooth muscles plays a role in glucocorticoid-induced hypertension [33].

Transplant renal artery stenosis is a potentially curable cause of post-transplant hypertension, allograft dysfunction, and graft loss. It usually occurs 3 months to 2 years after transplantation. The prevalence ranges widely from 1 to 23% in different series, reflecting the heterogeneous criteria used to establish the diagnosis [34]. With the development of more sophisticated doppler ultrasound techniques, the frequency of transplant renal artery stenosis diagnosis has been increasing with one study showing an increase in the rate of detection from 2.4% to 12.4% [35]. However, despite evidence of elevated systolic velocity, as would be caused by a stenotic lesion, there is no relationship with clinically and hemodynamically significant renal artery disease [36]. Some studies have shown that even with confirmation of transplant renal artery stenosis with angiography and treatment by angioplasty with or without stenting, the improvement in blood pressure control is not consistently achieved [37]. Many clinicians raise concern about angiography with contrast exposure and angioplasty with possible complications such as renal artery occlusion or dissection as well as the high incidence of restenosis especially with a single kidney [36,38]. Thus, decisions about intervention should be individualized carefully.

The overall influence of the native kidney on the pathogenesis of post-transplant hypertension is often debated. Prominent theories include overactivity of either the renin angiotensin system, the sympathetic nervous system or both. Thus, any hypertensive therapy needs to be targeted to these hormonal systems to facilitate better blood pressure control. Although bilateral native nephrectomy leads to better blood pressure control in most patients, it is by no means uniformly successful [39,40]. An interesting consideration may be whether renal denervation would be a strategy to treat this problem, but this would need to be studied more carefully.

MANAGEMENT OF POST-TRANSPLANT HYPERTENSION

Many factors are involved in controlling blood pressure post-transplantation. Lifestyle modifications including weight regulation, smoking cessation, and exercise remain important. Since the use of corticosteroids and calcineurin inhibitors cause a more salt sensitive form of hypertension, the importance of dietary salt modification, and or, the use of diuretics would be intuitive. Immunosuppression modification with lower doses of corticosteroids and calcineurin inhibitors or steroid avoidance may be helpful [41]. Some have even proposed calcineurin inhibitor discontinuation and using either an mTOR inhibitor, or belatacept as an alternative to facilitate better blood pressure control [42,43]. The benefits in blood pressure control must be weighed against the increased risk of rejection. Obstructive sleep apnea (OSA) is common in the ESRD population and may not improve after renal transplantation [44]. When present, it contributes to hypertension. However, the treatment of OSA has a beneficial effect based on blood pressure studies in the general population [45, 46].

The choice of appropriate medication should be based on tolerability, affordability, and utility in controlling the blood pressure. The majority of patients will require two or more antihypertensive medications. In addition, one also has to be worry about drug interactions and the dosing of medication based on renal function.

The most popular medications used in transplant patients include diuretics, calcium channel blockers, beta blockers, and drugs that block the renin angiotensin system.

Diuretics are often required for the reasons enumerated previously. Calcium channel blockers are also popular as they are powerful vasodilators and may counteract the vasoconstrictor effect of calcineurin inhibitors on the renal vasculature in the transplant kidney. Beta blocker use remains common in transplant patients given the cardiovascular disease risk profile of these patients, especially where there is known ischemic heart disease, congestive heart failure, or requirement for heart rate regulation.

Renin angiotensin system blockers and in particular, angiotensin converting enzyme (ACE) inhibitors, are equally effective in lowering blood pressure in transplant patients compared to other major classes [47]. The major interest in using these drugs stems from their proven benefits in large scale clinical trials of patients with established heart disease or kidney disease where they provide an approximate 20% relative risk reduction benefit for vascular events compared to other commonly used therapies [12,13]. Prospective clinical trials have been done to evaluate the effects of renin angiotensin system blockade on both kidney and cardiovascular outcomes in kidney transplant patients. The SECRET trial which intended to evaluate the effect of the angiotensin receptor blocker (ARB) candesartan on reducing the risk of the composite endpoint of death, graft loss and cardiovascular events had to be terminated prematurely due to lower-than-expected event rates after enrollment [48]. However the study provides evidence for the utility of candesartan, which showed good safety and tolerability, improved BP control, and decreased proteinuria in renal transplant recipients.

A double-blind, randomized, placebo-controlled trial to determine whether angiotensin II blockade prevents the expansion of the cortical interstitial compartment, the precursor of fibrosis was conducted by Ibrahim et al [49]. They randomly assigned 153 transplant recipients to receive losartan, 100 mg (n=77), or matching placebo (n=76) within 3 months of transplantation, continuing treatment for 5 years. Treatment with losartan did not lead to a statistically significant reduction in a composite of interstitial expansion or ESRD from interstitial fibrosis/tubular atrophy (IF/TA) in kidney transplant recipients. However the study showed that losartan was well tolerated with only one case of severe hyperkalemia (potassium level >6mEq/L).

A prospective European study showed that ACE-inhibitor/ARB use improved patient and graft survival over 10 years [50]. In a small randomized control trial, prolonged therapy with an ACE-inhibitor was associated with better general and cardiovascular outcomes [12]. However, other large data bases, when examined carefully, have failed to confirm the beneficial effect of an ACE inhibitor or an ARB on patient or allograft survival [51].

There is also clear evidence that drugs that block the renin angiotensin system are effective in reducing proteinuria in kidney transplant recipients. This has been confirmed in several studies including a recent meta-analysis [50]. It is quite likely that reducing proteinuria is of clinical relevance in these patients as it certainly will reduce the likelihood of developing nephrosis and associated lipoprotein abnormalities which lead to accelerated atherosclerosis. However, there are no studies demonstrating that reducing proteinuria in transplant patients improves long-term transplantation outcomes. Much of our suspicions for benefit is based on retrospective analyses from clinical trials in patients with native kidney disease, especially diabetic nephropathy [52,53]. Renin angiotensin system blockers, in particular ACE inhibitors, have demonstrated to be effective in reducing left ventricular hypertrophy in transplant recipients [54]. This also may prove to be a surrogate measure of benefit reducing cardiovascular events.

Despite all of the opportunities for utilizing renin angiotensin system blockade and particularly ACE inhibitors, post-transplantation, one must balance the benefits with the risks. On the benefits side, these drugs are extremely well tolerated and are similarly effective to other commonly used drugs in reducing blood pressure, and may specifically target the problems of an overactive renin angiotensin system which may be an important part of the hypertensive vascular process in many transplant recipients. In addition, these drugs also reduce proteinuria, regress left ventricular hypertrophy, and there is some suspicion that they may be helpful in delaying progression of interstitial fibrosis and tubular atrophy, and slowing progression of kidney and cardiovascular disease, much as they do in the general population. Yet, we know that these drugs cause a fall in glomerular filtration rate of approximately 20-30%. This can be further magnified if the patient is volume depleted. This acute change in serum creatinine, especially in the early period post-transplantation, may raise concerns about acute rejection, or possibly obstructive uropathy. Thus, many clinicians prefer not to introduce renin angiotensin system blockade until stable graft function has been established at least 2-3 months post-transplantation. By delaying the use of these drugs one can avoid unnecessary “fire drills”. In addition, it would also be preferred for the patients to be on stable doses of diuretics and immunosuppression agents.

Serum potassium can also increase with renin angiotensin system blocking drugs. Often this increase is of the order of 0.4-0.6 meq/L. However, when you combine this with the hyperkalemic effect of calcineurin inhibitors it can lead to serum potassium levels in the 5.5 to 6.5 range in selected patients. Thus, patients need to be monitored carefully, especially if there is any degree of graft dysfunction. Some studies have suggested that earlier use of renin angiotensin system inhibitors may reduce the incidence of delayed graft function an, improve graft survival, and all-cause mortality [50]. However, there may be some selection bias in these studies and, more importantly, a higher comfort level in using RAAS inhibition which may have limited the concern associated with acute changes in serum creatinine and potassium.

Renin angiotensin system blockers may also cause anemia. Studies have demonstrated that hemoglobin levels may be 5-15% lower on either ACE inhibitors or angiotensin receptor blockers. It is felt that reduction in hemoglobin may be related to erythropoietin-resistance caused by renin angiotensin system blockade. Thus, one needs to monitor hemoglobin when employing angiotensin system blockade.

Conclusion

Overall, the benefit to risk balance for using RAAS inhibitors and in particular ACE inhibitors, post-transplantation, is in favor of using these drugs. There does not appear to be any data to suggest that patients need to be placed on these drugs immediately post-transplantation. The authors of this review would suggest that once graft function and immunosuppression has been stabilized, that these medications be employed at about 2-3 months post-transplantation. At that point, serum creatinine and potassium can be monitored more capably and appropriate adjustments in dose and other medications can be considered. Renin angiotensin system blockers are well tolerated and are as effective as other commonly used drugs in lowering blood pressure. The likelihood that they would precipitate acute kidney injury in a patient with occult renin artery stenosis is remote. If it does occur, then these medications can be viewed as both diagnostic and therapeutic. What is not known is whether these drugs may prove to be an important contributor to better long-term graft function, either through reducing proteinuria or reducing interstitial fibrosis and tubular atrophy or simply, through their effects on lowering blood pressure, and perhaps glomerular capillary hypertension. Despite the controversial literature on the lack of confirmatory prospective randomized controlled trials, these drugs should be considered for use in the majority of transplant recipients as there is substantial convincing data in the general population that those individuals with established heart disease and kidney disease do derive a 20% relative risk reduction benefit for cardiovascular and renal events.

REFERENCES

[1] Curtis JJ: Cyclosporine and posttransplant hypertension. *J Am Soc Nephrol* 2:S243-S245, 1992.

[2] Kasiske BL, Anjum S, Shah R, Skogen J, Kandaswamy C, Danielson B, O'Shaughnessy EA, Dahl DC, Silkensen JR, Sahadevan M, Snyder JJ: Hypertension after kidney transplantation. *Am J Kidney Dis* 43:1071-1081, 2004.

[3] Mangray M, Vella JP: Hypertension after kidney transplant. *Am J Kidney Dis* 57:331-341, 2011.

[4] Mange KC, Cizman B, Joffe M, Feldman HI: Arterial hypertension and renal allograft survival. *JAMA* 283:633-638, 2000.

[5] Mange KC, Feldman HI, Joffe MM, Fa K, Bloom RD: Blood pressure and the survival of renal allografts from living donors. *J Am Soc Nephrol* 15:187-193, 2004.

[6] Morath C, Schmied B, Mehrabi A, Weitz J, Schmidt J, Werner J, Buchler MW, Morcos M, Nawroth PP, Schwenger V, Doehler B, Opelz G, Zeier M: Angiotensin-converting enzyme inhibitors and angiotensin II type 1 receptor blockers after renal transplantation. *Clin Transplant* 23 Suppl 21:33-36, 2009.

[7] Ojo AO: Cardiovascular complications after renal transplantation and their prevention. *Transplantation* 82:603-611, 2006.

[8] Opelz G, Wujciak T, Ritz E: Association of chronic kidney graft failure with recipient blood pressure. Collaborative Transplant Study. *Kidney Int* 53:217-222, 1998.

[9] Matas AJ, Gillingham KJ, Humar A, Kandaswamy R, Sutherland DE, Payne WD, Dunn TB, Najarian JS: 2202 kidney transplant recipients with 10 years of graft function: what happens next? *Am J Transplant* 8:2410-2419, 2008.

[10] Ojo AO, Hanson JA, Wolfe RA, Leichtman AB, Agodoa LY, Port FK: Long-term survival in renal transplant recipients with graft function. *Kidney Int* 57:307-313, 2000.

[11] Ponticelli C, Villa M, Cesana B, Montagnino G, Tarantino A: Risk factors for late kidney allograft failure. *Kidney Int* 62:1848-1854, 2002.

[12] Heinze G, Mitterbauer C, Regele H, Kramar R, Winkelmayer WC, Curhan GC, Oberbauer R: Angiotensin-converting enzyme inhibitor or angiotensin II type 1 receptor antagonist therapy is associated with prolonged patient and graft survival after renal transplantation. *J Am Soc Nephrol* 17:889-899, 2006.

[13] Hernandez D, Muriel A, Abraira V, Perez G, Porrini E, Marrero D, Zamora J, Gonzalez-Posada JM, Delgado P, Rufino M, Torres A: Renin-angiotensin system blockade and kidney transplantation: a longitudinal cohort study. *Nephrol Dial Transplant* 27:417-422, 2012.

[14] Pickering TG, Shimbo D, Haas D: Ambulatory blood-pressure monitoring. *N Engl J Med* 354:2368-2374, 2006.

[15] Prasad GV, Nash MM, Zaltzman JS: A prospective study of the physician effect on blood pressure in renal-transplant recipients. *Nephrol Dial Transplant* 18:996-1000, 2003.

[16] Stenehjem AE, Gudmundsdottir H, Os I: Office blood pressure measurements overestimate blood pressure control in renal transplant patients. *Blood Press Monit* 11:125-133, 2006.

[17] Bangash F, Agarwal R: Masked hypertension and white-coat hypertension in chronic kidney disease: a meta-analysis. *Clin J Am Soc Nephrol* 4:656-664, 2009.

[18] Clement DL, De Buyzere ML, De Bacquer DA, de Leeuw PW, Duprez DA, Fagard RH, Gheeraert PJ, Missault LH, Braun JJ, Six RO, Van Der Niepen P, O'Brien E: Prognostic value of ambulatory blood-pressure recordings in patients with treated hypertension. *N Engl J Med* 348:2407-2415, 2003.

[19] Haydar AA, Covic A, Jayawardene S, Agharazii M, Smith E, Gordon I, O'Sullivan H, Goldsmith DJ: Insights from ambulatory blood pressure monitoring: diagnosis of hypertension and diurnal blood pressure in renal transplant recipients. *Transplantation* 77:849-853, 2004.

[20] Paoletti E, Gherzi M, Amidone M, Massarino F, Cannella G: Association of arterial hypertension with renal target organ damage in kidney transplant recipients: the predictive role of ambulatory blood pressure monitoring. *Transplantation* 87:1864-1869, 2009.

[21] Toprak A, Koc M, Tezcan H, Ozener IC, Oktay A, Akoglu E: Night-time blood pressure load is associated with higher left ventricular mass index in renal transplant recipients. *J Hum Hypertens* 17:239-244, 2003.

[22] Wadei HM, Amer H, Taler SJ, Cosio FG, Griffin MD, Grande JP, Larson TS, Schwab TR, Stegall MD, Textor SC: Diurnal blood pressure changes one year after kidney transplantation: relationship to allograft function, histology, and resistive index. *J Am Soc Nephrol* 18:1607-1615, 2007.

[23] Agena F, Prado ES, Souza PS, da Silva GV, Lemos FB, Mion D, Jr., Nahas WC, David-Neto E: Home blood pressure (BP) monitoring in kidney transplant recipients is more adequate to monitor BP than office BP. *Nephrol Dial Transplant* 26:3745-3749, 2011.

[24] KDIGO clinical practice guideline for the care of kidney transplant recipients. *Am J Transplant* 9 Suppl 3:S1-155, 2009.

[25] European best practice guidelines for renal transplantation. Section IV: Long-term management of the transplant recipient. *Nephrol Dial Transplant* 17 Suppl 4:1-67, 2002.

[26] Delahousse M, Chaignon M, Mesnard L, Boutouyrie P, Safar ME, Lebret T, Pastural-Thaunat M, Tricot L, Kolko-Labadens A, Karras A, Haymann JP: Aortic stiffness of kidney transplant recipients correlates with donor age. *J Am Soc Nephrol* 19:798-805, 2008.

[27] Hoorn EJ, Walsh SB, McCormick JA, Zietse R, Unwin RJ, Ellison DH: Pathogenesis of calcineurin inhibitor-induced hypertension. *J Nephrol* 25:269-275, 2012.

[28] Lassila M: Interaction of cyclosporine A and the renin-angiotensin system; new perspectives. *Curr Drug Metab* 3:61-71, 2002.

[29] Melnikov S, Mayan H, Uchida S, Holtzman EJ, Farfel Z: Cyclosporine metabolic side effects: association with the WNK4 system. *Eur J Clin Invest* 41:1113-1120, 2011.

[30] Textor SC, Canzanello VJ, Taler SJ, Wilson DJ, Schwartz LL, Augustine JE, Raymer JM, Romero JC, Wiesner RH, Krom RA,: Cyclosporine-induced hypertension after transplantation. *Mayo Clin Proc* 69:1182-1193, 1994.

[31] Margreiter R: Efficacy and safety of tacrolimus compared with ciclosporin microemulsion in renal transplantation: a randomised multicentre study. *Lancet* 359:741-746, 2002.

[32] Vincenti F, Jensik SC, Filo RS, Miller J, Pirsch J: A long-term comparison of tacrolimus (FK506) and cyclosporine in kidney transplantation: evidence for improved allograft survival at five years. *Transplantation* 73:775-782, 2002.
[33] Taler SJ, Textor SC, Canzanello VJ, Schwartz L, Porayko M, Wiesner RH, Krom RA: Role of steroid dose in hypertension early after liver transplantation with tacrolimus (FK506) and cyclosporine. *Transplantation* 62:1588-1592, 1996.
[34] Goodwin JE, Zhang J, Geller DS: A critical role for vascular smooth muscle in acute glucocorticoid-induced hypertension. *J Am Soc Nephrol* 19:1291-1299, 2008.
[35] Bruno S, Remuzzi G, Ruggenenti P: Transplant renal artery stenosis. *J Am Soc Nephrol* 15:134-141, 2004.
[36] Wong W, Fynn SP, Higgins RM, Walters H, Evans S, Deane C, Goss D, Bewick M, Snowden SA, Scoble JE, Hendry BM: Transplant renal artery stenosis in 77 patients--does it have an immunological cause? *Transplantation* 61:215-219, 1996.
[37] Halimi JM, Al-Najjar A, Buchler M, Birmele B, Tranquart F, Alison D, Lebranchu Y: Transplant renal artery stenosis: potential role of ischemia/reperfusion injury and long-term outcome following angioplasty. *J Urol* 161:28-32, 1999.
[38] Hagen G, Wadstrom J, Magnusson M, Magnusson A: Outcome after percutaneous transluminal angioplasty of arterial stenosis in renal transplant patients. *Acta Radiol* 50:270-275, 2009.
[39] Curtis JJ, Luke RG, Diethelm AG, Whelchel JD, Jones P: Benefits of removal of native kidneys in hypertension after renal transplantation. *Lancet* 2:739-742, 1985.
[40] Voiculescu A, Schmitz M, Hollenbeck M, Braasch S, Luther B, Sandmann W, Jung G, Modder U, Grabensee B: Management of arterial stenosis affecting kidney graft perfusion: a single-centre study in 53 patients. *Am J Transplant* 5:1731-1738, 2005.
[41] Fricke L, Doehn C, Steinhoff J, Sack K, Jocham D, Fornara P: Treatment of posttransplant hypertension by laparoscopic bilateral nephrectomy? *Transplantation* 65:1182-1187, 1998.
[42] Knight SR, Morris PJ: Steroid avoidance or withdrawal after renal transplantation increases the risk of acute rejection but decreases cardiovascular risk. A meta-analysis. *Transplantation* 89:1-14, 2010.
[43] Vincenti F, Larsen C, Durrbach A, Wekerle T, Nashan B, Blancho G, Lang P, Grinyo J, Halloran PF, Solez K, Hagerty D, Levy E, Zhou W, Natarajan K, Charpentier B: Costimulation blockade with belatacept in renal transplantation. *N Engl J Med* 353:770-781, 2005.
[44] Ekberg H, Grinyo J, Nashan B, Vanrenterghem Y, Vincenti F, Voulgari A, Truman M, Nasmyth-Miller C, Rashford M: Cyclosporine sparing with mycophenolate mofetil, daclizumab and corticosteroids in renal allograft recipients: the CAESAR Study. *Am J Transplant* 7:560-570, 2007.
[45] Mavanur M, Sanders M, Unruh M: Sleep disordered breathing in patients with chronic kidney disease. *Indian J Med Res* 131:277-284, 2010.
[46] Marin JM, Agusti A, Villar I, Forner M, Nieto D, Carrizo SJ, Barbe F, Vicente E, Wei Y, Nieto FJ, Jelic S: Association between treated and untreated obstructive sleep apnea and risk of hypertension. *JAMA* 307:2169-2176, 2012.
[47] Hiremath S, Fergusson D, Doucette S, Mulay AV, Knoll GA: Renin angiotensin system blockade in kidney transplantation: a systematic review of the evidence. *Am J Transplant* 7:2350-2360, 2007.

[48] Philipp T, Martinez F, Geiger H, Moulin B, Mourad G, Schmieder R, Lievre M, Heemann U, Legendre C: Candesartan improves blood pressure control and reduces proteinuria in renal transplant recipients: results from SECRET. *Nephrol Dial Transplant* 25:967-976, 2010.

[49] Ibrahim HN, Jackson S, Connaire J, Matas A, Ney A, Najafian B, West A, Lentsch N, Ericksen J, Bodner J, Kasiske B, Mauer M: Angiotensin II blockade in kidney transplant recipients. *J Am Soc Nephrol* 24:320-327, 2013.

[50] Paoletti E, Bellino D, Marsano L, Cassottana P, Rolla D, Ratto E: Effects of ACE inhibitors on long-term outcome of renal transplant recipients: a randomized controlled trial. *Transplantation* 95:889-895, 2013.

[51] Opelz G, Zeier M, Laux G, Morath C, Dohler B: No improvement of patient or graft survival in transplant recipients treated with angiotensin-converting enzyme inhibitors or angiotensin II type 1 receptor blockers: a collaborative transplant study report. *J Am Soc Nephrol* 17:3257-3262, 2006.

[52] Fink HA, Ishani A, Taylor BC, Greer NL, MacDonald R, Rossini D, Sadiq S, Lankireddy S, Kane RL, Wilt TJ: Screening for, monitoring, and treatment of chronic kidney disease stages 1 to 3: a systematic review for the U.S. Preventive Services Task Force and for an American College of Physicians Clinical Practice Guideline. *Ann Intern Med.* 2012;156:570-581.

[53] Lewis EJ, Hunsicker LG, Bain RP, Rohde RD: The effect of angiotensin-converting-enzyme inhibition on diabetic nephropathy. The Collaborative Study Group. *N Engl J Med.* 1993;329:1456-1462.

[54] Paoletti E, Cassottana P, Amidone M, Gherzi M, Rolla D, Cannella G. ACE inhibitors and persistent left ventricular hypertrophy after renal transplantation: a randomized clinical trial. *Am J Kidney Dis.* 2007;50(1):133-42.

In: ACE Inhibitors. Volume 2
Editor: Macaulay Amechi Onuigbo

ISBN: 978-1-62948-422-8

Chapter 11

ACE INHIBITION AND RENAL ARTERY STENOSIS: WHAT LESSONS HAVE WE LEARNT? A 21ST CENTURY PERSPECTIVE

Mukesh Singh, MD MRCPI[1,2*], Daniela Filip Kovacs, MD FACC[1], Amteshwar Singh, MBBS[1], Prabhpreet Dhaliwal[1] and Sandeep Khosla, MD FACC[1].

[1]Chicago Medical School, Rosalind Franklin University of Medicine & Sciences, North Chicago, IL, US

[2]Department of Cardiology, Mt. Sinai Medical Center, Chicago, IL, US

ABSTRACT

Renal artery stenosis (RAS) may result in hypertension and/or ischemic nephropathy, eventually leading to end-stage renal disease. It is most commonly (90 % of all cases) caused by atherosclerotic disease referred to as atherosclerotic renal artery stenosis [ARAS]. The remaining 10% of the lesions include fibromuscular dysplasia [FMD], arteritis, and rare syndromes. Diagnosis and treatment have important implications for both BP control and preservation of renal function. Therapeutic modalities include medical therapy, percutaneous revascularization and surgical revascularization. The goals of therapy are BP control and preservation of renal function. Control of BP in renovascular hypertension may be achieved in most of cases with medical therapy alone, usually with a combination of antihypertensive drugs. Because the hypertension is often the result of activation of the rennin-angiotensin system, blocking this is particularly effective with either angiotensin converting enzyme inhibitors (ACEIs) or angiotensin receptor blockers (ARBs), and is considered a first-line therapy in hypertension coexisting with renal damage, due to renal protection exceeding the blood pressure–lowering effect. Both ACEIs and ARBs may slow the progression of renal function decline and, especially in patients with high cardiovascular risk, reduce the risk of cardiovascular events. In this chapter, we review

* Corresponding author: Mukesh Singh MD MRCPI; Email: drmukeshsingh@yahoo.com.

the role of renin-angiotensin system inhibition in the pathophysiology and management of renovascular hypertension.

BACKGROUND

Renal artery stenosis (RAS) is an anatomic diagnosis and the American Heart Association (AHA) in 2008 defined critical renal artery stenosis as a reduction by more than 60 % in renal artery diameter [1]. It is most commonly (90 % of all cases) caused by atherosclerotic disease referred to as atherosclerotic renal artery stenosis [ARAS]. The remaining 10 % of the lesions include fibromuscular dysplasia [FMD], arteritis, and rare syndromes, mostly reported in children [2–4]. ARAS typically involves the ostium and proximal third of the main renal artery whereas FMD classically involving the distal two-thirds of the renal artery with a characteristic beaded aneurysmal appearance. ARAS reflects a high atherosclerotic burden and is a strong predictor of subsequent cardiovascular events and cardiac mortality. The goals of therapy are to control blood pressure, stabilize renal function, and reduce cardiovascular complications. This article reviews the role of rennin-angiotensin system in pathophysiology and management of ARAS.

EPIDEMIOLOGY OF RAS

The true prevalence of ARAS is not known as it depends on the population examined, although general population autopsy studies had shown a prevalence of about 4%. The prevalence of end-stage renal disease (ESRD) in the United States is 372,407 patients per year, with approximately 100,000 new cases diagnosed each year [5]; 2.1% of these new cases are thought to be due to ARAS [6]. ARAS is reported in 0.5% to 5% of all hypertensive patients and 45% of patients with severe or malignant hypertension [7, 8]. The prevalence of ARAS increases with age, especially in patients with diabetes, hypertension, coronary artery disease, or aortoiliac occlusive disease [9]. In most cases of renal artery stenosis, one kidney is affected with the second kidney being essentially normal, hence the designation, "unilateral" disease. Individuals with high-grade stenosis to both kidneys, or to a solitary functioning kidney thereby affecting the entire functioning renal mass, are considered to have "bilateral" disease.

Atherosclerotic narrowing of the renal arteries generally occurs in older patients (>50 years of age) and is associated with systemic atherosclerosis. Cardiovascular health study was a multicenter, longitudinal cohort study of cardiovascular disease risk factors, morbidity, and mortality among free-living adults of more than 65 years of age. This study provided the first population-based estimate of the prevalence of ARAS among free-living, elderly black and white Americans and ARAS has been found to affect 6.8% of these patients [10]. The prevalence of ARAS is even higher in certain at-risk populations, including patients with poorly controlled hypertension (HTN) and systemic atherosclerosis [11,12]. Although isolated ARAS may be found, it is more commonly a manifestation of systemic atherosclerosis that involves other vascular beds including the aorta, coronary, cerebral, and peripheral arteries. The prevalence of ARAS is approximately 15% in patients with proven coronary artery disease and it is up to 40% in patients with end stage renal disease [13]. ARAS most often affects the aorto-ostial segment, including the proximal 1 cm of the main renal artery, that is, an intrinsic renal plaque extending to and contiguous with the aorta. Aortic and renal vascular calcification is often present [13-15].

Prognosis of ARAS

The natural history of ARAS is incompletely understood. ARAS reflects a high atherosclerotic burden and is a strong predictor of subsequent cardiovascular events including myocardial infarction, stroke, and cardiovascular death, [16-18] with bilateral ARAS conferring a worse prognosis than unilateral ARAS [18]. ARAS is often unrecognized as a contributor to refractory hypertension and renal dysfunction. When adjusted for baseline variables, ARAS remains an independent predictor of cardiovascular mortality, with a 4-year adjusted mortality rate of 25 to 40%. Factors associated with higher mortality include an elevated baseline creatinine level, more severe stenosis of renal arteries, worsening renal function, age, diabetes, other cardiovascular disease, and heart failure. ARAS is an important cause of or contributor to renal failure [19-22]. There is conflicting data about the correlation between severity of initial stenosis and progression to ESRD. In some studies, mortality rate and changes in serum creatinine over time were not correlated with baseline degree of stenosis [23,24]. In contrast, other studies have found that the severity of the stenosis predicted progression of disease, progression to occlusion, and renal atrophy [25,26]. At present, it remains unclear how many patients enter dialysis secondary to ARAS. ARAS also affects overall survival. Mailloux et al found that patients with renovascular disease as the cause of their renal failure had survival rates of 56% at 2 years [27]. In another series of about 4000 patients, screened for ARAS during cardiac catheterization, the 4-year survival rates were similarly much lower for patients with ARAS compared to those without (57% vs 89% without RAS, $P<0.001$) [28]. Moreover, anatomically severe lesions were associated with poor survival (70%, 68%, and 48% rates for 4-year survival for RAS lesions >50%, >75%, and >95% respectively). In patients with ARAS, survival rates fell as renal function declined, [29,30] with higher mortality among those who progressed to end-stage renal disease (ESRD) [27,28].

However, recent data on progression of atherosclerotic RAS suggest improvement of outcomes over last two decades. In earlier studies, progression of ARAS to occlusion had been observed in up to 16% of pharmacologically treated patients [31]. In the more recent Cardiovascular Health Study, no occlusion and 1.3% RAS progression per year were observed over an 8-year period [32]. It is generally believed that the wide use of statins and inhibitors of the renin-angiotensin system have improved the renal prognosis in patients with RAS. Recent data indicate that the decline of renal function in these patients had fallen by a factor of 10 compared with earlier studies [33, 34].

PATHOPHYSIOLOGY

Hypertension

The kidneys play a key role in the homeostatic regulation of blood pressure (BP) via pressure natriuresis and the renin-angiotensin-aldosterone system. Renovascular hypertension (hypertension induced by renal artery stenosis) is a form of secondary hypertension caused by over activation of the renin-angiotensin-aldosterone system by the ischemic kidney. In addition to renin-angiotensin-aldosterone system, several other mechanisms may contribute to the pathogenesis of hypertension, including activation of the sympathetic nervous system [35,36] endothelial dysfunction, oxidative stress [37], ischemic injury of the affected kidney, or hypertensive end-organ damage to the contralateral kidney [38]. Progressive stenosis of the renal artery leads to hypoperfusion of the juxtaglomerular apparatus, release of renin, and increased production of angiotensin II. This process causes increases in sympathetic nerve activity, intra-renal prostaglandin synthesis, aldosterone synthesis, and nitric oxide production, and decrease in renal sodium excretion that promote development of hypertension. Over time, the increased plasma renin activity falls as plasma volume expands, especially when chronic kidney disease is present, (most easily modeled in animal experiments by a prior contralateral nephrectomy, which has been called the one-kidney, one-clip Goldblatt model). During the chronic phase, both BP and intravascular volume can be reduced by angiotensin II antagonists or by relief of the arterial stenosis [39].

Renal Failure

Glomerular filtration rate (GFR) is determined by renal blood flow and glomerular capillary hydrostatic pressure. When renal perfusion pressure is decreased downstream due to RAS, intrarenal compensatory mechanisms are activated to maintain the GFR. These include dilatation of the afferent arteriole mediated by vasodilatory prostaglandins and constriction of the efferent arteriole mediated by angiotensin II, both of which result in increased filtration pressure. This autoregulation can maintain GFR and renal blood flow despite reduction in renal perfusion pressure by up to 40% [40]. Studies in humans with unilateral renal artery stenosis demonstrate that, despite the reduction in filtration in the stenotic kidney, the total GFR is usually well maintained due to a roughly equivalent rise in filtration in the contralateral kidney following the removal of angiotensin II-induced vasoconstriction [41]. A modest elevation in the serum creatinine concentration can occur in selected cases, a change that may be due to intrarenal vascular disease (nephrosclerosis) in the contralateral kidney that has been exposed to high systemic pressures [42,43]. A more significant reduction in renal function has been described in elderly patients with a baseline GFR less than 50 mL/min per 1.73 m^2 [44].

Other Cardiovascular Effects

ARAS has been implicated in pathophysiology of cardiac disturbance syndromes (recurrent unexplained congestive heart failure, refractory angina, and "flash" pulmonary edema). It has been proposed that alterations in circulatory homeostasis can be prominent in individuals with significant RAS and may provoke exacerbations of coronary ischemia and/or congestive heart failure due to peripheral arterial vasoconstriction, direct effects of angiotensin II on the myocardium, and/or volume overload [14]. Renovascular disease may also complicate the long-term management of certain group of patients with hypertension and/or left ventricular systolic dysfunction, by preventing administration of angiotensin antagonist therapies. Individuals with RAS may experience sudden-onset or "flash" pulmonary edema [45-52]. Patients with hemodynamically severe bilateral or solitary RAS lack normal renal function to respond to pressure natriuresis and, thus, are prone to have acute volume overload [51, 52]. Patients with unilateral RAS may also experience pulmonary edema due to increased left ventricular afterload secondary to angiotensin-mediated vasoconstriction. Unilateral RAS may contribute to the development of unstable coronary syndromes by causing sudden increases in myocardial oxygen demand in patients with coronary disease secondary to peripheral vasoconstriction; this mechanism is distinct from the plaque rupture causing acute coronary syndromes [53, 54].

Management of RAS

Patients with atherosclerotic renovascular disease have a high rate of systemic atherosclerosis and are at increased risk for adverse cardiovascular outcomes. As a result, they are considered to have a coronary artery disease equivalent and should be treated according to current guidelines for secondary prevention of cardiovascular disease. The goals of therapy are to control blood pressure, stabilize and preserve renal function, and reduce cardiovascular complications. Treatment of RAS involves medical therapy, revascularization, or both. Medical therapy is the cornerstone of treatment for RAS either alone or in combination with revascularization. The majority of evidence supporting current medical therapies is derived from studies conducted in patients with hypertension, diabetes, CKD, CAD, or heart failure rather than RAS specifically.

BP Control

Medical therapy thus far has focused on BP control and control of BP in renovascular hypertension may be achieved in most of cases with medical therapy alone, usually with a combination of antihypertensive drugs. Although it is well known that lowering BP can prevent adverse cardiovascular events, the ideal BP target that confers maximal cardiovascular protection is not known. Current blood pressure reduction target as recommended by Joint National Committee VII guidelines is below 140/90 mm Hg or below 130/80 mm Hg for patients with diabetes or CKD [55]. However, the evidence base for lower

BP targets is not strong and recent trials indicate a target pressure less than 140/90mm Hg is probably right [56,57]. Current ACC/AHA guidelines recommend angiotensin-converting enzyme inhibitors (ACEIs) (class I, LOE A), angiotensin receptor blockers (ARBs) (class I, LOE B), and calcium-channel blockers (class I, LOE A) for the treatment of hypertension in unilateral RAS; and β-blockers (class I, LOE A) are recommended for the treatment of hypertension in patients with RAS in general [14].

Multiple studies have now shown that ACEIs and calcium-channel blockers are effective in the treatment of hypertension in the presence of RAS [58-62]. Since the introduction of ACEIs, several authors reported successful BP control in 82%–96% of patients with renovascular hypertension [63]. Also, there is some evidence that ACEIs have the most potent BP-lowering effect in these patients [64]. These results address primarily the treatment of hypertension, but diminution in the progression of renal disease has also been demonstrated. Because the hypertension is often the result of activation of the rennin-angiotensin system, blockers of rennin-angiotensin system are particularly effective and rennin-angiotensin system blockade with ACEIs is considered a first-line therapy in hypertension coexisting with renal damage, due to renal protection exceeding the blood pressure–lowering effect. ARBs can be used as alternative agents.

Preservation of Renal Function

RAS is often suspected in patients with unexplained impairment in renal function, especially in hypertensive patients. RAS initially results in activation of the rennin-angiotensin-aldosterone system in response to autoregulatory pathways but in long-term this results in activation of inflammatory and profibrogenic pathways, production of reactive oxygen species leading to oxidative stress, and sympathetic nerve activation [65-67]. Thus, high levels of angiotensin II may contribute to vascular hypertrophy, proliferation of smooth muscle cells, and progressive glomerular sclerosis. Thus, antagonizing the rennin-angiotensin-aldosterone system appears to be a good target to stabilize or improve renal function and for reducing cardiovascular events recognized in ARAS. Moreover, ACEIs have been shown to preserve the renal blood flow and GFR in the kidney with RAS [68]. In patients with ARAS and advanced renal disease (chronic renal failure, proteinuria [>1 g/d]), diffuse intrarenal vascular disease, and renal atrophy), medical therapy is preferred to revascularization [69].

Cardiovascular Risk Reduction

ARAS reflects a high atherosclerotic burden and is a strong predictor of subsequent cardiovascular events. These patients must receive comprehensive therapy to reduce cardiovascular risk [70]. Medical therapy includes lipid-lowering therapy, smoking cessation, glycemic control in patients with diabetes mellitus, and antiplatelet medications in addition to hypertension treatment. Recent studies have established the benefit of ARBs and ACEIs in patients with coronary artery disease, congestive heart failure, or chronic renal disease. ACEIs use was independently associated with survival benefit in nonrandomized studies of patients with RAS, regardless of revascularization [71,72]. Losito et al [71] assessed the role of comorbid conditions, and pharmacological treatment on survival, and on renal function in 64 patients with diffuse atherosclerotic vascular and renovascular disease (RVD). The patients were followed for an average period of 37.3+/-20.4 months. At the end of the follow-up we found a cumulative survival at 5 years of 60%+/-10. Cerebrovascular and cardiovascular diseases were responsible for 92% of deaths. A decrease in creatinine clearance >10 ml/min at 5 years was found in 65% of patients, 3 of whom ended in dialysis. Multivariate analysis of predictors of survival showed that treatment with ACEIs was significantly associated with a favorable outcome ($p = 0.019$). Authors concluded that ACEIs have a beneficial effect on survival without affecting renal function in patients with RVD due to unilateral renal stenosis [71]. Hackam et al studied the association of renin-angiotensin system inhibition with prognosis in a population-based cohort comprising 3,570 patients with RVD in Ontario, Canada; slightly more than half (n = 1,857, 53%) were prescribed angiotensin inhibitors. The primary outcome was the composite of death, myocardial infarction, or stroke. Secondary outcomes included individual cardiovascular and renal events. Patients receiving angiotensin inhibitors had a significantly lower risk for the primary outcome during follow-up (10.0 vs 13.0 events per 100 patient-years at risk, multivariable adjusted hazard ratio [HR] 0.70, 95% CI 0.59-0.82). In addition, hospitalization for congestive heart failure (HR 0.69, 95% CI 0.53-0.90), chronic dialysis initiation (HR 0.62, 95% CI 0.42-0.92), and mortality (HR 0.56, 95% CI 0.47-0.68) was lower in treated patients [73].

Safety of RAAS Blockers in ARAS

The use of ACEIs and ARBs is sometimes limited in patients with RAS over concerns of precipitating acute renal failure. With hemodynamically significant ARAS, renal artery perfusion pressure is reduced distal to the stenosis that can cause precipitous declines in glomerular filtration pressure and filtration rate. Inhibiting the autoregulatory compensatory response (previously described in pathophysiology section) with an ACEIs or ARBs can lower GFR in the ischemic kidney, even though the associated decrease in renal vascular resistance may preserve renal blood flow [42,74]. A decline in GFR is less common with other antihypertensive agents, which do not preferentially decrease the resistance at the efferent arteriole. However, when vascular stenosis reaches a "critical" level, reduction in perfusion pressure with any antihypertensive agent can lower GFR, which will be clinically evident in patients who have bilateral disease [75]. However, available evidence suggests that the actual incidence of acute kidney injury with renin-angiotensin blocking drugs in patients with ARAS is quite low, affecting fewer than 5% of patients. A decline in renal function after initiation of an ACEI or ARB is often associated with bilateral RAS but is neither a sensitive nor a specific finding [76]. Hackam et al [77] suggest that these concerns may be overstated and may be applicable only to a specific subset of patients with RAS. In their retrospective analysis of about 10, 000 patients referred to a large hypertension clinic, including >400 patients with renovascular hypertension, authors found only 18 patients with acute renal failure with angiotensin blockade and all were reversible with discontinuation of renin angiotensin blockers. van de Ven et al [78] prospectively evaluated the renal function after initiation of enalapril in 93 patients with ARAS and used an increase in serum creatinine of ≥20% from baseline as the threshold for discontinuation of the medication. The study showed that all patients with severe bilateral RAS (≥50%) could not tolerate ACEIs because of increases of serum creatinine beyond the established threshold. On the other hand, most (63%) patients with unilateral RAS or lesser degrees of bilateral RAS (>50%) showed no significant increase in serum creatinine. All elevations in serum creatinine induced by initiation of ACEIs in this study were reversible with discontinuation of the medication, and no cases of renal failure were seen [78]. Current evidence suggests that acute deterioration in renal function is mainly confined to cases in which the entire renal mass is subject to renovascular obstruction [76,78-82]. Additional risk factors for acute renal failure in this setting include severe congestive heart failure, use of high-dose loop diuretics, volume contraction, and poor baseline renal function [81-83]. These results suggest that treatment with ACEIs can be safely initiated in patients with RAS as long as it is performed with careful supervision. If elevations in serum creatinine of ≥20% from baseline do occur, the medication should be promptly discontinued; and further investigation to the severity of their RAS may be warranted.

Renal Revascularization

Revascularization using angioplasty with or without stent in combination with medical therapy has been compared with medical therapy alone in seven randomized trials that included patients with unilateral ARAS [31,84-89]. These trials have failed to demonstrate any superiority of renal revascularization over medical therapy, with regard to attained blood pressure [31,33], change in renal function, or the incidence of heart failure, stroke, or total mortality [33,85]. There are limited data concerning renal stenting and cardiovascular outcomes. Nonrandomized cohort studies have suggested cardiovascular survival benefits in patients with RAS revascularized with surgery [90] or stents [91,92]. More recently, an impressive survival advantage was demonstrated for patients with CKD stage IV or V who were treated with revascularization compared to those treated with medical therapy [93]. The DRASTIC, EMMA and Scottish studies [31,88,89] used balloon angioplasty without stenting, and significantly less frequent use of renin-angiotensin system blockade compared with current practice. The STAR [85] and ASTRAL [34] were more contemporary trials, utilizing current guidelines for medical treatment but they also failed to demonstrate any benefit of revascularization on top of medical therapy. However, these trials had significant limitations and it has been suggested that in selected high-risk patients, renal revascularization may still have an important role. In brief, for patients with unilateral atherosclerotic renal artery stenosis who have characteristics similar to those enrolled in the STAR and ASTRAL trials, current data suggests that percutaneous renal revascularization provides no additional benefit to medical therapy and increases the risk of adverse events. Unfortunately, neither the STAR nor ASTRAL trial was powered to assess cardiovascular endpoints.

Renal Revascularisation Allows ACEI Use

A potential benefit of revascularization is the possibility of using ACEIs or ARBs in patients who previously did not tolerate renin-angiotensin blockade [94,95]. As the evidence base for the benefits of ACEI treatment accumulates, it is becoming clear that nearly all patients with ARAS will have some indication for ACEI use, because of CAD, impaired left ventricular function, cerebrovascular disease, or renal impairment with proteinuria [96,97]. In patients with bilateral ARAS it is usually impossible to use ACEI treatment without unacceptable loss of renal function. It is, however, usually possible to re-introduce ACEI treatment after successful renal revascularisation. Chrysochou et al [94] prospectively studied 621 patients with atherosclerotic renovascular disease. Mean age (SD) of the cohort was 71.3 (8.8) years, median (interquartile range) follow-up 3.1 (2.1, 4.8), range 0.2-10.61 years. Seventy-four patients had intolerance to angiotensin blockade at study entry. When utilized prospectively, renin-angiotensin blockade was tolerated in 357 of 378 patients (92%), and this was even seen in 54/69 (78.3%) patients with bilateral >60% renal artery stenosis (RAS) or occlusion. Patients (4/21) who were intolerant of renin-angiotensin blockade during follow-up (and 12 retrospectively intolerant), underwent renal revascularization which facilitated safe use of these medications post-procedure. On multivariate time-adjusted analysis, patients receiving renin-angiotensin blockade were significantly less likely to die (P=0.02). Authors concluded all atherosclerotic RVD patients be considered for renin-angiotensin blockade therapy unless an absolute contra-indication exists. Intolerance of these agents due to renal dysfunction should be considered an emerging indication for renal revascularization to facilitate their re-introduction [94]. We evaluated the safety of ACEI therapy in patients with bilateral RAS following successful revascularization using renal artery stenting [95]. We retrospectively analyzed 25 patients, from a larger prospective registry of 132 consecutive patients, who underwent bilateral renal artery stenting (bilateral renal artery stenting, 24; stenting of solitary kidney, 1) for refractory hypertension and had a strong clinical indication for long-term ACEI use (left ventricular dysfunction or diabetes). Patients were treated with ACEIs if the postprocedure serum creatinine level was < 2.0 mg/dL and the mean interval between stent revascularization and initiation of therapy was 11 ± 9 days. Eighteen of the 25 patients (72%) were safely maintained on a target dose of ACEIs, 2 of the 25 were treated with angiotensin receptor blockers due to cough with a mean follow-up of 26 ± 14 months. This indicates that patients with bilateral renal artery stenoses that have been successfully revascularized using renal stenting may be safely treated with long-term ACEI therapy [95]. These observations suggest that we should intervene not simply to improve blood pressure control or prevent progression of renal disease, but to switch off over activity in the renin-angiotensin system and thereby reduce cardio- and cerebrovascular morbidity and mortality. The renin-angiotensin system probably remains overactive after revascularization because of almost inevitable co-existent intrarenal vascular and parenchymal damage, and the extra benefit seen with aldosterone antagonism on top of renin-angiotensin system inhibition in trials may be due to suppressing the phenomenon of aldosterone escape [98].

CONCLUSION

RAS is caused by a heterogeneous group of diseases with varying pathophysiology, clinical manifestations and courses, treatments, and outcomes. ARAS and fibromuscular dysplasia are the most common causes of RAS. ARAS is prevalent and has potential serious medical consequences, and treatment options include medical and interventional therapies. Optimal medical therapy is the backbone of treatment for ARAS, whether intervention is required or not. The goals of therapy are to control blood pressure, stabilize renal function, and reduce cardiovascular complications. ACEIs are of particular benefit for patients with ARAS, and their use is supported by societal guidelines. ARBs can be used as an alternative. Although a renin–angiotensin–aldosterone system inhibitor may induce acute renal failure in some patients with ARAS, it is generally seen with bilateral severe stenosis, high-grade stenosis in one kidney, or advanced chronic kidney disease [76], the probability of this complication appears to be low, and in most cases, it is reversible with the discontinuation of treatment. Moreover, recent data from a large cohort of patients with renal-artery stenosis suggested a reduced risk of death among patients treated with an ACEI [99]. The available data from randomized trials have not shown a benefit of revascularization plus medical therapy with respect to blood-pressure control and renal function; however, these trials had methodological limitations, and were not powered for the assessment of cardiovascular outcomes.

REFERENCES

[1] Rocha-Singh KJ, Eisenhauer AC, Textor SC, et al. Atherosclerotic Peripheral Vascular Disease Symposium II: intervention for renal artery disease. *Circulation.* 2008;118(25):2873–8.

[2] Safian RD, Textor SC. Renal-artery stenosis. *N Engl J Med.* 2001;344(6):431–42.

[3] Tullus K, Brennan E, Hamilton G, et al. Renovascular hypertension in children. *Lancet.* 2008;371(9622):1453–63.

[4] Slovut DP, Olin JW. Fibromuscular dysplasia. *Curr Treat Options Cardiovasc Med.* 2005;7(2):159–69.

[5] McCullough PA: Cardiorenal risk: an important clinical intersection. *Rev Cardiovasc Med* 3(2):71–76, 2002.

[6] Fatica RA, Port FK, Young EW: Incidence trends and mortality in end-stage renal disease attributed to renovascular disease in the United States. *Am J Kidney Dis* 37(6):1184–1190, 2001.

[7] Mann SJ, Pickering TG: Detection of renovascular hypertension. State of the art: 1992. *Ann Intern Med* 117(10):845–853, 1992.

[8] Derkx FH, Schalekamp MA. Renal artery stenosis and hypertension. *Lancet* 194;344:237-9.

[9] Crowley JJ, Santos RM, Peter RH, et al: Progression of renal artery stenosis in patients undergoing cardiac catheterization. *Am Heart J* 136(5):913–918, 1998.

[10] Hansen KJ, Edwards MS, Craven TE, et al. Prevalence of renovascular disease in the elderly: a population-based study. *J Vasc Surg* 2002;36:443-451.

[11] Davis RP, Pearce JD, Craven TE, et al. Atherosclerotic renovascular disease among hypertensive adults. *J Vasc Surg* 2009;50:564-570.

[12] Olin JW, Melia M, Young JR, Graor RA, Risius B. Prevalence of atherosclerotic renal artery stenosis in patients with atherosclerosis elsewhere. *Am J Med* 1990;88:46N-51N.

[13] de Mast Q, Beutler JJ: The prevalence of atherosclerotic renal artery stenosis in risk groups: a systematic literature review. *J Hypertens* 2009, 27(7):1333–1340.

[14] Hirsch AT, Haskal ZJ, Hertzer NR, et al. ACC/AHA 2005 guidelines for the management of patients with peripheral arterial disease (lower extremity, renal, mesenteric, and abdominal aortic): executive summary of a collaborative report from the American Association for Vascular Surgery/Society for Vascular Surgery, Society for Cardiovascular Angiography and Intervention, Society for Vascular Medicine and Biology, Society of Interventional Radiology, and the ACC/AHA Task Force on Practice Guidelines for the Management of Patients With Peripheral Arterial Disease) endorsed by the American Association of Cardiovascular and Pulmonary Rehabilitation; National Heart, Lung, and Blood Institute; Society for Vascular Nursing; TransAtlantic Inter-Society Consensus; and Vascular Disease Foundation. *J Am Coll Cardiol* 2006;47:1239-312.

[15] Mui KW: Incidental Renal Artery Stenosis Is an Independent Predictor of Mortality in Patients with Peripheral Vascular Disease. *J Am Soc Nephrol* 2006, 17(7):2069–2074.

[16] Garovic V, Textor SC. Renovascular hypertension: current concepts. *Semin Nephrol* 2005;25:261-71.

[17] Garovic VD, Textor SC. Renovascular hypertension and ischemic nephropathy. *Circulation* 2005;112:1362-74.

[18] Conlon PJ, Little MA, Pieper K, Mark DB. Severity of renal vascular disease predicts mortality in patients undergoing coronary angiography. *Kidney Int* 2001;60:1490-7.

[19] Rimmer JM, Gennari FJ. Atherosclerotic renovascular disease and progressive renal failure. *Ann Intern Med* 1993;118:712-9.

[20] Harjai K, Khosla S, Shaw D, et al. Effect of gender on outcomes following renal artery stent placement for renovascular hypertension. *Cathet Cardiovasc Diagn* 1997;42:381-6.

[21] Tuttle KR. Ischemic nephropathy. *Curr Opin Nephrol Hypertens* 2001;10:167-73.

[22] Tuttle KR. Toward more rational management of ischemic nephropathy: the need for clinical evidence. *Am J Kidney Dis* 2000;36:863-5.

[23] Iglesias JI, Hamburger RJ, Feldman L, Kaufman JS. The natural history of incidental renal artery stenosis in patients with aortoiliac vascular disease. *Am J Med* 2000;109:642-647.

[24] Williamson WK, Abou-Zamzam AM Jr, Moneta GL, et al. Prophylactic repair of renal artery stenosis is not justified in patients who require infrarenal aortic reconstruction. *J Vasc Surg* 1998;28:14-20.

[25] Caps MT, Zierler RE, Polissar NL, et al. Risk of atrophy in kidneys with atherosclerotic renal artery stenosis. *Kidney Int* 1998;53:735-742.

[26] Schreiber MJ, Pohl MA, Novick AC. The natural history of atherosclerotic and fibrous renal artery disease. *Urol Clin North Am* 1984;11:383-392.

[27] Mailloux LU, Napolitano B, Bellucci AG, et al. Renal vascular disease causing end-stage renal disease, incidence, clinical correlates, and outcomes: a 20-year clinical experience. *Am J Kidney Dis* 1994;24:622-9.

[28] Eggers PW, Connerton R, McMullan M. The Medicare experience with end-stage renal disease: trends in incidence, prevalence, and survival. *Health Care Financ Rev* 1984;5:69-88.

[29] Dorros G, Jaff M, Mathiak L, et al. Four-year follow-up of Palmaz-Schatz stent revascularization as treatment for atherosclerotic renal artery stenosis. *Circulation* 1998;98:642-7.

[30] Kalra PA, Chrysochou C, Green D, et al. The benefit of renal artery stenting in patients with atheromatous renovascular disease and advanced chronic kidney disease. *Catheter Cardiovasc Interv* 2010;75:1-10.
[31] van Jaarsveld BC, Krijnen P, Pieterman H, et al; Dutch Renal Artery Stenosis Intervention Cooperative Study Group. The effect of balloon angioplasty on hypertension in atherosclerotic renal-artery stenosis. *N Engl J Med.* 2000;342(14): 1007-1014.
[32] Pearce JD, Craven BL, Craven TE, et al. Progression of atherosclerotic renovascular disease: a prospective populationbased study. *J Vasc Surg.* 2006;44(5):955-962, discussion 962-963.
[33] Wheatley K, Ives N, Gray R, et al; ASTRAL Investigators. Revascularization versus medical therapy for renal-artery stenosis. *N Engl J Med.* 2009;361(20):1953-1962.
[34] Harden PN, MacLeod MJ, Rodger RS, et al. Effect of renal-artery stenting on progression of renovascular renal failure.*Lancet.* 1997;349(9059):1133-1136.
[35] Johansson M, Elam M, Rundqvist B, et al. Increased sympathetic nerveactivity in renovascular hypertension. *Circulation* 1999;99:2537-42.
[36] Petersson MJ, Rundqvist B, Johansson M, et al. Increased cardiac sympathetic drive in renovascular hypertension. *J Hypertens* 2002;20:1181-7.
[37] Higashi Y, Sasaki S, Nakagawa K, et al. Endothelial function and oxidative stress in renovascular hypertension. *N Engl J Med* 2002;346:1954-62.
[38] Korner PI. Cardiovascular hypertrophy and hypertension: causes and consequences. *Blood Press Suppl* 1995;2:6-16.
[39] Elliott WJ. Secondary hypertension: Renovasculat hypertension. Hypertension: A Companion to Braunwald's Heart Disease. ISBN: 978-1-4777-2766-1.
[40] Textor SC, Wilcox CS. Ischemic nephropathy/azotemic renovascular disease. *Semin Nephrol* 2000;20:489-502.
[41] Hollenberg NK. The treatment of renovascular hypertension: surgery, angioplasty, and medical therapy with converting-enzyme inhibitors. *Am J Kidney Dis.* 1987;10(1 Suppl 1):52.
[42] Hricik DE, Dunn MJ. Angiotensin-converting enzyme inhibitor-induced renal failure: causes, consequences, and diagnostic uses. *J Am Soc Nephrol.* 1990;1(6):845.
[43] Franklin SS, Smith RD. Comparison of effects of enalapril plus hydrochlorothiazide versus standard triple therapy on renal function in renovascular hypertension. *Am J Med.* 1985;79(3C):14.
[44] Onuigbo MA, Onuigbo NT. Worsening renal failure in older chronic kidney disease patients with renal artery stenosis concurrently on renin angiotensin aldosterone system blockade: a prospective 50-month Mayo-Health-System clinic analysis. *QJM.* 2008;101(7):519.
[45] Pickering TG, Herman L, Devereux RB, et al. Recurrent pulmonary oedema in hypertension due to bilateral renal artery stenosis: treatment by angioplasty or surgical revascularization. *Lancet* 1988;2:551-2.
[46] Messina LM, Zelenock GB, Yao KA, et al. Renal revascularization for recurrent pulmonary edema in patients with poorly controlled hypertension and renal insufficiency: a distinct subgroup of patients with arteriosclerotic renal artery occlusive disease. *J Vasc Surg* 1992;15:73-80; discussion 80-2.

[47] Weatherford DA, Freeman MB, Regester RF, et al. Surgical management of flash pulmonary edema secondary to renovascular hypertension. *Surg Gynecol Obstet* 1997;174:160-3.

[48] Mansoor S, Shah A, Scoble JE. 'Flash pulmonary oedema'—a diagnosis for both the cardiologist and the nephrologist? *Nephrol Dial Transplant* 2001;16:1311-3.

[49] Planken II, Rietveld AP. Rapid onset pulmonary edema (flash edema) in renal artery stenosis. *Neth J Med* 1998;52:116-9.

[50] Gray BH, Olin JW, Childs MB, et al. Clinical benefit of renal artery angioplasty with stenting for the control of recurrent and refractory congestive heart failure. *Vasc Med* 2002;7:275-9.

[51] Azizi M, Lavergne T, Day M, et al. Renal artery stenosis and congestive heart failure. *Lancet* 1993;342(8866):302.

[52] Missouris CG, Buckenham T, Vallance PJ, et al. Renal artery stenosis masquerading as congestive heart failure. *Lancet* 1993; 341:1521-2.

[53] Tami LF, McElderry MW, al-Adli NM, et al. Renal artery stenosis presenting as crescendo angina pectoris. *Cathet Cardiovasc Diagn* 1995;35:252-6.

[54] Gross CM, Kramer J, Waigand J, et al. Ostial renal artery stent placement for atherosclerotic renal artery stenosis in patients with coronary artery disease. *Cathet Cardiovasc Diagn* 1998;45:1-8.

[55] Chobanian AV, Bakris GL, Black HR, et al: The seventh report of the Joint National Committee on Prevention, Detection, Evaluation, and Treatment of High Blood Pressure: the JNC 7 report. *JAMA* 2003; 289: 2560-2572.

[56] Hansson L, Zanchetti A, Carruthers SG, et al. Effects of intensive bloodpressure lowering and low-dose aspirin in patients with hypertension: principal results of the Hypertension Optimal Treatment (HOT) randomized trial: HOT Study Group. *Lancet* 1998; 351:1755–1762.

[57] Meier P, Maillard MP, Meier JR, et al. Combining blockers of the renin-angiotensin system or increasing the dose of an angiotensin II receptor antagonist in proteinuric patients: a randomized triple-crossover study. *J Hypertens* 2011; 29:1228–1235.

[58] Plouin PF, Chatellier G, Darne B, et al. Blood pressure outcome of angioplasty in atherosclerotic renal artery stenosis: a randomized trial. Essai Multicentrique Medicaments vs Angioplastie (EMMA) Study Group. *Hypertension* 1998;31:823-9.

[59] Webster J, Marshall F, Abdalla M, et al. Randomized comparison of percutaneous angioplasty vs continued medical therapy for hypertensive patients with atheromatous renal artery stenosis. Scottish and Newcastle Renal Artery Stenosis Collaborative Group. *J Hum Hypertens* 1998;12:329-35.

[60] Nordmann AJ, Woo K, Parkes R, et al. Balloon angioplasty or medical therapy for hypertensive patients with atherosclerotic renal artery stenosis? A meta-analysis of randomized controlled trials. *Am J Med* 2003;114:44-50.

[61] Plouin PF. Stable patients with atherosclerotic renal artery stenosis should be treated first with medical management. *Am J Kidney Dis* 2003;42:851-7.

[62] Hollenberg NK. Medical therapy of renovascular hypertension: efficacy and safety of captopril in 269 patients. *Cardiovasc Rev Repl* 1983;4:852-76.

[63] Textor SC. ACE inhibitors in renovascular hypertension. *Cardiovasc Drugs Ther* 1990; 4:229–235.

[64] Tullis MJ, Caps MT, Zierler RE, et al. Blood pressure, antihypertensive medication, and atherosclerotic renal artery stenosis. *Am J Kidney Dis* 1999;33:675-81.

[65] Meier P, Rossert J, Plouin PF, Burnier M. Atherosclerotic renovascular disease: beyond the renal artery stenosis. *Nephrol Dial Transplant* 2007; 22:1002–1006.

[66] Textor SC, Lerman L, McKusick M. The uncertain value of renal artery interventions: where are we now? *JACC Cardiovasc Interv* 2009; 2:175–182.

[67] Seddon M, Saw J. Atherosclerotic renal artery stenosis: review of pathophysiology, clinical trial evidence, and management strategies. *Can J Cardiol* 2011.

[68] Gloviczki ML, Glockner JF, Lerman LO, et al. Preserved oxygenation despite reduced blood flow in poststenotic kidneys in human atherosclerotic renal artery stenosis. *Hypertension* 2010; 55:961–966.

[69] Bokhari SW, Faxon DP. Current advances in the diagnosis and treatment of renal artery stenosis. *Rev cardiovasc Med.* 2004;5(4):204-215.

[70] Reich SB. Renal-artery stenosis. *N Engl J Med* 2001;345:221.

[71] Losito A, Gaburri M, Errico R, Parente B, Cao PG. Survival of patients with renovascular disease and ACE inhibition. *Clin Nephrol* 1999;52: 339-43.

[72] Losito A, Errico R, Santirosi P, et al. Long-term follow-up of atherosclerotic renovascular disease. Beneficial effect of ACE inhibition. *Nephrol Dial Transplant* 2005;20:1604-9.

[73] Hackam DG, Duong-Hua ML, Mamdani M, et al. Angiotensin inhibition in renovascular disease: a population-based cohort study. *Am Heart J* 2008;156:549-55.

[74] Schoolwerth AC, Sica DA, Ballermann BJ, Wilcox CS, Council on the Kidney in Cardiovascular Disease and the Council for High Blood Pressure Research of the American Heart Association. Renal considerations in angiotensin converting enzyme inhibitor therapy: a statement for healthcare professionals from the Council on the Kidney in Cardiovascular Disease and the Council for High Blood Pressure Research of the American Heart Association. *Circulation*. 2001 Oct;104(16):1985-91.

[75] Textor SC, Novick AC, Tarazi RC, Klimas V, Vidt DG, Pohl M. Critical perfusion pressure for renal function in patients with bilateral atherosclerotic renal vascular disease. *Ann Intern Med.* 1985;102(3):308.

[76] Hricik DE, Browning PJ, Kopelman R, Goorno WE, Madias NE, Dzau VJ. Captopril-induced functional renal insufficiency in patients with bilateral renal-artery stenoses or renal-artery stenosis in a solitary kidney. *N Eng J Med* 1983;308(7):373-376.

[77] Hackam DG, Spence D, Garg AX, et al. Role of renin-angiotensin system blockade in atherosclerotic renal artery stenosis. *Hypertension* 2007;50:998-1003.

[78] van de Ven PJ, Beuttler JJ, Kaatee R, et al. Angiotensin converting enzyme inhibitor–induced renal dysfunction in atherosclerotic renovascular disease. *Kidney Int* 1998;53:986-93.

[79] O'Donnell D. Renal failure due to enalapril and captopril in bilateral renal artery stenosis: greater awareness needed. *Med J Aust*. 1988;148: 525–527.

[80] Silas JH, Klenka Z, Solomon SA, Bone JM. Captopril induced reversible renal failure: a marker of renal artery stenosis affecting a solitary kidney. *BMJ* (*Clin Res Ed*). 1983;286:1702–1703.

[81] Jackson B, Matthews PG, McGrath BP, Johnston CI. Angiotensin converting enzyme inhibition in renovascular hypertension: frequency of reversible renal failure. *Lancet*. 1984;1:225–226.

[82] Jackson B, McGrath BP, Matthews PG, Wong C, Johnston CI. Differential renal function during angiotensin converting enzyme inhibition in renovascular hypertension. *Hypertension*. 1986;8:650–654.

[83] Maillard JO, Descombes E, Fellay G, Regamey C. Repeated transient anuria following losartan administration in a patient with a solitary kidney. *Ren Fail*. 2001;23:143–147.

[84] ASTRAL Investigators, Wheatley K, Ives N, Gray R, Kalra PA, Moss JG, Baigent C, Carr S, Chalmers N, Eadington D, Hamilton G, Lipkin G, Nicholson A, Scoble J. Revascularization versus medical therapy for renal-artery stenosis. *N Engl J Med*. 2009;361(20):1953.

[85] Bax L, Woittiez AJ, Kouwenberg HJ, Mali WP, Buskens E, et al. Stent placement in patients with atherosclerotic renal artery stenosis and impaired renal function: a randomized trial. *Ann Intern Med*. 2009;150(12):840-848, W150-151.

[86] Marcantoni C, Zanoli L, Rastelli S, Tripepi G, Matalone M, Mangiafico S, Capodanno D, Scandura S, Di Landro D, Tamburino C, Zoccali C, Castellino P. Effect of renal artery stenting on left ventricular mass: a randomized clinical trial. *Am J Kidney Dis*. 2012;60(1):39.

[87] Kumbhani DJ, Bavry AA, Harvey JE, de Souza R, Scarpioni R, Bhatt DL, Kapadia SR. Clinical outcomes after percutaneous revascularization versus medical management in patients with significant renal artery stenosis: a meta-analysis of randomized controlled trials. *Am Heart J*. 2011;161(3):622.

[88] Plouin PF, Chatellier G, Darné B, Raynaud A. Blood pressure outcome of angioplasty in atherosclerotic renal artery stenosis: a randomized trial. Essai Multicentrique Medicaments vs Angioplastie (EMMA) Study Group. *Hypertension*. 1998;31(3):823-829.

[89] Webster J, Marshall F, Abdalla M, Dominiczak A, Edwards R, Isles CG, Loose H, Main J, Padfield P, Russell IT, Walker B, Watson M, Wilkinson R. Scottish and Newcastle Renal Artery Stenosis Collaborative Group. Randomized comparison of percutaneous angioplasty vs continued medical therapy for hypertensive patients with atheromatous renal artery stenosis. *J Hum Hypertens*. 1998;12(5):329-335.

[90] Hunt JC, Sheps SG, Harrison EG Jr, Strong CG, Bernatz PE. Renal and renovascular hypertension. A reasoned approach to diagnosis and management. *Arch Intern Med* 1974;133:988-99.

[91] Dorros G, Jaff M, Mathiak L, et al. Four-year follow-up of Palmaz-Schatz stent revascularization as treatment for atherosclerotic renal artery stenosis. *Circulation* 1998;98:642-7.

[92] Pizzolo F, Mansueto G, Minniti S, et al. Renovascular disease: effect of ACE gene deletion polymorphism and endovascular revascularization. *J Vasc Surg* 2004;39:140-7.

[93] Kalra PA, Chrysochou C, Green D, et al. The benefit of renal artery stenting in patients with atheromatous renovascular disease and advanced chronic kidney disease. *Catheter Cardiovasc Interv* 2010;75:1-10.

[94] Chrysochou C, Foley RN, Young JF, Khavandi K, Cheung CM, Kalra PA. Dispelling the myth: the use of renin-angiotensin blockade in atheromatous renovascular disease. *Nephrol Dial Transplant*. 2012;27(4):1403-1409.

[95] Khosla S, Ahmed A, Siddiqui M, et al. Safety of angiotensin converting enzyme inhibitors in patients with bilateral renal artery stenosis following successful renal artery stent revascularization. *Am J Ther*. 2006;13(4):306-308.

[96] Lewis EJ, Hunsicker LG, Clarke WR, et al. Renoprotective effect of the angiotensin receptor antagonist irbesartan in patients with nephropathy due to type 2 diabetes. *N Engl J Med* 2001;345:851–60.

[97] Lip GYH, Beevers DG. More evidence on blocking the renin-angiotensin- aldosterone system in cardiovascular disease and the long-term treatment of hypertension: data from recent clinical trials (CHARM, EUROPA, ValHEFT, HOPE-TOO and SYST-EUR2). *J Hum Hypertens* 2003;17:747–50.

[98] Epstein M. Aldosterone receptor blockade and the role of eplerenone: evolving perspectives. *Nephrol Dial Transplant* 2003;18:1984–92.

[99] Hackam DG, Duong-Hua ML, Mamdani M, et al. Angiotensin inhibition *in renovascular disease: a population-based cohort study.* Am Heart J 2008;156:549-55.

In: ACE Inhibitors. Volume 2
Editor: Macaulay Amechi Onuigbo
ISBN: 978-1-62948-422-8

Chapter 12

ANGIOTENSIN-CONVERTING ENZYME INHIBITORS IN RENAL DISEASE: A EUROPEAN PERSPECTIVE

Nicolas Roberto Robles, MD*
Institute of Cardiovascular Risk, Faculty of Medicine,
University of Salamanca, Salamanca, Spain
Unidad de Hipertensión Arterial. Servicio de Nefrologia,
Hospital Infanta Cristina, Badajoz, Spain

ABSTRACT

Current clinical guidelines for management of hypertension recommend the use of renin-angiotensin axis blocking drugs, either angiotensin-receptor blockers (ARBs) or angiotensin-converting enzyme inhibitors (ACEIs) for the treatment of renal disease associated to high blood pressure. The presence of proteinuria is a well-known risk factor for both the progression of renal disease and cardiovascular morbidity and mortality, and decreases in urine protein excretion level were associated with a slower decrease in renal function and decrease in risk of cardiovascular events. Most reports suggest that ACEIs reduce proteinuria, and delayed progression of chronic kidney disease. The reduction in urinary protein excretion seems to be in part independent of the reduction in blood pressure and it may depend on the activity of the renin–angiotensin system which induces vasodilatation of both afferent glomerular and efferent glomerular arterioles, thereby reducing simultaneously systemic and intraglomerular blood pressure. Contrariwise, impaired renal function has been associated with ACEIs use. This review tries to provide an extended summary of current basic and clinical evidence regarding the rationale for recommended use of ACE inhibitors in renal patients.

INTRODUCTION

Current clinical guidelines for management of hypertension recommend the use of renin-angiotensin axis blocking drugs, either angiotensin-receptor blockers (ARBs) or angiotensin-

* Corresponding author: Email: nrrobles@yahoo.es.

converting enzyme inhibitors (ACEIs) for the treatment of renal disease associated with high blood pressure. The presence of proteinuria is a well-known risk factor for both the progression of renal disease and cardiovascular morbidity and mortality, and decreases in urine protein excretion level were associated with a slower decrease in renal function and decrease in risk of cardiovascular events. Most reports suggest that ACEIs reduce proteinuria and delay the progression of chronic kidney disease. The reduction in urinary protein excretion seems to be in part independent of the reduction in blood pressure and it may depend on the activity of the renin–angiotensin (RAS) system which induces vasodilatation of both afferent glomerular and efferent glomerular arterioles, thereby reducing simultaneously systemic and intraglomerular blood pressure. Contrariwise, impaired renal function has been associated to ACEIs use. This review tries to provide an extended summary of current basic and clinical evidence regarding the rationale for recommended use of ACEIs in renal patients.

The Experimental Basis of ACEIs Nephroprotection

Kidney and Blood Pressure

The extent to which the kidney sustains damage from hypertension is proportional to the degree of its BP exposure. Therefore, it is not systemic BP *per se* that determines the severity of renal damage but the degree to which it is transmitted to the renal microvasculature. As long as the normally efficient renal auto regulatory mechanisms are intact, as is the case in the vast majority of patients with essential hypertension, the transmission of systemic BP elevations, episodic or sustained, to the renal microvasculature is expected to be largely prevented [1,2]. In fact, the systolic BP serves as a trigger for the myogenic auto regulatory response [3]. As a protective adaptation, chronic hypertension tends to shift the curve to the right to preserve the glomeruli. However, if BP elevations become severe as to exceed the range of auto regulatory protection (MAP >160 mmHg), then acute disruptive vascular and glomerular injury could ensue. By contrast, if renal auto regulation is impaired, as is observed after severe nephron loss, the BP threshold for glomerular injury is reduced with transmission of even modest and transient systemic BP elevations to the glomerular capillaries [4-6]. It is important to note that even more modest reductions in functional renal mass, such as after uninephrectomy, do result in preglomerular vasodilatation and increased fractional glomerular BP transmission, [7], however, the increase is relatively small.

Studies using a variety of approaches demonstrated that the afferent arteriole is the primary site at which renal blood flow (RBF) is regulated and auto regulated [8]. Conceptually, the regulators of renal blood flow can be classified into three classes. The first class consists of systemic mechanisms, both neural and hormonal, that transfer information from the rest of the organism to the kidney. These include the endocrine renin-angiotensin system, efferent sympathetic nerve activity, vasopressin, and the family of natriuretic peptides. Although these systems can have profound effects on RBF, their actions are not directionally consistent with auto regulation; nor are they consistent with its autonomous operation. The second class consists of paracrine mechanisms including the intrarenal renin-angiotensin system, nitric oxide, endothelin, and eicosanoids that transfer information from one part of the kidney to another. These agonists can affect RBF [9], but are ruled out as mediators by the rapid kinetics of myogenic auto regulation that effectively preclude all but electromechanical coupling of pressure to contraction [10]. At the end, blood pressure alone (or more correctly renal perfusion pressure) forms the third and more important class of RBF regulators [11,12]. Tubulo-glomerular feedback (TGF) has a sensor ([Cl^-] at the macula densa), which detects altered preglomerular conductance, and attempts to increase early distal delivery and transport to decrease conductance by vasodilatation of preglomerular arterioles [13]. By the way, this might provide metabolic stabilization to the kidney because reducing RBF inevitably reduces tubular work.

Figure 1 shows the interrelation of high blood pressure and the RAS system in the pathogenesis of renal disease. Pathogenesis of renal disease is like an "ourobouros", the snake who bite its tail. Renal damage induces nephron loss and this, in turn, increases both high blood pressure and intraglomerular pressure which produces glomerulosclerosis and proteinuria. Glomerulosclerosis worsens nephron loss and proteinuria induces interstitial inflammation, thus perpetuating renal damage. Angiotensin II interacts with the above processes, thus amplifying both the increments in blood pressure as well as the pathological changes produced by the higher systemic and intraglomerular blood pressures.

Antihypertensive treatment, particularly ACEIs, can have a beneficial effect on progression of glomerular damage including sclerosis associated with severe reduction in renal mass [14-16]. When the glomeruli are protected from increased pressure by preglomerular vasoconstriction, as in the spontaneously hypertensive rat, the hypertensive effects on the kidney are less evident or are prevented [17,18]. As a matter of fact, lowering systemic blood pressure prevents renal injury and this is a common protective mechanism for all kinds of antihypertensive drugs [19-21].

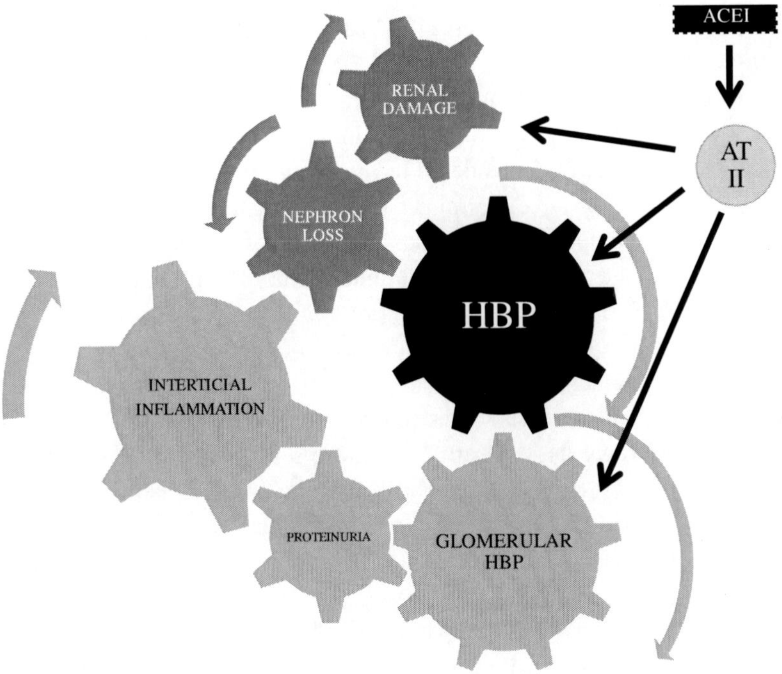

Figure 1. The figure shows the feed back of renal disease and hypertension as well as the participation of AT-II in the pathogenesis of renal disease. [HBP: High blood pressure. AT-II: Angiotensin II].

Moreover, ACEIs, but not other class of antihypertensives (diuretics, beta blockers, calcium antagonists) can normalize glomerular capillary hydraulic pressure by efferent glomerular arteriolar vasodilatation (Figure 2). In turn, these changes may inhibit or lessen later development of glomerular sclerosis in experimental kidney disease [22,23]. But the mechanisms whereby ACEIs ameliorates glomerular sclerosis might be beyond these hemodynamic effects. The structural and functional effects of ACEIs seems to be separable; the earlier effects on proteinuria do not correlate with the late effects on glomerular sclerosis [24,25].The benefit appears to represent a combination of short-term hemodynamic effects and potentially the inhibition of a variety of growth factors (i.e. platelet derived growth factor, PGDF) interacting with angiotensin II that can lead to overproduction of proteins and extracellular matrix, as well as mesangial cells hypertrophy [26-28].

Last but not the least, ACE inhibition independent of angiotensin II can cause prolongation of the half-life of bradykinin and the secondary increase in nitric oxide in body tissues, which may have additional anti-inflammatory effects [29]. Inhibition of nitric oxide synthetase via administration of *N*G-monomethyl-L-arginine accelerates the process of glomerular ischemia or sclerosis in nonimmune renal models and enhances the protein synthesis induced by angiotensin II in vascular smooth muscle [30]. Since these changes are strikingly similar to those observed after the infusion or endogenous generation of angiotensin II, the collateral action of ACEIs prolonging bradykinin activity may also contribute to its nephroprotective effects.

Clinical Use of ACEIs in Renal Disease

Most trials have focused on the effects of ACEIs on proteinuria and/or microalbuminuria. The normal rate of albumin excretion is less than 20 mg/day. Microalbuminuria is associated with increased risk of progressive renal deterioration, cardiovascular disease, and mortality [31]. Persistent albuminuria between 30 and 300 mg/day is referred to as microalbuminuria. Albuminuria above 300 mg/day is considered to represent clinical proteinuria. Proteinuria has been shown to have a strong adverse impact on the progression of renal disease and the likelihood of adverse outcomes [32-35]. It has been suggested that there is an independent role for proteinuria in the mediation of tubular injury and nephron loss (Figure 1); furthermore, there is considerable evidence that proteinuria also may serve as a biomarker for glomerular susceptibility to hypertensive injury. While a wide variety of heterogeneous mechanisms, including increased glomerular capillary pressure, can result in glomerular capillary wall injury and proteinuria, it is likely that the barrier properties of an altered (diseased) capillary wall, regardless of cause, are more sensitive to small changes in capillary pressure [36,37]. In this way, those patients with the most pronounced initial antiproteinuric response to ACEIs showed less deterioration of renal function, estimated from the slope of the inverse serum creatinine value in time [38]. The antiproteinuric effect is persistent and is not reduced by heavy proteinuria [39,40].

A number of clinical trials have compared the efficacy of ACEIs with other classes of antihypertensive agents in slowing the progression of nondiabetic CKD. Already in 1985, Taguma et al. described the antiproteinuric effect of ACEIs in diabetic patients in a small study [41]. The largest studies were the ACE Inhibition in Progressive Renal Insufficiency

(AIPRI) Study [42], and the Ramipril Efficacy in Nephropathy (REIN) Study [43]. The AIPRI was a three-year trial involving 583 patients with renal insufficiency caused by various disorders, 300 patients received benazepril and 283 received placebo. The primary end point was a doubling of the base-line serum creatinine concentration or the need for dialysis. In the benazepril group, the reduction in the risk of reaching the end point was 53 percent overall among the patients with mild renal insufficiency, and 46 percent among those with moderate renal insufficiency. Diastolic pressure decreased by 3.5 to 5.0 mm Hg in the benazepril group and increased by 0.2 to 1.5 mm Hg in the placebo group. The REIN study found that in a sample of 97 patients with chronic nephropathies and proteinuria of 3 g or more per 24 h, ramipril safely reduced the rate of decline of the GFR and halved the combined risk of doubling of serum creatinine or end-stage renal failure (ESRD), as compared with placebo plus conventional antihypertensive drugs at the same level of blood pressure control. Even patients previously treated with antihypertensive drugs other than ACEIs benefited from switching to ramipril. The findings of African American Study of Kidney Disease and Hypertension (AASK) also corroborated that ACEIs were more efficacious than other antihypertensive agents in slowing progression of CKD in hypertensive nephrosclerosis, which is typically not associated with heavy albuminuria [44].

In patients with type 1 diabetic nephropathy, the Collaborative Study showed an overall approximately 50% relative risk reduction for doubling of serum creatinine and/or ESRD in the ACEIs group as compared with the placebo group, with a significant relative risk reductions (approximately 70%) in patients with entry serum creatinine of $\geq$1.5 mg/dl [45]. Although the placebo group had significantly higher proteinuria at baseline (3.0 *versus* 2.5 g/24 h; $P < 0.02$), the relative risk reductions were not significantly altered by adjustment for this difference using proportional hazards regression analysis.

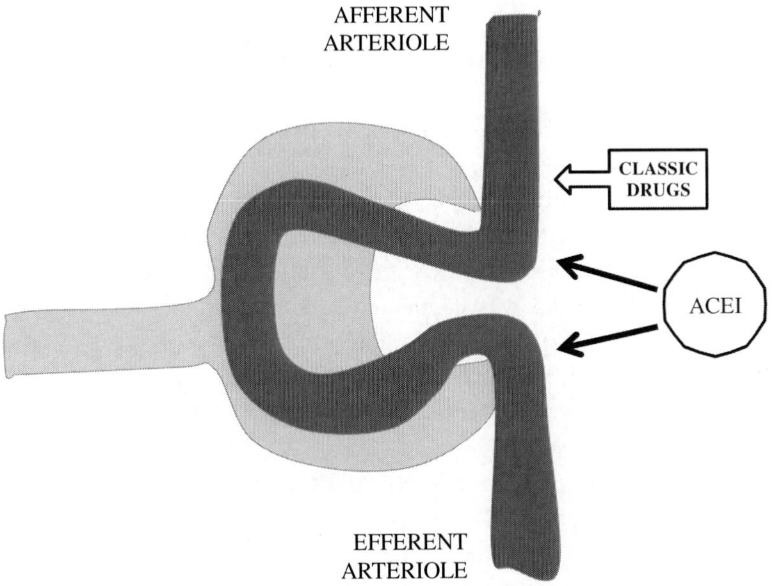

Figure 2. ACEIs (ACE-I) have dual effects. They reduce intraglomerular blood pressure by inhibiting pre- and postglomerular arterioles constriction. Other antihypertensive drug classes do not have this effect.

IS THERE AN EFFECT BEYOND BLOOD PRESSURE CONTROL?

Long-term ACEIs treatment may be beneficial in normotensive patients with nephrotic-range proteinuria, not only to reduce the symptoms of a nephrotic syndrome, but also to prevent further renal damage. The Heart Outcomes Prevention Evaluation (HOPE) substudy data may be relevant to such issues. The MICRO-HOPE investigated whether ramipril could lower risk for renal disease in patients with diabetes. The study included 3577 people with diabetes, aged 55 years or older, who had a previous cardiovascular event or at least one other cardiovascular risk factor, no clinical proteinuria, and who were not taking ACEIs. These subjects were randomly assigned to ramipril (10 mg/day) or placebo. High blood pressure was not needed to be recruited and most of patients were normotensive. Ramipril lowered the risk of overt nephropathy by 24%. After adjustment for the changes in systolic (2.4 mm Hg) and diastolic (1.0 mm Hg) blood pressures, ramipril still lowered the risk of the combined primary outcome by 25% [46]. Nevertheless, another substudy of the HOPE trial showed BP reductions of 3/2 mmHg in clinic pressures in a subset of 38 ramipril-treated patients, similar to that in the parent study, translated into a reduction of 10/4 mmHg in the average 24-h ambulatory BP in the same patients because of a large decrease in nocturnal BP of 17/8 mmHg (ramipril was dosed in the evening) [47]. Although the sample in which BP was monitored was very small and not related to the microalbuminuria subgroup, these results cast some doubts on the real “beyond the blood pressure” effects of blocking RAS.

In the same way, the Blood Pressure Lowering Treatment Trialists’ Collaboration (BPLTTC), using data from 29 prospectively designed randomized trials involving 162,341 subjects, demonstrated that ACEIs reduced blood pressure to a lesser extent than calcium antagonists or diuretics [48]. In spite of this reduced antihypertensive effect there were no differences in the incidence of total major cardiovascular events with the other classes of antihypertensives.

Evidence from studies of advanced proteinuric kidney disease also indicates that ACEIs have effects independent of blood pressure. In patients with type 1 diabetes, captopril treatment was associated with a 50% reduction in the risk of the combined end point of death, dialysis, and transplantation compared with placebo [45]. This reduction was independent of the difference in blood pressure between the groups. The African American Study of Kidney Disease and Hypertension (AASK) trial revealed that ramipril conferred greater benefit than metoprolol in black patients with nephrosclerosis, although blood pressure control was similar with both drugs. The trial was conducted in 1,094 patients with hypertensive renal disease (GFR of 20–65 mL/min) who were studied for 3–6.4 years [49]. Analysis revealed that compared with metoprolol, ramipril treatment resulted in a slower decrease in GFR and delayed the onset of a significant decrease in GFR, ESRD, or death, and decreased urinary protein excretion.

A small trial had investigated the relation of ACEIs to renal prognosis in CKD patients in a retrospective cohort. The objectives were patients with non-diabetic CKD of stage 4 or below receiving monotherapy with calcium channel blockers (CCBs), ACEIs, or ARBs, and combination therapy. Analyzed patients comprised 131 males and 117 females, with mean age of 47.8 years. Patients were observed for 44.2 months and CCBs, ACEIs, and ARBs types were administered to 93, 85, and 127 patients, respectively. In the multivariate analysis extracted, common prognostic factors included the baseline GFR and final proteinuria, the odds ratio of which was 0.876 (every increase by 1 ml/min of GFR) and 2.229 (every increase by 1 g of proteinuria), respectively. Among drugs in use, ACEIs were an independent prognostic factor, whose odds ratio was 0.147. This study suggests that ACEIs use is a prognostic factor independent of its hypotensive action in CKD patients [50].

META-ANALYSES ON RENOPROTECTIVE EFFECTS OF ACEIS

Methods for reviewing the evidence have matured over the years as groups have gained experience in developing evidence-based guidelines. Systematic searches of multiple bibliographic research databases may help to ensure thorough and unbiased identification of the relevant literature. Predetermined selection criteria are supposed to minimize bias and improve the efficiency of reviewing that literature. Quality criteria developed by methodologists guide judgments of weaknesses and strengths of individual research studies. In this way and looking at internal validity quality rating, meta-analyses are considered the best level of evidence [51,52]. On the other hand, meta-analyses do not to necessarily represent the top level of evidence. Indeed, although meta-analyses have a greater statistical power than individual trials, and may provide useful average measurements of treatment effects, they also have limitations. By definition, they are post-hoc analyses, the choice of the trials to be included is often arbitrary, the trials included are frequently not homogeneous, with differences not always susceptible to being assessed by statistical tests. Therefore, meta-analysis should also be reviewed critically, as have all other sources of information.

A number of meta-analyses on the nephroprotective effects of ACEIs have been published (Table 1). They selected different populations and so they can be classified as follows.

Table 1. Meta-Analises on ACEIs in Renal Disease

First author	Patients	Objective	Risk Reduction	BP Decrease*
Casas	37 089	SCr duplication/ ESRD	0.87 (0.75-0.99)	-1.0/+0.2
Daien	33 240	Changes in SCr	OR:1.05 (0.89-1.25)	
Giatras	1 594	ESRD	0.70 (0.51-0.97)	-4.9/-1.2
Jafar	1 860	SCr duplication/ ESRD	0.67 (0.53-0.84)	-4.5/-2.3
Gansevoort	1 124	Proteinuria	0.76 (0.71-0.81)	-0.5% #
Maione	21 708	Albuminuria/ESRD	0.67 (0.54–0.84)	No data
Sarafidis	10 598	SCr Duplication**	0.79 (0.68-0.91)	No data
Vejakama	134 912	SCr Duplication€	0.66 (0.52-0.83)	-2.4/-0.5
Kshirsagar	1 456	Proteinuria/ ESRD	0.60 (0.49-0.63)	-0.5% #

* mmHg. $Not significant.

Mean Blood Pressure.

SCr, Serum creatinine.

ESRD: End-stage renal disease.

** No effects on ESRD incidence was found.

€ No significant effects on albuminuria progression.

Hypertensive Patients without CKD

Casas et al. performed a meta-analysis on the renoprotective effects ACEIs and ARBs. Comparisons of ACEIs or ARBs with other antihypertensive drugs yielded a relative risk of 0.71 for doubling of creatinine and 0.87 for ESRD. Analysis of the results by study size showed a smaller benefit in large studies. In patients with diabetic nephropathy, no benefit was seen in comparative trials of ACEIs or ARBs. Placebo-controlled trials of ACEIs or ARBs showed greater benefits than comparative trials on all renal outcomes, but were accompanied by substantial reductions in blood pressure in favor of ACEIs or ARBs, this was interpreted as the benefits of ACEIs or ARBs on renal outcomes in placebo-controlled trials were probably result from a blood-pressure-lowering effect. This report cast some doubts on the renoprotective effects of these kinds of drugs in patients with diabetes [53].

More recently a second meta-analysis was aimed to determine whether inhibitors of the RAS reduced the incidence of renal dysfunction when compared to other antihypertensive treatments in patients with essential hypertension and no pre-existent renal disease. In all, 33,240 patients met the inclusion criteria for studies with a dichotomous outcome and 10,634 patients for studies with a continuous outcome. The mean follow-up was 42 ± 13 months. Patients randomized to RAS inhibitors did not show any significant reduction in the risk of developing renal dysfunction as compared to other antihypertensive strategies (OR = 1.05; 95%CI 0.89-1.25; P = 0.54). There was no significant difference in change of serum creatinine between groups. The conclusion was that, in patients with essential hypertension and without pre-existent renal disease, prevention of renal dysfunction was not significantly different with RAS inhibitors when compared to other antihypertensive agents [54].

Non-Diabetic CKD

Giatras et al. focused on the effect of ACEIs in slowing the decline in renal function in non-diabetic renal disease. All randomized studies that compared ACEIs with other antihypertensive agents and had at least 1 year of planned follow-up were selected. Studies of diabetic renal disease were excluded. A total of 1594 patients in 10 studies were included. Among 806 patients receiving ACEIs, the pooled relative risks were 0.70 for ESRD, and this difference was statistically significant. The decreases in weighted mean systolic and diastolic blood pressures during follow-up were 4.9 and 1.2 mm Hg greater respectively in the patients who received ACEIs. Although ACEIs were more effective than other antihypertensive agents in reducing the development of ESRD in non-diabetic renal disease, it could not be determined whether this beneficial effect was due to the greater decline in blood pressure or to other effects of ACE inhibition [55].

A second meta-analysis has examined the efficacy of ACEIs for the treatment of non-diabetic renal disease. It included 11 randomized controlled trials comparing the efficacy of antihypertensive regimens including ACEIs to the efficacy of regimens without ACEIs in predominantly non-diabetic renal disease. Data on 1860 non-diabetic patients were analyzed. Patients in the ACEIs group had a greater mean decrease in systolic and diastolic blood pressure and urinary protein excretion. Relative risk in the ACEIs group was 0.69 for ESRD. Patients with greater urinary protein excretion at baseline benefited more from ACEIs therapy. The authors concluded that ACEIs were more effective than other antihypertensive drugs in slowing the progression of non-diabetic renal disease; this effect could be mediated by other factors in addition to decreasing blood pressure and urinary protein excretion [56]. Using the same data the authors studied the levels of blood pressure and urine protein excretion associated with the lowest risk for progression of chronic kidney disease during antihypertensive therapy with and without ACEIs. Systolic blood pressure of 110 to 129 mm Hg and urine protein excretion less than 2.0 g/d were associated with the lowest risk for kidney disease progression. Nevertheless, ACEIs treatment remained beneficial after adjustment for blood pressure and urine protein excretion [57].

Proteinuria

Gansevoort et al. studied the efficacy of ACEIs to lower proteinuria; the secondary objective was whether there was any difference between diabetic and non-diabetic patients in antiproteinuric response to blood pressure reduction. It included 41 studies, comprising 1124 patients, of which 558 had non-diabetic renal disease. The mean antiproteinuric effect of ACEIs was significantly greater than that of their comparator drugs and the blood pressure lowering effect was equal. Thus it was concluded that ACEIs conferred an antiproteinuric effect beyond that attributable to their blood pressure lowering effect [58].

A recently published clinical trial examined the benefits and risks of ACEIs and ARBs in people with micro- or macroalbuminuria and one or more cardiovascular risk factors. Eighty-five trials (21 708 patients) were included. There was no significant reduction in the risk of all-cause mortality or fatal cardiac–cerebrovascular outcomes with ACEIs versus placebo, ARBs versus placebo, ACEIs versus ARBs or with combined therapy versus monotherapy. There was a significant reduction in the risk of nonfatal cardiovascular events with ACEIs versus placebo but not with ARBs versus placebo, ACEIs versus ARBs or with combined therapy with ACEIs plus ARBs versus monotherapy. Development of ESRD and progression of microalbuminuria to macroalbuminuria were reduced significantly with ACEIs versus placebo and ARBs versus placebo but not with combined therapy versus monotherapy [59].

Diabetic Patients

Sarafidis et al. evaluated the effect of ACEIs and ARBs in patients with diabetic nephropathy. Of the 1,028 originally identified studies, 24 fulfilled the inclusion criteria (20 using ACEIs and 4 using ARBs). Use of ACEIs was associated with a trend toward reduction of ESRD incidence (RR 0.70; 95%CI 0.46-1.05) and use of ARBs with significant reduction of ESRD risk (RR 0.78; 95%CI 0.67-0.91). Both drug classes were associated with reduction in the risk of doubling serum creatinine (RR 0.71; 95%CI 0.56-0.91 for ACEIs and RR 0.79; 95%CI 0.68-0.91 for ARBs) but none affected all-cause mortality. These findings are added to the evidence of a renoprotective role of RAS blockers in such patients [60].

Another meta-analysis aimed to compare the renal outcomes between ACEIs /ARBs and other antihypertensive drugs or placebo in type 2 diabetes. Of 673 studies identified, 28 were eligible (n = 134,912). In direct meta-analysis, ACEIs/ARBs had significantly lower risk of serum creatinine doubling (RR 0.66, 95% CI 0.52-0.83) and macroalbuminuria (RR 0.70, 95% CI 0.50-1.00), but a higher incidence of albuminuria regression (RR 1.16, 95% CI 1.00,

1.39) than other antihypertensive drugs, mainly CCBs. Although the risks of ESRD and microalbuminuria were lower in the ACEIs/ARBs group, the differences were not statistically significant. The ACEIs/ARBs benefit over placebo was significant for all outcomes except microalbuminuria. Lack of differences in BP decrease between ACEIs/ARBs and active comparators suggest that this benefit is not simply due to the antihypertensive effect [61].

Kshirsagar et al. reported a third meta-analysis on the effect of ACEIs in diabetic and non-diabetic chronic renal disease. In nine trials of subjects with diabetic nephropathy and microalbuminuria, the relative risk for developing macroalbuminuria was significantly lower for individuals treated with an ACEI compared with placebo. In seven trials of subjects with overt proteinuria and renal insufficiency from a variety of causes (30% diabetes, 70% non-diabetic), the relative risk for doubling of serum creatinine concentration or developing ESRD was also lower for individuals treated with ACEIs compared with placebo. The conclusion was that treatment of individuals with chronic renal insufficiency with ACEIs delays the progression of disease compared with placebo across a spectrum of disease causes and renal dysfunction. Mean arterial pressure was not significantly decreased (-0.5 mmHg), thus again the renoprotective effect was attributed to an effect different from blood pressure control [62].

Cardiovascular Outcomes

Balamuthusamy et al. did not address the renoprotective effect of ACEIs. Their meta-analysis was aimed to examine the role of RAS blockade in improving CV outcomes in patients with CKD. Twenty-five trials (n = 45,758) were used for analysis. RAS blockade decreased the risk for heart failure in patients with diabetic nephropathy when compared with placebo 0.78 (95% CI 0.66-0.92, P = .003) and control therapy (0.63, 95% CI 0.47-0.86, P = .003). The risk for major adverse cardiovascular events was decreased with RAS blockade (0.56, 95% CI 0.47-0.67, P < .001) in non-diabetic nephropathy patients with CKD when compared with control therapy. There was also a significant reduction of CV outcomes (0.84, 95% CI 0.78-0.91, P < .0001), myocardial infarction (0.78, 95% CI 0.65-0.97, P = .03), and heart failure (0.74, 95% CI 0.58-0.95, P = .02) with RAS blockade compared to placebo, when all the patients with CKD were pooled. There were also benefits with RAS blockade in reducing the risk of CV outcomes and heart failure in patients with diabetic nephropathy when compared with placebo [63].

Taken all data altogether, the evidence suggests a higher renoprotective effect of ACEIs in renal disease, either diabetic or non-diabetic, compared with other antihypertensive drugs. The relationship between renoprotection and blood pressure reduction remains to be settled but an effect of blocking RAS beyond the blood pressure control cannot be definitively discarded. Contrariwise, a superior preventive effect on renal dysfunction due to chronic hypertension could not be demonstrated.

Combination of ACEIs and ARBs in Renal Disease

Several authors have reported a superior effect of the combination of ACEIs and ARBs on microalbuminuria and on clinical proteinuria in patients with primary nephropathies [64-

68], and in type 1 and type 2 diabetic patients [69,70]. A systematic review and meta-analysis has addressed this issue suggesting that concomitant therapy with an ARB and an ACEI leads to greater reductions in proteinuria than monotherapy [71]. The renal results of ONTARGET trial were separately reported. The primary renal outcome was a composite of dialysis, doubling of serum creatinine, and death. Seven hundred and eighty four patients permanently discontinued randomised therapy during the trial because of hypotensive symptoms (406 on combination therapy, 149 on ramipril, and 229 on telmisartan). The number of events for the composite primary outcome was similar for telmisartan (13.4%) and ramipril (13.5%), but was slightly increased with combination therapy (14.5%; p=0·037). The secondary renal outcome, dialysis or doubling of serum creatinine, was similar with telmisartan (2.21%) and ramipril (2.03%) and slightly more frequent with combination therapy (2.49%, p=0.038). Estimated glomerular filtration rate declined less with ramipril compared with telmisartan (−2·82 mL/min/1·73 m^2 vs −4·12, p<0·0001) or combination therapy (−6·11, p<0·0001). Conversely, the increase in urinary albumin excretion was smaller with telmisartan (p=0·004) or with combination therapy (p=0·001) than with ramipril [72]. Nevertheless, the results of the ONTARGET were difficult to translate. Most of the true renal patients had high blood pressure and proteinuric non-vascular renal disease. Contrariwise, the patients recruited in ONTARGET were not hypertensive at recruitment and, as its antecedents suggest, they had renal microvascular disease highly sensitive to changes in blood pressure levels. Other reports suggest that in proteinuric renal disease, the dual blockade of RAS could be useful and secure in most patients even in stage III CKD; moreover according to KDOQI Guidelines, renal function in these patients should be closely monitored [73].

Recently Fernandez Juarez et al. [74], reported the results of a multicenter open-label randomized controlled trial to compare the efficacy of combining the ACEI, lisinopril, and the ARB, irbesartan, with that of each drug in monotherapy (at both high and equipotent doses) in slowing the progression of type 2 diabetic nephropathy. There were no significant differences in proteinuria reduction or blood pressure control between the groups. The number of adverse events, including hyperkalemia, was similar in all 3 groups. They were unable to show any benefit of the combination of lisinopril and irbesartan compared to either agent alone at optimal high doses on the risk of progression of type 2 diabetic nephropathy. Therefore, presently, we can only assume that dual blockade of RAS using an ACEI and an ARB may get a further decrease in proteinuria but there is no evidence in the long run that this combination will retard CKD progression any better than with monotherapy alone.

To date, several meta-analyses have evaluated the efficacy of combined ACEIs and ARBs therapy in proteinuric renal disease and the main findings of these studies have been summarized in three systematic reviews. The combination of an ACEI and an ARB reduces BP by ~4/3 mmHg when compared with an ACEI or an ARB administered as monotherapy, hence demonstrating that combined RAS blockade confers little advantage over monotherapy with an ACEI or an ARB as far as additive effects on BP are concerned. Combined RAS blockade gets a deeper reduction in proteinuria compared with monotherapy with ACEIs or ARBs [76,77]. Nevertheless, a third meta-analysis found that development of end-stage kidney disease and progression of microalbuminuria to macroalbuminuria were reduced significantly with ACEIs versus placebo and ARBs versus placebo but not with combined therapy with ACEIs plus ARBs versus monotherapy [78].

ACEIs or ARBs for Renal Disease?

A comprehensive review of available evidence shows that ACEIs and ARBs have similar effects on blood pressure control but that ACEIs have higher rates of untoward effects (specifically cough) than ARBs [79]. Unfortunately, data regarding renal disease are limited. This review identified 19 studies with renal outcomes (a resume of these trials has been showed in table 2). Fifteen of these studies described changes in creatinine level or glomerular filtration rate. They did not consistently demonstrate differential effects related to renal function with the use of ACEIs versus ARBs. Nevertheless, most of these studies were not specifically designed to demonstrate protective effects on renal function; the recruited samples were small and follow up time too short to show statistical differences.

Due to the high similarities between the properties of ACEIs and ARBs, the incremental benefits of newer treatments are expected to be small, so that these conditions implies an important increase of the required sample and/or a very much longer follow-up. These two factors have led some investigators to design trials to show that the new treatment has an effect similar to that of the standard, rather than outright superiority. One example is the Diabetics Exposed to Telmisartan And EnalaprIL (DETAIL). This trial was designed to address the absence of comparative data on the long-term effects of telmisartan *versus* enalapril on renoprotection and survival in 250 patients with hypertension and early type 2 diabetic nephropathy. The primary purpose of this 5-yr double-blind, double-dummy, randomized study was to establish whether 40 to 80 mg of telmisartan conferred similar (i.e., non-inferior) renoprotection to 10 to 20 mg of enalapril as determined by the change from baseline in GFR, measured by the plasma clearance of iohexol. Secondary end points included the emergence of ESRD and all-cause mortality. Telmisartan was not inferior to enalapril in reducing the decline in GFR: Mean annual declines in GFR were 3.7 and 3.3 ml/min per 1.73 m^2 with telmisartan and enalapril, respectively. During the 5-yr study period, no patient developed a serum creatinine >200 μmol/L, and none required dialysis. There were only six deaths in each treatment group during the study, with half being due to cardiovascular events [80].

A number of studies described changes in urine albumin level or protein excretion. Taken altogether they demonstrated no differential effects between ACEIs and ARBs related to the reduction of urinary protein or albumin excretion among patients with essential hypertension. As an example the CALM (CAndesartan and Lisinopril Microalbuminuria) study tried to assess and compare the effects of candesartan or lisinopril, or both, on blood pressure and urinary albumin excretion in patients with microalbuminuria, hypertension, and type 2 diabetes. Patients were treated during 12 weeks with either candesartan 16 mg once daily or lisinopril 20 mg once daily [70]. At 12 weeks, reductions in urinary albumin/creatinine ratios were 30% and 46% for candesartan and lisinopril, respectively. Thus, lisinopril was effective as candesartan in reducing microalbuminuria in hypertensive patients with type 2 diabetes.

In conclusion, regarding renal disease, the effects of ACEIs and ARBs are closely similar and no different results on renal end points could be drawn through the available studies. It is interesting to note that in studies where a head-to-head comparison of an ACEI and an ARB with regard to reduction of proteinuria was possible, regression of proteinuria favored the ACEIs. The most obvious explanation could be that without dose titration it is difficult to assess dose equivalence of the two compounds. Alternatively it is possible that ACEIs and ARBs may have different effects beyond modulation of the RAS [81].

SAFE USE IN PATIENTS WITH RENAL FAILURE

Epidemiological data from all over the world point to the increasing incidence of renal failure encompassing acute kidney injury (AKI), CKD and ESRD. In the USA, between 1996 and 2003, the incidence of non-dialysis requiring community-based AKI increased from 322.7/100,000 to 522.4/100,000 person years. Equally, the incidence of dialysis-requiring AKI increased from 19.5/100,000 to 29.5/100,000 person years [82]. Hospital incidence for AKI per 10,000 population in the USA increased from 1.8 in 1980 to a shocking 36.5 in 2005 [83]. Simultaneously, in 2008, a US Centers for Disease Control and Prevention report showed an acceleration of CKD prevalence up to 16.5% among the US population in the period 1999–2004, representing a 15.9% increase in CKD prevalence when compared to the 1988–1994 period [84]. As a result of some of these foregoing themes, Onuigbo has hypothesized that RAS blocking drugs, may be responsible for some of the observed increasing CKD/ESRD/AKI incidence currently observed in the US [85,86]. In this regard, a subgroup analysis of the ALLHAT diabetic population revealed that more patients in the lisinopril group progressed to ESRD compared to the chlorthalidone group—25/1563 vs. 26/2755 (P = 0.05; RR 1.74; 95% CI: 1.00–3.01) [87], in spite of the theoretic beneficial effects of ACEIs in diabetic kidney disease which have been discussed above.

In this way, Suissa et al. presented a population-based study suggesting that ACEIs do not appear to decrease the long-term risk of ESRD in diabetes. This study was based on a registry of medication prescription, including diabetic patients who were prescribed antihypertensive agents from 1982 to 1986. The 6,102 patients were followed to the end of 1997 with respect to the development of ESRD, which occurred in 102 patients, of whom 21 had been treated with an ACEI within the initial 3 years of follow-up. The adjusted rate ratio for renal failure was 2.5 in patients initially treated with ACEIs compared with patients treated with diuretics, when compared with the control patients [88]. This study has several limitations which need to be taken into consideration. First, there was no information on the indication for the medication in the patients, making bias by indication a major problem since it is possible that the ACEIs were given to patients at particularly high risk for development of ESRD. No information regarding well-known risk factors for development of ESRD due to diabetes were available, such as proteinuria/albuminuria, presence of retinopathy, lipids, smoking, blood pressure or glycemic control. In addition, the development of renal failure requiring dialysis for at least 6 weeks was the endpoint, without any information regarding the cause for ESRD, which could be due to numerous renal and non-renal conditions [89]. Most importantly, there was no information on the doses of ACEIs used. When captopril was introduced, potentially nephrotoxic doses were used irrespective of renal function (a dose of captopril 450 mg per day was usual) [90]. Unfortunately, the study gives no information regarding this issue, or on the use of the combination of diuretics with ACEIs.

Table 2.

	n	Objective	ACE-I	ARB	Favours
Avanza et al.[1]	31	Renal function	Enalapril	Losartan	None
Barnett et al.[77]	250	Renal function/AER	Enalapril	Telmisartan	None
De Rosa et al.[2]	50	Renal function	Enalapril	Losartan	ARB
Derosa et al.[3]	96	AER	Perindopril	Candesartan	None
Elliott et al.[4]	528	Renal function	Enalapril	Eprosartan	None
Fogari et al.[5]	86	Renal function	Perindopril	Losartan	None
Kagvaci et al.[6]	33	Renal function/AER	Fosinopril	Losartan	ACEI
Lacourciere et al.[7]	92	Renal function/AER	Enalapril	Losartan	None
Matsuda et al.[8]	27	Renal function/ Proteinuria	Trandolapril or Perindopril	Losartan or candesartan	ACEI
Mimram et al.[9]	200	Renal function	Enalapril	Irbesartan	None
Mogensen et al.[10]	199	AER	Lisinopril	Candesartan	None
Rosei et al.[11]	118	Renal function/AER	Enalapril	Candesartan	None
Schram et al.[12]	70	AER	Lisinopril	Candesartan	None
Shand[13]	29	Renal function	Enalapril	Losartan	None
Uchiyama et al.[14]	57	Renal function	Quinapril	Losartan	None
Verdecchia et al.[15]	88	Renal function	Enalapril	Losartan	None
Tikkanen et al.[16]	407	Renal function/ AER	Enalapril	Losartan	None
Roca-Cusachs et al.[17]	396	Renal function	Captopril	Losartan	None
Sato et al.[18]	49	AER	Several	Candesartan	None
Mann et al.[72]	25,620	Renal function/AER	Ramipril	Telmisartan	See note
Fernandez et al.[74]	133	Renal function/AER	Lisinopril	Irbesartan	None

AER: Albumin excretion rate.

* Estimated glomerular filtration rate declined least with ramipril compared with telmisartan. The increase in urinary albumin excretion was lesser with telmisartan than with ramipril.

Many physicians are worried about the use of ACEIs in patients with renal insufficiency for fear that either serum creatinine or potassium levels will rise. Nevertheless, the rate of hyperkalemia has been very low in the major trials in patients with chronic heart failure, whereas in unselected outpatients, 10% developed hyperkalemia during 1 year of therapy with ACEIs [91]. On the other hand, it has been described, a close dose–effect relationship between therapy with ACEIs and serum potassium, and this effect is most pronounced in patients with lower GFR. There is a strong inverse relation between GFR and serum potassium. In patients with decreasing renal function several mechanisms impair the excretion of potassium: (i) decreased delivery of sodium to the distal nephron, (ii) aldosterone deficiency and (iii) abnormal function of the cortical collecting ducts. In addition, hyporeninemic hypoaldosteronism and metabolic acidosis may contribute to hyperkalemia in diabetic patients [92]. The effect of ARBs seemed to be much milder and no interaction with kidney function was found for ARBs, which is consistent with earlier trials with this kind of drug. One explanation for this difference may be that many ACEIs accumulate in renal failure, whereas ARBs are usually eliminated by the liver [93]. In the clinical setting, the therapeutic approach is based on the appropriate use of dietetic counseling (specifically, to avoid excessive fruit and tomato intake) and/or diuretics use; these measures may help prevent profound increases in serum potassium. Thus, withdrawal of an ACEI in such patients should occur only when hyperkalemia develops, i.e., serum potassium level of 6 mmol/L or greater. When persistent hyperkalemia is found in diabetic patients in spite of these maneuvers, metabolic acidosis should be ruled out and an ion exchange resin could be helpful.

A usual question when renal failure occurs in patients on concurrent ACEI or ARB therapy, is whether ACEIs/ARBs withdrawal would lead to improved renal function. The impact of discontinuation of RAS blocking drugs in patients with advanced kidney disease was evaluated in a small sample of patients with advanced CKD (stages 4 and 5, mean GFR 16.38 ml/min). Patients were followed for at least 12 months before and after ACEIs/ARBs were stopped. After discontinuation of treatment GFR increased significantly to 26.6 ml/min/ 1.73 m2 ($p = 0.0001$). 61.5% of patients had more than a 25% increase in GFR, whilst 36.5% had an increase exceeding 50%. There was a significant decline in the eGFR slope −0.39 in the 12 months preceding discontinuation and this negative slope was reversed +0.48 ($p = 0.0001$), but overall proteinuria was not affected. Therefore, discontinuation of ACEIs/ARBs has undoubtedly delayed the onset of renal replacement therapy in this study [94]. Contrariwise, Hou et al. enrolled 422 non-diabetic patients in a randomized, double-blind study comparing benazepril treatment with placebo [95]. One hundred and four patients with serum creatinine levels of 1.5 to 3.0 mg/dl received 20 mg of benazepril per day, whereas 224 patients with serum creatinine levels of 3.1 to 5.0 mg/dl were randomly assigned to receive 20 mg of benazepril per day (112 patients) or placebo (112 patients) and then followed for a mean of 3.4 years. The primary outcome was the composite of a doubling of the serum creatinine level, ESRD, or death. As compared with placebo, benazepril was associated with a 43% reduction in the risk of the primary end point in patients with higher baseline serum creatinine levels treated with benazepril. In all, benazepril therapy was associated with a 52 percent reduction in the level of proteinuria and a reduction of 23 percent in the rate of decline in renal function [95].

A strong association exists between acute increases in serum creatinine of up to 30% to 35% after initiating ACEIs therapy and long-term preservation of renal function. This association is predominantly present in people with a baseline serum creatinine of up to 3 mg/dL and usually stabilizes within 2 to 3 months of therapy, given that blood pressure is reduced to goal [96]. Higher increments of serum creatinine, in absence of hypotensive states or simultaneous non-steroidal anti-inflammatory drugs administration, should mandate a search to rule out symptomatic renal artery stenosis [97]. In these cases, ACEIs treatment must be stopped; but, if there is not recovery of renal function, especially in proteinuric patients, ACEIs could be restarted with close monitoring of serum creatinine levels.

Although ACEIs seem to be renoprotective, patient selection with reference to age, baseline kidney function, presence of co-morbidities and exposure to other nephrotoxins should be taken into account. In elderly CKD patients, the recommendation with reference to dosing of ACEIs (and obviously ARBs) would be to ‘start low and go slow’ with dose titration, combined with very close and indefinite monitoring of serum creatinine, potassium and GFR [85].

References

[1] Bidani, AK; Griffin, KA. Long-term renal consequences of hypertension for normal and diseased kidneys. *Curr Opin Nephrol Hypertens*, 2002, 11, 73–80.

[2] Bidani, AK; Griffin, KA. Pathophysiology of hypertensive renal damage: Implications for therapy. *Hipertensión*, 2004, 44, 595 –601.

[3] Loutzenhiser, R; Griffin, KA; Williamson, G; Bidani, AK. Renal autoregulation: New perspectives regarding the protective and regulatory roles of the underlying mechanisms. *Am J Physiol Regul Integr Comp Physiol*, 2006, 290, R1153 –R1167.

[4] Pelayo, JC; Westcott, JY. Impaired autoregulation of glomerular capillary hydrostatic pressure in the rat remnant nephron. *J Clin Invest*, 1991, 88, 101 –105.

[5] Bidani, AK; Hacioglu, R; Abu-Amarah, I; Williamson, GA; Loutzenhiser, R; Griffin, KA. 'Step' vs 'dynamic' autoregulation: Implications for susceptibility to hypertensive injury. *Am J Physiol*, 2003, 285, F113 –F120.

[6] Griffin, KA; Picken, MM; Bidani, AK. Blood pressure lability and glomerulosclerosis after normotensive 5/6 renal mass reduction in the rat. *Kidney Int*, 2004, 65, 209 –218.

[7] Neuringer, JR; Brenner, BM. Hemodynamic theory of progressive renal disease, A 10-year update in brief review. *Am J Kidney Dis*., 1993, 22, 98 –104.

[8] Cupples, WA; Braam, B. Assessment of renal autoregulation. *Am J Physiol Renal Physiol*, 2007, 292, 1105-1123.

[9] Navar, LG. Renal autoregulation, perspectives from whole kidney and single nephron studies. *Am J Physiol Renal Fluid Electrolyte Physiol*, 1978, 234, F357–F370.

[10] Loutzenhiser, R; Bidani, A; Chilton L. Renal myogenic response: kinetic attributes and physiological role. *Circ Res*, 2002, 90, 1316–1324.

[11] Loutzenhiser, R; Bidani, A; Chilton, L. Renal myogenic response: kinetic attributes and physiological role. *Circ Res*., 2002, 90, 1316–1324,

[12] Navar, LG. Integrating multiple paracrine regulators of renal microvascular dynamics. *Am J Physiol Renal Physiol*, 1998, 274, F433–F444.

[13] Vallon, V. Tubuloglomerular feedback and the control of glomerular filtration rate. *News Physiol Sci*., 2003, 18, 169–174.

[14] Brunner, HR. ACEIs in renal disease. *Kidney Int*., 1992, 42, 463-479.

[15] Neugarten, J; Kaminetsky, B; Feiner, H; Schacht, RG; Liu, DT; Baldwin, DS. Nephrotoxic serum nephritis with hypertension, amelioration by antihypertensive therapy. *Kidney Int*., 1985, 28, 135-139.

[16] Anderson, S; Meyer, TW; Rennke, HG; Brenner, BM. Control of glomerular hypertension limits glomerular injury in rats with reduced renal mass. *J Clin Invest*., 1985, 76, 612-619.

[17] Raij, L; Azar, S; Keane, WF. Role of hypertension in progressive glomerular immune injury. Hypertension., 1985, 7(3 Pt 1), 398-404.

[18] Stein, HD; Sterzel, RB; Hunt, JD; Pabst, R; Kashgarian, M. No aggravation of the course of experimental glomerulonephritis in spontaneously hypertensive rats. *Am J Pathol*., 1986, 122, 520-530.

[19] Parving, HH; Andersen, AR; Smidt, UM; Svendsen, PA. Early aggressive antihypertensive treatment reduces rate of decline in kidney function in diabetic nephropathy. *Lancet*, 1983, 1, 1175-1179.

[20] Bergstrom, J; Alvestrand, A; Bucht, H; Gutierrez, A. Stockholm clinical study on progression of chronic renal failure--an interim report. *Kidney Int Suppl.*, 1989, 27, S110-S114.
[21] Hartford, M; Wendelhag, I; Berglund, G; Wallentin, I; Ljungman, S; Wikstrand, J. Cardiovascular and renal effects of long-term antihypertensive treatment. *JAMA.*, 1988, 259, 2553-2557.
[22] Anderson, S; Diamond, JR; Karnovsky, MJ; Brenner, BM. Mechanisms underlying transition from acute glomerular injury to late glomerular sclerosis in a rat model of nephrotic síndrome. *J. Clin. Invest.*, 1988, 82, 1757-1768.
[23] Anderson, S; Brenner, BM. Therapeutic benefit of converting-enzyme inhibition in progressive renal disease. *Am J Hypertens.*, 1988, 1(4 Pt 2), 380S-383S.
[24] Tanaka, R; Kon, V; Yoshioka, T; Ichikawa, I; Fogo, A. Angiotensin converting enzyme inhibitor modulates glomerular function and structure by distinct mechanisms. *Kidney Int.*, 1994, 45, 537-543.
[25] Ritz, E; Orth, S; Weinreich, T; Wagner, J. Systemic hypertension versus intraglomerular hypertension in progresión. *Kidney Int.*, 1994, 45, 438-442.
[26] Fogo, A; Yoshida, Y; Glick, AD; Homma, T; Ichikawa I. Serial micropuncture analysis of glomerular function in two rat models of glomerular sclerosis. *J Clin Invest.*, 1988, 82, 322-330.
[27] Lax, DS; Benstein, JA; Tolbert, E; Dworkin, LD. Effects of salt restriction on renal growth and glomerular injury in rats with remnant kidneys. *Kidney Int.*, 1992, 41, 1527-1534.
[28] Hsueh, WA; Do, YS; Anderson, PW; Law, RE. Angiotensin II in cell growth and matrix production. *Adv Exp Med Biol.*, 1995, 377, 217-223.
[29] Vanhoutte, PM. Endothelial dysfunction and inhibition of converting enzyme. *Eur Heart J.*, 1998, 19 Suppl J, J7-J15.
[30] Zatz, R; Fujihara, CK. Mechanisms of progressive renal disease: role of angiotensin II, cyclooxygenase products and nitric oxide. *J Hypertens Suppl.*, 2002, 20, S37-S44.
[31] Basi, S; Lewis, JB. Microalbuminuria as a target to improve cardiovascular and renal outcomes in diabetic patients. *Curr Diab Rep.*, 2007, 7, 439-442.
[32] Gruppo Italiano di Studi Epidemiologici in Nefrologia (GISEN): Randomized placebo-controlled trials of effect of ramipril on decline in glomerular filtration rate and risks of terminal renal failure in proteinuric, non-diabetic nephropathy. *Lancet.*, 1997, 349, 1857 –1863.
[33] Ruggenenti, P; Perna, A; Gherardi, G; Garini, G; Zoccali, C; Salvadori, M; Scolari, F; Schena, FP; Remuzzi, G: Renoprotective properties of ACE-inhibition in non-diabetic nephropathies with non-nephrotic proteinuria. *Lancet.*1999, 354, 359 –367.
[34] Lea, J; Greene, T; Hebert, L; Liphowitz, M; Massry, S; Middleton, J; Rostand, SG; Miller, E; Smith, W; Bakris, GL. for the African American Study of Kidney Disease and Hypertension Study Group: The relationship between magnitude of proteinuria reduction and risk of end-stage renal disease. *Arch Intern Med.*, 2005, 165, 947 –953.
[35] Khosla, N; Bakris, G. Lessons learned from recent hypertension trials about kidney disease. *Clin J Am Soc Nephrol*, 2006, 1, 229 –235.
[36] Kriz, W; Elger, M; Mundel, P; Lemley, KV. Structure-stabilizing forces in the glomerular tuft. *J Am Soc Nephrol*, 1995, 51, 1731 –1739.

[37] Pavenstadt, H; Kriz, W; Kretzler, M. Cell biology of the glomerular podocyte. *Physiol Rev.*, 2003, 83, 253 –307.

[38] Gansevoort, RT; de Zeeuw, D; de Jong, PE. Long-term benefits of the antiproteinuric effect of angiotensin-converting enzyme inhibition in nondiabetic renal disease. *Am J Kidney Dis.*, 1993, 22, 202-206.

[39] Nosrati, SM; Khwaja, S; el-Shahawy, M; Massry SG. Effect of angiotensin converting enzyme inhibition by perindopril on proteinuria of primary renal diseases. *Am J Nephrol.*, 1997, 17, 511-517.

[40] Coppo, R; Amore, A; Gianoglio, B; Cacace, G; Picciotto, G; Roccatello, D; et al. Angiotensin II local hyperreactivity in the progression of IgA nephropathy. *Am J Kidney Dis.*, 1993, 21, 593-602.

[41] Taguma, Y; Kitamoto, Y; Futaki, G; Ueda, H; Monma, H; Ishizaki, M; et al. Effect of captopril on heavy proteinuria in azotemic diabetics. *N Engl JMed*, 1985, 313, 1617–1620.

[42] Maschio, G; Alberti, D; Janin, G; Locatelli, F; Mann, JF; Motolese, M; et al. Effect of the angiotensin-converting-enzyme inhibitor benazepril on the progression of chronic renal insufficiency. The Angiotensin-Converting-Enzyme Inhibition in Progressive Renal Insufficiency Study Group. *N Engl J Med*, 1996, 334, 939-945

[43] Ruggenenti, P; Perna, A; Gherardi, G; Gaspari, F; Benini, R; Remuzzi, G. Renal function and requirement for dialysis in chronic nephropathy patients on longterm ramipril: REIN follow-up trial. Gruppo Italiano di Studi Epidemiologici in Nefrologia (GISEN). Ramipril Efficacy in Nephropathy. *Lancet*, 1998, 352, 1252-1256

[44] Agodoa, LY; Appel, L; Bakris, GL; Beck, G; Bourgoignie, J; Briggs, JP; et al. African American Study of Kidney Disease and Hypertension (AASK) Study Group. Effect of ramipril vs amlodipine on renal outcomes in hypertensive nephrosclerosis: a randomized controlled trial. *JAMA*, 2001, 285, 2719-2728.

[45] Lewis, EJ; Hunsicker, LG; Bain, RP. Rohde RD for the Collaborative Study Group, a clinical trial of an angiotensin converting enzyme inhibitor in the nephropathy of insulin-dependent diabetes mellitus. *N. Engl. J. Med.*, 1993, 329, 1456-1462.

[46] Effects of ramipril on cardiovascular and microvascular outcomes in people with diabetes mellitus: results of the HOPE study and MICRO-HOPE substudy. Heart Outcomes Prevention Evaluation Study Investigators. *Lancet.*, 2000, 355, 253-259.

[47] Svensson, P; de Faire, U; Sleight, P; Salim, Yusuf, S; Ostergren, J. Comparison of the effects of ramipril on ambulatory and office blood pressures. *A HOPE substudy. Hypertension*, 2001, 38, E28–E32.

[48] Turnbull, F. Blood Pressure Lowering Treatment Trialists' Collaboration. Effects of different blood-pressure-lowering regimens on major cardiovascular events: results of prospectively-designed overviews of randomised trials. *Lancet*, 2003, 362, 1527–1535.

[49] Wright, JT; Bakris, G; Greene, T; Agodoa, LY; Appel, LJ; Charleston, J; Cheek, D; Douglas-Baltimore, JG; Gassman, J; Glassock, R; et al.: for the African American Study of Kidney Disease and Hypertension Study Group. Effect of blood pressure lowering and antihypertensive drug class on progression of hypertensive kidney disease: results from the ASSK trial. JAMA, 2002, 288, 2421–2431

[50] Omae, K; Ogawa, T; Nitta, K. Therapeutic advantage of angiotensin-converting enzyme inhibitors in patients with proteinuric chronic kidney disease. Heart Vessels., 2010, 25, 203-8.

[51] Harris, RP; Helfand, M; Woolf, SH; Lohr, KN; Mulrow, CD; Teutsch, SM; Atkins, D. Methods Work Group, Third US Preventive Services Task Force. Current methods of the US Preventive Services Task Force: a review of the process. *Am J Prev Med.*, 2001 20(Suppl3), 21-35.

[52] Canadian Task Force on Preventive Health Care. Canadian Guide to Clinical Preventive Health Care. Ottawa (ON), Canada Communications Group, 1994.

[53] Casas, JP; Chua, W; Loukogeorgakis, S; Vallance, P; Smeeth, L; Hingorani, AD; MacAllister, RJ. Effect of inhibitors of the renin-angiotensin system and other antihypertensive drugs on renal outcomes: systematic review and meta-analysis. *Lancet.*, 2005, 366, 2026-2033.

[54] Daien, V; Duny, Y; Ribstein, J; du, Cailar, G; Mimran, A; Villain, M; et al. Treatment of hypertension with renin-angiotensin system inhibitors and renal dysfunction: a systematic review and meta-analysis. *Am J Hypertens.*, 2012, 25, 126-32.

[55] Giatras, I; Lau, J; Levey, AS, for the Angiotensin-Converting-Enzyme Inhibition and Progressive Renal Disease Study Group: Effect of angiotensin-converting-enzyme inhibitors on the progression of nondiabetic renal disease: a metaanalysis of randomized trials. *Ann Intern Med*, 1997, 127, 337-345.

[56] Jafar, TH; Schmid, CH; Landa, M; Giatras, I; Toto, R; Remuzzi, G. for the ACE Inhibition in Progressive Renal Disease Study Group, Angiotensin-converting enzyme inhibitors and progression of nondiabetic renal disease. A meta-analysis of patient-level data. *Ann Intern Med*, 2001, 135, 73-87.

[57] Jafar, TH; Stark, PC; Schmid, CH; Landa, M; Maschio, G; de Jong, PE; de Zeeuw, D; Shahinfar, S; Toto, R; Levey, AS. for the AIPRD Study Group, Progression of chronic kidney disease, The role of blood pressure control, proteinuria, and angiotensin-converting enzyme inhibition. A patient level meta-analysis. *Ann Intern Med.*, 2003, 139, 244–252.

[58] Gansevoort, RT; Sluiter, WJ; Hemmelder, MH; de Zeeuw, D; de Jong, PE. Antiproteinuric effect of blood-pressure-lowering agents: A meta-analysis of comparative trials. *Nephrol Dial Transplant*, 1995, 10, 1963-1974.

[59] Maione, A; Navaneethan, SD; Graziano, G; Mitchell, R; Johnson, D; Mann, JF; et al. Angiotensin-converting enzyme inhibitors, angiotensin receptor blockers and combined therapy in patients with micro- and macroalbuminuria and other cardiovascular risk factors: a systematic review of randomized controlled trials. *Nephrol Dial Transplant.*, 2011, 26, 2827-47.

[60] Sarafidis, PA; Stafylas, PC; Kanaki, AI, Lasaridis, AN. Effects of renin-angiotensin system blockers on renal outcomes and all-cause mortality in patients with diabetic nephropathy: an updated meta-analysis. *Am J Hypertens.*, 2008, 21, 922-9.

[61] Vejakama, P; Thakkinstian, A; Lertrattananon, D; Ingsathit, A; Ngarmukos, C; Attia, J. Reno-protective effects of renin-angiotensin system blockade in type 2 diabetic patients: a systematic review and network meta-analysis. *Diabetologia.*, 2012, 55, 566-78.

[62] Kshirsagar, AV; Joy, MS; Hogan, SL; Falk, RJ; Colindres, RE. Effect of ACEIs in diabetic and nondiabetic chronic renal disease: A systematic overview of randomised placebocontrolled trials. *Am J Kidney Dis.*, 2000, 35, 695-707.

[63] Balamuthusamy, S; Srinivasan, L; Verma, M; Adigopula, S; Jalandhara, N; Hathiwala, S; et al. Renin angiotensin system blockade and cardiovascular outcomes in patients

with chronic kidney disease and proteinuria: a meta-analysis. *Am Heart J.*, 2008, 155, 791-805.

[64] Russo, D; Minutolo, R; Pisani, A; Esposito, R; Signorello, G; Andreucci, M; et al. Coadministration of losartan and enalapril exerts additive antiproteinuric effect in IgA nefropathy. *Am. J. Kidney Dis.*, 2001, 38, 18-25.

[65] Ruilope, LM; Aldigier, JC; Ponticelli, C; Oddou-Stock, P; Botteri, F; Mann, JF. Safety of the combination of valsartan and benazepril in patients with chronic renal disease. European Group for the Investigation of Valsartan in Chronic Renal Disease. *J. Hypertens*, 2000, 18, 89-95.

[66] Luño, J; Barrio, V; Goicoechea, MA; Gonzalez, C; Garcia, de Vinuesa, S; Gomez, F; et al. Effects of dual blockade of the renin-angiotensin system in primary proteinuric nephropathies. *Kidney Int.*, 2002, 62 (Suppl. 82), S47–S52.

[67] Robles, NR; Ruiz Jiménez, B; Hernandez Gallego, R; Ruiz Calero, R; Sanchez Casado, E; Cubero, JJ. Dual renin-angiotensin system blockade in patients with single functioning kidey and proteinuria. *Eur. J. Intern. Med.*, 2009, 20, 186-189.

[68] Robles, NR; Fernandez-Carbonero, E; Romero, B; Sanchez, Casado, E; Cubero, JJ., Long-term antiproteinuric effect of dual renin-angiotensin system blockade. Cardiovasc. *Ther*, 2009, 27, 101-107.

[69] Jacobsen, P; Andersen, S; Rossing, K; Hansen, BV; Parving, HH. Dual blockade of the renin-angiotensin system in type 1 patients with diabetic nephropathy. *Nephrol Dial Transplant.*, 2002, 17, 1019-1024.

[70] Mogensen, CE; Neldam, S; Tikkanen, I; Oren, S; Viskoper, R; Watts, RW; Cooper, ME. for the C. A. L. M. study group. Randomised controlled trial of dual blockade of reninangiotensin system in patients with hypertension, microalbuminuria, and non-insulin dependent diabetes: the candesartan and lisinopril microalbuminuria (C. A. L. M.) study. *B. M. J.*, 2000, 321, 1440–1444.

[71] Kunz, R; Friedrich, C; Wolbers, M; Mann, JFE. Meta-analysis, Effect of Monotherapy and Combination Therapy with Inhibitors of the Renin–Angiotensin System on Proteinuria in Renal Disease. *Ann. Intern. Med.*, 2008, 148, 30-48.

[72] Mann, JFE; Schmieder, RE; McQueen, M; Dyal, L; Shumacher, H; Pogue, J; et al. Renal outcomes with telmisartan, ramipril, or both, in people at high vascular risk (the ONTARGET study), a multicentre, randomised, double-blind, controlled trial. *Lancet.*, 2008, 372, 547-553.

[73] Robles, NR; Cancho, B; Barroso, S; Martin, MV; Sanchez, Casado, E. Untoward effects of dual rennin-angiotensis system blockade: Influence of previous chonic renal failure. *Intl. J. Clin. Pract.*, 2006, 60, 1035-1039.

[74] Fernandez, Juarez, G; Luño, J; Barrio, V; de, Vinuesa, S; G; Praga, M; Goicoechea, M; et al. P. R. O. N. E. D. I. Study Group. Effect of Dual Blockade of the Renin-Angiotensin System on the Progression of Type 2 Diabetic Nephropathy: A Randomized Trial. *Am. J. Kidney Dis.*, 2012 Aug. 28. [Epub ahead of print].

[75] Doulton, TW; He, FJ; MacGregor, GA. Systematic review of combined angiotensin-converting enzyme inhibition and angiotensin receptor blockade in hypertension. *Hypertension*, 2005, 45, 880–886.

[76] MacKinnon, M; Shurraw, S; Akbari, A; Knoll, GA; Jaffey, J; Clark, HD. Combination therapy with an angiotensin receptor blocker and an ACE inhibitor in proteinuric renal

disease: A systematic review of the efficacy and safety data. *Am. J. Kidney Dis.*, 2006, 48, 8–20.

[77] Kunz, R; Friedrich, C; Wolbers, M; Mann, JFE. Meta-analysis, Effect of Monotherapy and Combination Therapy with Inhibitors of the Renin–Angiotensin System on Proteinuria in Renal Disease. *Ann Intern Med.*, 2008, 148, 30-48.

[78] Maione, A; Navaneethan, SD; Graziano, G; Mitchell, R; Johnson, D; Mann, JF; et al. Angiotensin-converting enzyme inhibitors, angiotensin receptor blockers and combined therapy in patients with micro- and macroalbuminuria and other cardiovascular risk factors: a systematic review of randomized controlled trials. *Nephrol Dial Transplant.*, 2011, 26, 2827-47.

[79] Matchar, DB; McCrory, DC; Orlando, LA; Patel, MR; Patel, UD; Patwardhan, MB; et al. Systematic Review: Comparative Effectiveness of Angiotensin-Converting Enzyme Inhibitors and Angiotensin II Receptor Blockers for Treating Essential Hipertensión. *Ann Intern Med.*, 2008, 148, 16-29.

[80] Barnett, AH; Bain, SC; Bouter, P; Karlberg, B; Madsbad, S; Jervell, J; Mustonen J. Diabetics exposed to telmisartan and enalapril study group, Angiotensin-receptor blockade versus converting-enzyme inhibition in type 2 diabetes and nephropathy. *N Engl J Med.*, 2004, 351, 1952 –1961,

[81] Ferrari, P. Prescribing angiotensin-converting enzyme inhibitors and angiotensin receptor blockers in chronic kidney disease. *Nephrology.*, 2007, 12, 81–89.

[82] Hsu, CY; McCulloch, CE; Fan, D; Ordoñez, JD; Chertow, GM; Go, AS. Community-based incidence of acute renal failure. *Kidney Int*, 2007, 72, 208–212.

[83] Eachempati, SR; Wang, JC; Hydo, LJ; Shou, J; Barie, PS. Acute renal failure in critically ill surgical patients: persistent lethality despite new modes of renal replacement therapy. *J Trauma*, 2007, 63, 987–993.

[84] Centers for Disease Control and Prevention (CDC): Prevalence of chronic kidney disease and associated risk factors – United States,, 1999–2004. *MMWR Morb Mortal Wkly Rep*, 2007, 56, 161–165.

[85] Onuigbo, MAC. Reno-prevention vs. reno-protection: a critical re-appraisal of the evidence-base from the large RAAS blockade trials after ontarget—a call for more circumspection. *Q Med J.*, 2009, 102, 155-157.

[86] Onuigbo, MAC. Can ACE Inhibitors and Angiotensin Receptor Blockers Be Detrimental in CKD Patients? *Nephron Clin Pract*, 2011, 118, c407–c419.

[87] Rahman, M; Pressel, S; Davis, BR; Nwachuku, C; Wright, JT Jr; Whelton, PK; et al. Renal outcomes in high-risk hypertensive patients treated with an angiotensin-converting enzyme inhibitor or a calcium channel blocker vs a diuretic: a report from the Antihypertensive and Lipid-Lowering Treatment to Prevent Heart Attack Trial (ALLHAT). *Arch Intern Med.*, 2005, 165, 936–46.

[88] Suissa, S; Hutchinson, T; Brophy, JM; Kezouh, A. ACE-inhibitor use and the long-term risk of renal failure in diabetes. *Kidney Int.*, 2006, 69, 913–919.

[89] Rossing, P; Parving, HH; de Zeeuw, D. Renoprotection by blocking the RAAS in diabetic nephropathy—fact or fiction?. *Nephrol Dial Transplant*, 2006, 21, 2354-2357.

[90] Hoorntje, SJ; Kallenberg, CG; Weening, JJ; Donker, AJ; The, TH; Hoedemaeker, PJ. Immune-complex glomerulopathy in patients treated with captopril. *Lancet*, 1980, 1, 1212–1215.

[91] Reardon, LC; Macpherson, DS. Hyperkalemia in outpatients using angiotensin-converting enzyme inhibitors. How much should we worry? *Arch Intern Med.*, 1998, 158, 26–32.

[92] Palmer, BF. Managing hyperkalemia caused by inhibitors of the reninangiotensin-aldosterone system. *N Engl J Med*, 2004, 351, 585–592.

[93] Henz, S; Maeder, MT; Huber, S; Schmid, M; Loher, M; Fehr, T. Influence of drugs and comorbidity on serum potassium in 15 000 consecutive hospital admissions. *Nephrol Dial Transplant.*, 2008, Jul 9. [Epub ahead of print].

[94] Ahmed, AK; Kamath, NS; Kossi, El; M, El; Nahas, AM. The impact of stopping inhibitors of the renin-angiotensin system in patients with advanced chronic kidney disease. *Nephrol Dial Transplant.*, 2010, 25, 3977-82.

[95] Hou, FF; Zhang, X; Zhang, GH; Xie, D; Chen, PY; Zhang, WR; Jiang, JP; et al. Efficacy and safety of benazepril for advanced chronic renal insufficiency. *N Engl J Med.*, 2006, 354, 131-40.

[96] Mangrum, AJ; Bakris, GL. Angiotensin-converting enzyme inhibitors and angiotensin receptor blockers in chronic renal disease: safety issues. *Semin Nephrol.*, 2004, 24, 168-175.

[97] Onuigbo, MA; Onuigbo, NT. Renal failure and concurrent RAAS blockade in older CKD patients with renal artery stenosis: an extended Mayo Clinic prospective 63-month experience. *Ren Fail*, 2008, 30, 363–71.

[98] Avanza, AC, Jr El; Aouar, LM; Mill, JG. Reduction in left ventricular hypertrophy in hypertensive patients treated with enalapril, losartan or the combination of enalapril and losartan. *Arq Bras Cardiol.*, 2000, 74, 103-117.

[99] De, Rosa, ML; Cardace, P; Rossi, M; Baiano, A; de Cristofaro, A. Comparative effects of chronic ACE inhibition and AT1 receptor blocked losartan on cardiac hypertrophy and renal function in hypertensive patients. *J Hum Hypertens.*, 2002, 16, 133-140.

[100] Derosa, G; Cicero, AF; Ciccarelli, L; Fogari, R. A randomized, double-blind, controlled, parallel-group comparison of perindopril and candesartan in hypertensive patients with type 2 diabetes mellitus. *Clin Ther.*, 2003, 25, 2006-2021.

[101] Elliott, WJ. Double-blind comparison of eprosartan and enalapril on cough and blood pressure in unselected hypertensive patients. Eprosartan Study Group. *J Hum Hypertens.*, 1999, 13, 413-417.

[102] Fogari, R; Mugellini, A; Zoppi, A; Corradi, L; Preti, P; Lazzari, P; et al. Losartan and perindopril effects on plasma plasminogen activator inhibitor-1 and fibrinogen in hypertensive type 2 diabetic patients. *Am J Hypertens.*, 2002, 15, 316-320.

[103] Kavgaci, H; Sahin, A; Onder, Ersoz, H; Erem, C; Ozdemir, F. The effects of losartan and fosinopril in hypertensive type 2 diabetic patients. *Diabetes Res Clin Pract.*, 2002, 58, 19-25.

[104] Lacourciere, Y; Be´langer, A; Godin, C; Halle´, JP; Ross, S; Wright, N; et al. Long-term comparison of losartan and enalapril on kidney function in hypertensive type 2 diabetics with early nephropathy. *Kidney Int.*, 2000, 58, 762-769.

[105] Matsuda, H; Hayashi, K; Saruta, T. Distinct time courses of renal protective action of angiotensin receptor antagonists and ACEIs in chronic renal disease. *J Hum Hypertens.*, 2003, 17, 271-276.

[106] Mimran, A; Ruilope, L; Kerwin, L; Nys, M; Owens, D; Kassler-Taub, K; et al. A randomised, double-blind comparison of the angiotensin II receptor antagonist,

irbesartan, with the full dose range of enalapril for the treatment of mild-to moderate hypertension. *J Hum Hypertens.*, 1998, 12, 203-208.

[107] Mogensen, CE; Neldam, S; Tikkanen, I; Oren, S; Viskoper, R; Watts, RW; et al. Randomised controlled trial of dual blockade of renin-angiotensin system in patients with hypertension, microalbuminuria, and non-insulin dependent diabetes, the candesartan and lisinopril microalbuminuria (CALM) study. *BMJ.*, 2000, 321, 1440-1444.

[108] Rosei, EA; Rizzoni, D; Muiesan, ML; Sleiman, I; Salvetti, M; Monteduro, C; et al. CENTRO (CandEsartaN on aTherosclerotic Risk factors) Study Investigators. Effects of candesartan cilexetil and enalapril on inflammatory markers of atherosclerosis in hypertensive patients with non-insulin-dependent diabetes mellitus *J Hypertens.*, 2005, 23, 435-444.

[109] Schram, MT; van, Ittersum, FJ; Spoelstra-de Man, A; van Dijk, RA; Schalkwijk, CG; Ijzerman, RG; et al. Aggressive antihypertensive therapy based on hydrochlorothiazide, candesartan or lisinopril as initial choice in hypertensive type II diabetic individuals, effects on albumin excretion, endothelial function and inflammation in a double-blind, randomized clinical trial. *J Hum Hypertens.*, 2005, 19, 429-437.

[110] Shand, BI. Haemorheological effects of losartan and enalapril in patients with renal parenchymal disease and hypertension. *J Hum Hypertens.*, 2000, 14, 305-309.

[111] Uchiyama-Tanaka, Y; Mori, Y; Kishimoto, N; Fukui, M; Nose, A; Kijima, Y; et al. Comparison of the effects of quinapril and losartan on carotid artery intimamedia thickness in patients with mild-to-moderate arterial hypertension. *Kidney Blood Press Res.*, 2005, 28, 111-116.

[112] Verdecchia, P; Schillaci, G; Reboldi, GP; Sacchi, N; Bruni, B; Benemio, G; et al. Long-term effects of losartan and enalapril, alone or with a diuretic, on ambulatory blood pressure and cardiac performance in hypertension, a case-control study. *Blood Press Monit.*, 2000, 5, 187-193.

[113] Tikkanen, I; Omvik, P; Jensen, HA. Comparison of the angiotensin II antagonist losartan with the angiotensin converting enzyme inhibitor enalapril in patients with essential hypertension. *J Hypertens.*, 1995, 13, 1343-1351.

[114] Roca-Cusachs, A; Oigman, W; Lepe, L; Cifkova, R; Karpov, YA; Harron, DW. A randomized, double-blind comparison of the antihypertensive efficacy and safety of once-daily losartan compared to twice-daily captopril in mild to moderate essential hypertension. *Acta Cardiol.*, 1997, 52, 495-506.

[115] Sato, A; Tabata, M; Hayashi, K; Saruta, T. Effects of the angiotensin II type 1 receptor antagonist candesartan, compared with angiotensin-converting enzyme inhibitors, on the urinary excretion of albumin and type IV collagen in patients with diabetic nephropathy. *Clin Exp Nephrol.*, 2003, 7, 215-220.

In: ACE Inhibitors. Volume 2
Editor: Macaulay Amechi Onuigbo

ISBN: 978-1-62948-422-8

Chapter 13

ANGIOTENSIN-CONVERTING ENZYME INHIBITORS IN HEART FAILURE

Kaushik Guha, MD[1,2*] and R. Sharma, MD[1,2]

[1] Dept of Cardiology, Royal Brompton Hospital, London, UK

[2] National Heart and Lung Institute, Imperial College London, London, UK

ABSTRACT

The pharmacological management of patients with left ventricular systolic dysfunction has gradually evolved over the last few decades. Whereas once the treatment options were limited to digitalis extract and mercurial diuretics, currently there has been introduced the incorporation of multiple agents which are neuro-hormonal inhibitors. The discovery of the role of the renin-angiotensin-aldosterone system in the pathobiology of heart failure initiated the impetus to investigate the actions of these novel neuro-hormonal inhibitors. The realization, and importantly, the adept clinical testing in small and large clinical trials of the inhibitors of the renin-angiotensin-aldosterone system has rapidly established angiotensin converting enzyme inhibitors as a cornerstone of modern heart failure pharmacotherapy. This short report intends to provide a brief synopsis of the area.

LIST OF ABBREVIATIONS

LVSD	Left Ventricular Systolic Dysfunction
RAAS	Rennin –Angiotensin –Aldosterone System
NYHA	New York Heart Association
HF	Heart Failure

* Corresponding Author: Kaushik Guha MD; Email: kguha@doctors.org.uk.

INTRODUCTION

Heart failure treatment has evolved over the last thirty years with several landmark studies that have demonstrated prognostic and clinical benefits of pharmacological agents primarily aimed at modulating the effects of neurohormonal activation. There is now a clearly established treatment algorithm for patients with left ventricular systolic dysfunction (LVSD) with the emphasis being on the introduction and uptitration of such evidence based therapies [1, 2].

However prior to the modern era, heart failure though clinically recognised for the preceding two centuries was treated with either mercurial diuretics or digoxin (digitalis extract). This remained the status quo for most of the last century until the recognition that activation of the renin –angiotensin- aldosterone system (RAAS) was implicated in the pathophysiology of heart failure and thus could be targeted with selective inhibition. This led to the development of the first strategies which were able to modify the natural history of the disease with substantial implications on patient survival and morbidity.

HISTORY OF RAAS SYSTEM

The first part of the pathway; renin; was investigated in the mid-late 19th century. Following clinical observation that patients with renal disease displayed elevated blood pressures, Tigerstedt et al in 1898 demonstrated that the injection of renal extracts from rabbits induced a vasopressor response [3]. The findings were overlooked for approximately forty years until the publication from several groups which reproduced the original findings and went on to conclude that renin did not directly exert a vasopressor effect but that this was due to rennin's effects on another substance named Angiotensin [4-6].

Further work by Skeggs, Elliott and Peart in 1956 showed that the results of cleavage of the decapeptide, angiotensin resulted in an active octapeptide angiotensin I [7, 8]. The nomenclature of angiotensin converting enzyme and angiotensin I and angiotensin II were derived from thess series of experiments.

Around this time period others concentrated their efforts on the identification of an agent which would antagonise the effect of ACE or angiotensin II which was recognised to be a potent vasoconstrictor in the cardiac, renal and cerebral circulation.

Ferreira in 1965 published what was to become a seminal paper in the field – with the notification that venom from a Brazilian viper could potentiate the effects of bradykinin [9]. Previous work had shown an agent which inactivated bradykinin and it was also later discovered that peptides from the same venom could inhibit ACE [10]. This resulted in the first ACE inhibitor teprotide. This led ultimately to the first oral ACE inhibitor, captopril.

Captopril was then evaluated in small case series and shown to have positive haemodynamic effects in patients with heart failure with reductions in pulmonary wedge pressure, right atrial pressures and subsequent rises in cardiac index [11, 12]. The beneficial effects of ACE inhibitors were then evaluated in a trial whereby enalapril showed a positive effect on survival as compared to other vasodilators. This formed the basis for the landmark study performed in Scandinavia.

Clinical Trials

The Co-operative North Scandinavian Enalapril Survival Study (CONSENSUS) was created to study the clinical impact of Enalapril in a highly symptomatic cohort (NYHA Class IV) of patients with LVSD [13]. 253 participants were enrolled into a randomised double blind placebo controlled trial. The entire cohort was pre-treated with diuretics and digoxin and the study endpoint was all cause mortality.

The trial was halted early by the ethics committee due to a significant reduction in deaths in the treatment arm with significant reductions at 6 months and 1 year. The overall relative risk reduction was 27% (p=0.003). Following the initial publication the study was allowed to run on an open basis with the effect of Enalapril found to be long lasting and ultimately leading to a 50% increase in life expectancy (521 days versus 781 days) [14, 15].

CONSENSUS was hailed as a landmark trial due to the notable effect of Enalapril. For the first time in a cohort with advanced heart failure, Enalapril, an ACE inhibitor had been demonstrated to have prognostic disease modifying benefit.

The success of Enalapril and CONSENSUS led to further studies. These are summarised in Table 1. A number of ACE inhibitors were investigated within heart failure including the most widely used currently (Lisinopril, Enalapril, Ramipril and Perindropril). All of the agents were proven to be effective at reducing morbidity and mortality within patients with significant LVSD. Beyond their effects upon symptoms, reducing HF hospitalisation and increasing longevity, they have also shown to be effective in asymptomatic populations with LVSD.

Several of the agents were trialled in the acute period following myocardial infarction and were shown to have preventive effects on adverse left ventricular remodelling. Hence ACE inhibitors have become important agents in the post infarction period with particular focus on those patients who have post infarct LVSD.

The continuous stream of studies has created a clear evidence base for ACE inhibitors in heart failure. They have now become a cornerstone of HF pharmacotherapy and are advocated as first line agents where LVSD has been confirmed by cardiac imaging. National and international guidance suggest the introduction of these agents with low dose and careful uptitration with accompanying clinical review, blood pressure, electrolytes and renal function [1, 2]. The collection of studies dictates the optimal dose for which healthcare professionals should be aiming for. It is noteworthy that despite the clear evidence base and guidance about the usage of ACE inhibitors that they remain along with other HF therapeutic agents remain underutilised. One such example is the recent data from the national HF audit data based within England and Wales. This covers data for admissions for patients with heart failure [16]. The rates of prescription of ACE inhibitors varied depending on discharge ward between 76% and 87%.

Conclusion

The use of ACE inhibitors in heart failure represented a clear example of successful translation of bench to bedside medicine. Following the successful characterisation of the RAAS system, the stream of several large randomised controlled trials has established a clear evidence base for the class and they have now become a cornerstone of pharmacotherapy for left ventricular systolic dysfunction. The challenge that now faces modern healthcare teams and infrastructure is how to ensure that such patients are commenced on appropriate therapy.

Table 1. Summary of key randomised controlled trials using ACE inhibitors

Name of Study	n	Year of Publication	Agent	Outcome
CONSENSUS	253	1987	Enalapril	All Cause Mortality (P=0.003)
SOLVD	2568	1991	Enalapril	All Cause Mortality (P=0.003)
SAVE	2231	1992	Captopril	All Cause Mortality (P=0.014)
AIRE	2006	1993	Ramipril	All Cause Mortality (P=0.002)
GISSI-3	19,394	1994	Lisinopril	All Cause Mortality (12% relative Risk reduction)
ATLAS	3164	1999	Lisinopril	All cause Mortality and hospitalisation + HF hospitalisation (P=0.002)

TRIALS

[1] The CONSENSUS Trial Study group. Effects of Enalapril on mortality in severe heart failure. *N Engl J Med*;1987;316;1429-1435.

[2] SOLVD Investigators; Effects of enalapril on survival in patients with reduced left ventricular ejection fraction and congestive heart failure. *N Engl J Med*;1191;325;293-302

[3] Pfeffer MA, Braunwald E, Moye LA et al. Effect of captopril on mortality and morbidity in patients with left ventricular dysfunction after myocardial infarction: Results of the Survival and Ventricular Enlargement Trial. *N Engl J Med*;1992;327;685-691.

[4] AIRE Investigators: Effect of Ramipril on mortality and morbidity of survivors of acute myocardial infarction with clinical evidence of heart failure. *Lancet*;1993; 342;821-828

[5] GISSI-3 Investigators: Effects of lisinopril and transdermal glyceryl trinitrate singly and together on 6-week mortality and ventricular function after acute myocardial infarction. Gruppo Italiano per lo Studio della Sopravvivenza nell'infarto Miocardico. *Lancet*;1994;343;1115-1122.

[6] Packer M, Poole-Wilson PA, Armstrong PW et al. Comparative effects of low and high doses of the angiotensin-converting enzyme inhibitor, lisinopril on morbidity and mortality in chronic heart failure. (ATLAS Study). *Circulation*;1999;100;2312-2318.

FURTHER READING

[1] Cleland SJ, Reid JL. The rennin-angiotensin system and the heart: a historical review. *Heart*;1996; (Suppl 3); 76;7-12.

REFERENCES

[1] McMurray JJ, Adamopoulos S, Anker SD, et al. ESC guidelines for the diagnosis and treatment of acute and chronic heart failure 2012: The Task Force for the Diagnosis and Treatment of Acute and Chronic Heart Failure 2012 of the European Society of Cardiology. Developed in collaboration with the Heart Failure Association (HFA) of the ESC. *Eur J Heart Fail* 2012 Aug;14(8):803-69.

[2] Al-Mohammad A, Mant J, Laramee P, et al. Diagnosis and management of adults with chronic heart failure: summary of updated NICE guidance. *BMJ* 2010;341:c4130.

[3] Tigerstedt R, Bergman PG. Niere und kreislauf. *Scand Arch Physiol* 1898;8:223-70.

[4] Landis EM, Montgomery H, Sparkman D. The Effects Of Pressor Drugs And Of Saline Kidney Extracts On Blood Pressure And Skin Temperature

[5] 24. *J Clin Invest* 1938 Mar;17(2):189-206.

[6] Braun-Menendez E, Fasciolo JC, Leloir LF, et al. The substance causing renal hypertension. *J Physiol* 1940 Jul 24;98(3):283-98.

[7] Pickering GW. The role of the kidney in acute and chronic hypertension following renal artery constriction in the rabbit. *Clin Sci* 1945;5(3-4):229-47.

[8] ELLIOTT DF, Peart WS. Amino-acid sequence in a hypertensin. *Nature* 1956 Mar 17;**177**(4507):527-8.

[9] Skeggs LT, Jr., Kahn JR, Shumway NP. The preparation and function of the hypertensin-converting enzyme. *J Exp Med* 1956 Mar 1;103(3):295-9.

[10] Ferreira SH. A Bradykinin-Potentiating Factor (Bpf) Present In The Venom Of Bothrops Jararca. *Br J Pharmacol Chemother* 1965 Feb;24:163-9.

[11] Erdos EG, Sloane EM. An enzyme in human blood plasma that inactivates bradykinin and kallidins. *Biochem Pharmacol* 1962 Jul;11:585-92.

[12] Davis R, Ribner HS, Keung E, et al. Treatment of chronic congestive heart failure with captopril, an oral inhibitor of angiotensin-converting enzyme. *N Engl J Med* 1979 Jul 19;301(3):117-21.

[13] Turini GA, Brunner HR, Gribic M, et al. Improvement of chronic congestive heart-failure by oral captopril. *Lancet* 1979 Jun 9;1(8128):1213-5.

[14] Swedberg K, Kjekshus J. Effects of enalapril on mortality in severe congestive heart failure: results of the Cooperative North Scandinavian Enalapril Survival Study (CONSENSUS). *Am J Cardiol* 1988 Jul 11;62(2):60A-6A.

[15] Swedberg K, Kjekshus J, Snapinn S. Long-term survival in severe heart failure in patients treated with enalapril. Ten year follow-up of CONSENSUS I. *Eur Heart J* 1999 Jan;20(2):136-9.

[16] Cleland JG, McDonagh T, Rigby AS, et al. The national heart failure audit for England and Wales 2008-2009. *Heart* 2011 Jun;97(11):876-86.

In: ACE Inhibitors. Volume 2
Editor: Macaulay Amechi Onuigbo
ISBN: 978-1-62948-422-8

Chapter 14

RAAS Blockade in Ethnic Minorities with Chronic Kidney Disease: A United Kingdom Perspective

Conor Byrne, MD[1,2] and Muhammad Magdi Yaqoob,* MD PhD[1,2]
[1]Barts Health NHS Trust & William Harvey Research Institute,
Queen Mary College, University of London, UK
[2]Renal Unit, Royal London Hospital, Whitechapel, London, UK

Abstract

Chronic Kidney disease (CKD), with and without diabetes, represents a growing public health problem in the UK where 8% of the population are of Black and South Asian origin. Ethnicity has been identified as a risk factor for diabetes mellitus, hypertension and concomitant CKD. In line with these observations, as in USA, ethnic minorities are over represented on renal replacement therapy (RRT) programmes.

Blockade of the renin-angiotensin system (RAS) is accepted as the first-line strategy for the treatment of hypertension, endorsed by numerous national and international guidelines. The role of RAS blockade (RB) is especially emphasised for primary and secondary prevention of cardiovascular disease and CKD. The preference for RAS blockers in these conditions is based on their neutral metabolic actions and their direct cardiac and renoprotective properties, independent of the BP-lowering, so called pleiotropic effects.

In the UK, the risk of developing CKD and cardiovascular complications of hypertension and DM is significantly greater amongst black and minority ethnic (BME) communities. However, no specific randomised controlled trials focused on these high risk groups for superior RB benefits exist. Instead BME groups are treated with RAS blockers based on evidence derived from predominantly white patients.

In our own observational studies, we have been unable to show a beneficial effect of RB compared to other antihypertensive agents in BME patients with CKD, managed in either primary care or a tertiary specialist facility. A comprehensive meta-analysis of the effects of RB and other anti-hypertensive drugs on renal outcomes concluded that the

* Corresponding author: Muhammad Magdi Yaqoob MD PhD; Email: m.m.yaqoob@qmul.ac.uk.

benefits of RB in placebo controlled trials probably resulted solely from a BP-lowering effect. In addition, the renoprotective actions of RB in DM, independent of BP-lowering effect, remained unproven. Moreover, 6 large, recently published clinical trials, designed to demonstrate the beneficial effects of angiotensin receptor blockers (ARB) over placebo, in patients at high cardiovascular risk, failed to demonstrate any cardiovascular protection. Two trials revealed higher cardiovascular mortality in patients treated with ARB. Their putative beneficial effect in the prevention of atrial fibrillation (highly prevalent in patients with CKD) was not confirmed in four major clinical studies specifically designed to investigate this effect. Furthermore, in various recent trials, treatment with ARB led to worse renal outcomes, such as an increased incidence of microalbuminuria, renal impairment and decreased GFR. The role of RB in the prevention of cardiovascular and renal disease should be re-examined in general and more importantly in high risk ethnic populations.

SUMMARY

Chronic Kidney disease (CKD), with and without diabetes, represents a growing public health problem in the UK where 12 % of the population are of Black and South Asian origin. Ethnicity has been identified as a risk factor for diabetes mellitus, hypertension and concomitant CKD. In line with these observations, ethnic minorities are over represented on renal replacement therapy (RRT) programmes in the UK.

Blockade of the renin-angiotensin system (RAS) is accepted as the first-line strategy for the treatment of hypertension and is endorsed by numerous national and international guidelines. The role of RAS blockade is especially emphasised for primary and secondary prevention of cardiovascular disease and CKD. The preference for RAS blockers in these conditions is based on their neutral metabolic actions and their putative direct cardiac and renoprotective properties, independent of blood pressure lowering, so called pleiotropic effects.

In the UK, the risk of developing CKD and cardiovascular complications of hypertension and DM is significantly greater amongst black, Asian and minority ethnic (BAME) communities. However, there are no specific randomised controlled trials focusing on these high-risk groups and comparing the effects of RAS blockade against either placebo or alternative agents. Instead BAME groups are treated with RAS blockers based on evidence derived predominantly from white patients.

In our own observational studies, we have been unable to show a beneficial effect of RAS blockade compared to other antihypertensive agents in BAME patients with CKD, managed in either primary care or a tertiary specialist centre. A comprehensive meta-analysis of the effects of inhibitors of RAS and other anti-hypertensive drugs on renal outcomes concluded that the benefits of RAS blockade in placebo controlled trials probably resulted solely from a BP lowering effect. In addition, the renoprotective actions of RAS blockade in DM, independent of BP lowering effect, remain unproven. Moreover, several recently published clinical trials, designed to demonstrate the beneficial effects of angiotensin receptor blockers (ARB) over placebo, in patients at high cardiovascular risk, failed to demonstrate any cardiovascular protection. Their putative beneficial effect in the prevention of atrial fibrillation (highly prevalent in patients with CKD) was not confirmed in four major clinical studies specifically designed to investigate this effect. Furthermore, in various recent trials, treatment with ARB led to worse renal outcomes, such as an increased incidence of microalbuminuria, renal impairment and decreased glomerular filtration rate. The role of RAS blockade in the prevention of cardiovascular and renal disease should be re-examined in general and more importantly in high-risk ethnic populations.

Ethnicity, Hypertension and CKD in the UK

The majority (86%) of the UK population is of White ethnicity. Persons of Black African, Black Caribbean and Chinese ethnicity account for approximately 3.5% of the population. However, The largest non-White ethnic group is made up of South Asians (accounting for roughly 7.5% of the UK population) [1] There are similar numbers of South Asians living in the UK as the US, although there are substantially more persons of Bangladeshi origin living in London alone than the entire United States.

Hypertension is a major risk factor for cardiovascular disease (CVD) and progression of chronic kidney disease (CKD) towards end stage kidney failure (ESKF) [2]. In the UK, both men and women of Afro-Caribbean (black) decent are more likely to be hypertensive then either those of white or South Asian decent [1,3] In addition, Afro-Caribbean's have more than 3 fold greater risk of mortality from acute stroke than whites or South Asians [2,4] However, paradoxically coronary heart disease (CHD) is lower in the black population than either the white or South Asian.

In the UK, as in other developed countries, the public health burden of CKD and ESKD has become a matter of national priority and the subject of recently published national CKD guidelines [5]. The latest reports JNC 7 and NKF KDOQI, [2,6] have identified patients with CKD as a high-risk group in which blood pressure control is especially important. Studies in the USA have identified that blood pressure control in CKD is frequently sub-optimal and that risk factors for poor blood pressure control in patients with CKD include non-Hispanic Black ethnicity, albuminuria and age >75 [7].

As in the USA, black and minority ethnic (BME) groups are over represented amongst the UK chronic kidney disease population. Data collection, in respect of acceptance rates to dialysis programmes by ethnicity, is less robust in the UK compared to the US. However, available data suggests that around 10.5% of incident dialysis patients in the UK are of South Asian ethnicity and 6.8% black ethnicity [8]. Which approximates to 1.5 and double the expected rate based on proportion of population. Similarly, 17.8% of the prevalent ESKF population are from a BAME background (compared to 11% of the overall UK population).

The introduction in 2004 of performance related pay for general practice in the UK, the quality and outcomes framework (QOF), [9], has contributed to an improvement in hypertension control. Moreover, there is also evidence that inequalities in performance between affluent and deprived areas have diminished [10,11]. However there remains room for improvement, especially in high-risk groups such as individuals with CKD.

In the UK, the effect of ethnicity on blood pressure control and associated CKD in a hypertensive population has not been studied in detail. Previous studies of primary care hypertension management in the UK have excluded or had very low numbers of patients with CKD, [10,12], or have had small ethnic minority populations [12,13]. Millet et alhave demonstrated disparities by ethnicity in blood pressure control in a London study, however this study had low reporting rates of CKD [10].

We recently analysed data from a large, multi-ethnic population (n=49,203) with hypertension and high recorded levels of self-reported ethnicity to examine the effect of ethnicity on the prevalence and management of hypertension and on the prevalence and severity of associated CKD [14]. The crude prevalence of hypertension was 9.5%, and by ethnicity was 8.2% for White, 11.3% for South Asian and 11.1% for Black groups. The prevalence of CKD stages 3-5 among those with hypertension was 22%. Stage 3 CKD was less prevalent in South Asian groups (OR 0.77, 95% CI 0.67 - 0.88) compared to Whites (reference population) with Black groups having similar rates to Whites. The prevalence of severe CKD (stages 4-5) was higher in the South Asian group (OR 1.53, 95% CI 1.17 - 2.0) compared to Whites, but did not differ between Black and White groups [14].

Our results confirmed a higher prevalence of hypertension amongst South Asian and Black groups compared to the White population. In the whole hypertension cohort, achievement of a less stringent target blood pressure (<140/90 mmHg) was better in South Asian (OR 1.43, 95% CI 1.28 - 1.60) and worse in Black groups (OR 0.79, 95% CI 0.74 - 0.84) compared to White patients. However, blood pressure control for a high risk CKD population remained suboptimal. In patients with an eGFR <60 ml/min/1.73m^2, a recommended blood pressure of <130/80 mmHg, [2], was achieved in <50% of all patients and <30% of Black patients. These findings are comparable with a previous study of diabetic patients with CKD in East London, and a study of patients with CKD in the USA [7,15]. The putative renoprotective benefits of ACE-I and ARB's have resulted in numerous international and national societies advocating them as first line therapy in patients with CKD, in this respect the UK is no different [7]. However nearly 40% of patients with CKD in our study did not receive an ACE-I or ARB, and Black patients were significantly less likely to be prescribed these medications than other ethnic groups in contrast to the findings of the recent AASK study which demonstrated the benefits of these medications in this patient group [16]. Interestingly, there was no difference between the prevalence of CKD and degree of BP control in patients with and without usage of ACE-I and or ARBs in our cohort.

Racial disparities in blood pressure (BP) control are well documented and possibly in part explained by worse medication adherence, more discrimination, and more concerns about high blood pressure and medications among ethnic minorities compared with whites. It is our impression that equalizing patients' health beliefs, medication adherence, and experiences with care could ameliorate disparities in BP control.

Geographic variations in cardiovascular mortality at a similar blood pressure level are well documented [17]. Despite better blood pressure control, South Asians had high prevalence of severe CKD. The universal blood pressure targets recommended in hypertension guidelines may paradoxically disadvantage some ethnic groups in whom the ambient BP of the general population is lower than in other ethnic groups. For example if the normal mean blood pressure of South Asians is lower than for Black or White groups, a "one size fits all" blood pressure target may be too high to achieve optimal renal protection in South Asian patients.

Ethnicity, Diabetes and CKD in the UK

Diabetes mellitus (DM) is a huge global public health problem [18-20]. As the number of individuals with type 2 DM grows, the prevalence of CKD is expected to rise sharply [21,22]. Many ethnic minority groups have both a greater risk of developing DM and increased chance of adverse outcomes from cardiovascular disease, [23,24], the most common complication of CKD.

Data on the prevalence of DM and associated CKD in the ethnic minority populations of the UK is sparse. We recently analysed data from a large, multi-ethnic population (n=34,359) with DM and high recorded levels of self-reported ethnicity, in order to examine the effect of ethnicity on the prevalence and severity of diabetes mellitus and associated CKD. The prevalence of DM was 3.5% for Whites, 11% for South Asians and 8% for Black groups. The prevalence of CKD (stages 3–5) among diabetics was 18%. CKD stage 3 was more prevalent in Whites compared to South Asians (OR 0.79, 95% CI: 0.71–0.87) and Blacks (OR 0.49, 95% CI: 0.43–0.57). Among all CKD patients, severity (CKD stages 4, 5) was associated with Black (OR 1.39, 95% CI: 1.06–1.81) and South Asian (OR 1.54, 95% CI: 1.26–1.88) ethnicity compared to Whites. Less than 50% of diabetics with CKD achieved the recommended target blood pressure (BP) of 130/80 mmHg. The prevalence of a blood pressure >150/90mmHg in diabetics with CKD was 15.6%, for South Asians, 13.9% White and, 21.8% for Black ethnicity (P<0.001). Proteinuria was present in 8.6% of all diabetic patients. However, this increased to 18.6% in patients with CKD, and was more frequent in Black (22.6%) and South Asian (21%) patients compared to White patients (14.1%) (P<0.001). Significant disparities exist between the major ethnic groups in both disease prevalence and management [15].

We further studied the effect of ethnicity, on both disease prevalence, management and on the progression of chronic kidney disease in people with diabetes managed in a community setting [25]. A 5-year retrospective, community-based cohort study including 3855 people with diabetes mellitus of white, black or South Asian ethnicity and an estimated glomerular filtration rate (eGFR) of <60 ml/min was undertaken. Using repeated-measures analysis, the annual decline in eGFR was calculated [25]. Comparisons between the rate of decline in the three main ethnic groups, with and without proteinuria at baseline, were made. The mean annual adjusted decline in eGFR for the entire cohort was 0.85 ml/min. The rate decline was statistically greater in the South Asian group (-1.01 ml/min) compared with the white group (–0.70 ml/min) (P = 0.001). As expected, for those individuals with proteinuria at baseline, the annual decline was greater at 2.05 ml/min, with both South Asian and black groups having a significantly faster rate of decline than the white group. Interestingly the rate of decline in GFR for patients with diabetes and chronic kidney disease managed in primary care, was less than previously thought and approximated to an age-related annual decline of 1 ml/min. Moreover, the rate of progression of CKD independent of ethnicity, in patients with DM treated with ACEi and or ARBs did not differ. However this study identified patients with proteinuria and those of South Asian and Black ethnicity as high-risk, who might benefit from additional monitoring in a specialist clinic [25].

In order to investigate the effect of specialist management on the rate of progression of CKD in patients with DM, stratified by ethnicity we undertook a prospective cohort study of patients managed in a tertiary hospital setting. All new patients referred with diabetic CKD between 2000 and 2007 were included. The primary outcome was annual decline in estimated glomerular filtration rate (eGFR). Secondary end points were the number of patients developing end stage kidney failure (ESKF), and all cause mortality. 329 patients (age 60 years ± 11.9, 208 men) were studied comprising 149 South Asian, 105 White and 75 Black patients. Follow up was until 2009, with mean follow up duration greater than 5 years, which was similar for all 3 ethnic groups. The overall annual decrease in eGFR was -1.69 in the total population. In the unadjusted linear regression analysis the annual decline in eGFR (ml/min) in white, black and South Asian groups was -1.78, -2.02 and -1.51 respectively. However, following adjustment for age at baseline, gender, presence or absence of vascular disease, drug treatment, presence or absence of proteinuria at baseline and baseline eGFR, no significant difference was observed in the rate of decline in eGFR between ethnic groups. In addition, there was no difference between ethnic groups in either all-cause mortality or the number of individuals developing ESKF. ACE-I or ARB use, and glycated haemoglobin (HbA1C) were similar at baseline and throughout the study period. Gender, severity of renal impairment and blood pressure control were the only independent predictors of progression. Interestingly, even on univariate analysis, ACE-I and/ or ARB use was not identified as a factor in the progression of CKD associated with DM. We concluded that ethnicity is not an independent risk factor for the progression of renal failure in patients with diabetic CKD if managed in a specialist clinic setting [26].

ETHNICITY, CKD AND RAS BLOCKADE

In the UK, the risk of developing CKD and cardiovascular complications of hypertension and DM is significantly greater amongst black, Asian and minority ethnic (BAME) communities. However, there are no specific randomised controlled trials focusing on these high-risk groups and comparing the effects of RAS blockade against either placebo or an alternative agent. Instead BAME groups are treated with RAS blockers based on evidence derived predominantly from white patients.

Nonetheless blockade of the renin-angiotensin system (RAS) is accepted as the first-line strategy for the treatment of hypertension, endorsed by numerous national and international guidelines. The role of RAS blockade is especially emphasized for primary and secondary prevention of cardiovascular disease and CKD [2,5,27-29]. The use of ACE inhibitors or ARBs in diabetes has been included in the new General Medical Services Contract for primary care in the UK, with financial remuneration linked to the prescription of these drugs for this indication. The preference for RAS blockers in these conditions is based on their neutral metabolic actions and for their direct cardiac and renoprotective properties, independent of the blood pressure lowering, so called pleiotropic effects [30-32]. There is an impression among some clinicians that overwhelming endorsement for RAS blockers in practically all guidelines is partly based on corporate bias, allied with massive commercial promotion. Pleiotropic effects RAS blockers on cardiovascular outcomes have been proposed based on the results of several large multicenter trials [33-36]. However, in placebo controlled trials it was difficult to tease out the blood pressure independent effects because the use of the active drug reduced blood pressure compared with the control group. However, when ACE-Is compared with an active comparator rather than placebo for cardiovascular effects, no significant advantage of ACE-Is has been seen over other classes of blood-pressure-lowering drugs [37].

The efficacy of ARB in the prevention of atrial fibrillation (a common complication in patients with CKD) was not confirmed by four large studies specifically designed to investigate this outcome. In the GISSI-atrial fibrillation trial, valsartan was completely ineffective in the prevention of recurrence of atrial fibrillation [38]. In the ACTIVE trial, irbesartan did not prevent atrial fibrillation diagnosed by electrocardiography or trans telephonic monitoring [39]. In the ANTIPAF trial, 1-year therapy with olmesartan did not reduce the number of episodes of atrial fibrillation in patients without structural heart disease [40]. Finally, in the Japanese J-RHYTHM II Study, candesartan and amlodipine did not influence the incidence of episodes of paroxysmal atrial fibrillation [41].

Similarly, the advocacy of ACE-Is and ARBs in renal disease is largely based on the results of placebo-controlled trials, often using surrogate markers such as proteinuria and GFR rather than renal survival [42-44]. A meta-analysis of trials comparing ACE-Is or ARBs with placebo or other antihypertensive drugs showed no beneficial effect on doubling of creatinine and a only a very modest reduction in the risk of ESKF (relative risk 0·87, 0·75–0·99). Likewise in patients with diabetic nephropathy, no benefit was seen in comparative trials of ACE-Is or ARBs on the doubling of creatinine or ESKF. Understandably placebo-controlled trials of ACE-Is or ARBs showed greater benefits than comparative trials on all renal outcomes, but were accompanied by substantial reductions in blood pressure in favour of ACE-Is or ARBs, [45], making assumptions of specific renoprotective effects, independent of better blood pressure, unrealistic. This meta-analysis generated a lot of controversy because the results from the Antihypertensive and Lipid Lowering treatment to prevent Heart Attack Trial (ALLHAT) study, [46], were included and were partly responsible for biasing the data against ACE-Is. The ALLHAT study, which was one of the largest RCT in hypertensive patients reported post hoc analysis for renal outcomes and lacked detail about proteinuria or serial renal function but it is extremely unlikely that the investigators missed ESKF, a very robust renal outcome measure.

In contrast to the lack of evidence for the superiority of ACE-Is and or ARBs over other anti- hypertensive agents, there is some evidence of direct harm resulting from the use of these agents. The authors of a Canadian cohort study, using a nested case control method, identified a 2.5 fold increased risk of ESKF over 10 years in patients with diabetes treated ACE-Is/ ARBs [47]. Despite the inherent weakness of any retrospective study such as lack of baseline data about renal function and proteinuria, this study calls for strict monitoring of patients whilst on ACE-Is. Similarly, concerns were raised in a recently published series of 100 consecutive CKD patients in which worsening azotemia in elderly patients was attributed to ACE-Is or ARBs as sustained improvement in eGFR often followed the discontinuation of these agents [48].

Moreover, some recent randomized control trails with ARB have suggested that these agents may have adverse effects on the kidneys. In the RAAS study, 285 normotensive patients with type 1 diabetes and normoalbuminuria were randomly assigned to receive losartan, enalapril or placebo [49]. After 5 years of follow-up, there was no differential change in mesangial fractional volume per glomerulus, the primary outcome. The 5-year cumulative incidence of microalbuminuria, a secondary outcome, was 6% in the placebo group, 4% in the enalapril group and 17% with losartan (p=0.01). The ROADMAP trial reported a slightly lower incidence of microalbuminuria in patients randomised to olmesartan than in patients randomised to placebo, but the reduction in glomerular filtration rate was higher in patients treated with olmesartan instead of placebo [50]. In the ACTIVE trial[38] the incidence of renal dysfunction leading to discontinuation of the drug almost doubled in patients treated with irbesartan (0.95%) versus placebo (0.53%). In the TRANSCEND trial, the decrease in glomerular filtration rate was greater with telmisartan than with placebo ($p<0.001$) [51].

In the same vein, the recent ONTARGET study, which ran between 2001-2007 and included over 25,000 subjects, demonstrated that dual blockade with ACE-Is and ARBs in high risk patients with atherosclerosis or diabetes was associated with worse renal outcomes (dialysis requirement, doubling of creatinine and annual decline of eGFR) compared to monotherapy with either ARBs or ACE-Is. These adverse renal outcomes were seen despite greater improvement in proteinuria with combination therapy compared to monotherapy [52]. It is thought that Renin and or aldosterone breakthrough also known as escape phenomenon and evident clinically by reappearance of baseline proteinuria may be important mechanisms involved in limiting the effects of ACE-Is and ARBs. This led to ALTITUDE (Cardiorenal End Points in a Trial of Aliskiren for Type 2 Diabetes) trial where addition of Aliskerin a direct renin inhibitor or placebo to ACE-I or ARBs was studied in over 8500 patients. The primary end point was a composite of the time to cardiovascular death or a first occurrence of cardiac arrest with resuscitation; nonfatal myocardial infarction; nonfatal stroke; unplanned hospitalization for heart failure; end-stage renal disease, death attributable to kidney failure, or the need for renal-replacement therapy with no dialysis or transplantation available or initiated; or doubling of the baseline serum creatinine level. The trial was stopped prematurely after the second interim efficacy analysis. After a median follow-up of 32.9 months, the primary end point had occurred in 18.3% assigned to aliskiren as compared with 17.1% assigned to placebo ($P=0.12$). Effects on secondary renal end points were similar despite lower systolic and diastolic blood pressure with and greater mean reduction in the urinary albumin-to-creatinine ratio with aliskerin. However, the proportion of patients with hyperkalemia was significantly higher in the aliskiren group as was the proportion with reported hypotension. It was concluded that the addition of aliskiren to standard therapy with renin–angiotensin system blockade in patients with type 2 diabetes who were at high risk for cardiovascular and renal events was not supported by study. However concerns were raised about potential harmful effects [53].

We also have our personal experiences in patients with stable non-progressive CKD developing sudden unexplained deterioration of renal function whilst being on long-term ACE-Is with improvement of renal function on withdrawal of the drug. In this regard the short term follow up of patients in practically all ACE-Is or ARBs trials with use of surrogate outcome measures may have concealed the deleterious effects of these drugs in the later stages of renal failure. In view of the currently available evidence, treatment decisions for hypertension should be based on the efficacy of blood pressure lowering effect, tolerability and more importantly the cost benefit ratio of antihypertensive drugs in the long-term. We support the quotations generated from the debate about the pros and cons of guidelines advocating the use of RAS blockers as first line agents in CKD patients that "guidelines are for the population and doctor is for an individual patient" and "one size does not fit all". Unfortunately no guidelines are detailed enough to include recommendations for individual patients with different types and severity of co-morbidities. We propose that guidelines should be viewed as desirables and should not replace a common sense clinical approach to patient care by an autonomously practicing competent clinician. Moreover, role of RAS blockade in the prevention of cardiovascular and renal disease should be re-examined in general and more importantly in high-risk ethnic populations.

REFERENCES

[1] 2011 Census: Office of National Statistics [Internet]. HM Government (UK); [cited 2013 Jul 10]. Available from: http://www.ons.gov.uk/ons/guide-method/census/2011/index.html

[2] Chobanian AV, Bakris GL, Black HR, Cushman WC, Green LA, Izzo JL, Jones DW, Materson BJ, Oparil S, Wright JT, Roccella EJ, National Heart, Lung, and Blood Institute Joint National Committee on Prevention, Detection, Evaluation, and Treatment of High Blood Pressure, National High Blood Pressure Education Program Coordinating Committee. The Seventh Report of the Joint National Committee on Prevention, Detection, Evaluation, and Treatment of High Blood Pressure: the JNC 7 report. JAMA. 2003; 289:2560–2572.

[3] Lane D, Beevers DG, Lip GY. Ethnic differences in blood pressure and the prevalence of hypertension in England. *J Hum Hypertens*. 2002; 16:267–273.

[4] Chaturvedi N, Fuller JH. Ethnic differences in mortality from cardiovascular disease in the UK: do they persist in people with diabetes? *J Epidemiol Community Health*. 1996; 50:137–139.

[5] Standards RA, Subcommittee A, Society BT, Nephrologists BAOP. Treatment of adults and children with renal failure: standards and audit measures. 2002;

[6] Part 1. Executive Summary. *American Journal of Kidney Diseases*. 2002; 39:S17–S31.

[7] Peralta CA, Hicks LS, Chertow GM, Ayanian JZ, Vittinghoff E, Lin F, Shlipak MG. Control of hypertension in adults with chronic kidney disease in the United States. *Hypertension*. 2005; 45:1119–1124.

[8] Byrne C, Ford D, Gilg J, Ansell D, Feehally J. UK Renal Registry 12th Annual Report (December 2009): chapter 3: UK ESRD incident rates in 2008: national and centre-specific analyses. *Nephron Clin Pract*. 2010; 115 Suppl 1:c9–39.

[9] Quality Outcomes Framework [Internet]. [cited 2013 Jul 10]. Available from: http://www.nhsemployers.org/payandcontracts/generalmedicalservicescontract/qof/Pages/QualityOutcomesFramework.aspx

[10] Millett C, Gray J, Bottle A, Majeed A. Ethnic disparities in blood pressure management in patients with hypertension after the introduction of pay for performance. *Ann Fam Med*. 2008; 6:490–496.

[11] Ashworth M, Medina J, Morgan M. Effect of social deprivation on blood pressure monitoring and control in England: a survey of data from the quality and outcomes framework. *BMJ*. 2008; 337:a2030.

[12] Falaschetti E, Chaudhury M, Mindell J, Poulter N. Continued improvement in hypertension management in England: results from the Health Survey for England 2006. *Hypertension*. 2009; 53:480–486.

[13] Primatesta P, Bost L, Poulter NR. Blood pressure levels and hypertension status among ethnic groups in England. *J Hum Hypertens*. 2000; 14:143–148.

[14] Hull S, Dreyer G, Badrick E, Chesser A, Yaqoob MM. The relationship of ethnicity to the prevalence and management of hypertension and associated chronic kidney disease. *BMC Nephrol.* 2011; 12:41.
[15] Dreyer G, Hull S, Aitken Z, Chesser A, Yaqoob MM. The effect of ethnicity on the prevalence of diabetes and associated chronic kidney disease. *QJM.* 2009; 102:261–269.
[16] Wright JT, Bakris GL, Greene T, Agodoa LY, Appel LJ, Charleston J, Cheek D, Douglas-Baltimore JG, Gassman J, Glassock R, Hebert L, Jamerson K, Lewis J, Phillips RA, Toto RD, Middleton JP, Rostand SG, African-American Study of Kidney Disease, and Hypertension Study Group. Effect of blood pressure lowering and antihypertensive drug class on progression of hypertensive kidney disease: results from the AASK trial. *JAMA.* 2002; 288:2421–2431.
[17] van den Hoogen PC, Feskens EJ, Nagelkerke NJ, Menotti A, Nissinen A, Kromhout D. The relation between blood pressure and mortality due to coronary heart disease among men in different parts of the world. Seven Countries Study Research Group. *N. Engl. J. Med.* 2000; 342:1–8.
[18] Coresh J, Astor BC, Greene T, Eknoyan G, Levey AS. Prevalence of chronic kidney disease and decreased kidney function in the adult US population: Third National Health and Nutrition Examination Survey. *Am J Kidney Dis.* 2003; 41:1–12.
[19] Stevens PE, O'Donoghue DJ, de Lusignan S, Van Vlymen J, Klebe B, Middleton R, Hague N, New J, Farmer CKT. Chronic kidney disease management in the United Kingdom: NEOERICA project results. *Kidney Int.* 2007; 72:92–99.
[20] Arogundade FA, Barsoum RS. CKD Prevention in Sub-Saharan Africa: A Call for Governmental, Nongovernmental, and Community Support. *American Journal of Kidney Diseases.* 2008; 51:515–523.
[21] New JP, Middleton RJ, Klebe B, Farmer CKT, de Lusignan S, Stevens PE, O'Donoghue DJ. Assessing the prevalence, monitoring and management of chronic kidney disease in patients with diabetes compared with those without diabetes in general practice. *Diabet Med.* 2007; 24:364–369.
[22] Ritz E, Orth SR. Nephropathy in patients with type 2 diabetes mellitus. *N. Engl. J. Med.* 1999; 341:1127–1133.
[23] Saunders E, Ofili E. Epidemiology of atherothrombotic disease and the effectiveness and risks of antiplatelet therapy: race and ethnicity considerations. *Cardiology in Review.* 2008; 16:82–88.
[24] Gunarathne A, Patel JV, Potluri R, Gammon B, Jessani S, Hughes EA, Lip GYH. Increased 5-year mortality in the migrant South Asian stroke patients with diabetes mellitus in the United Kingdom: the West Birmingham Stroke Project. *International Journal of Clinical Practice.* 2008; 62:197–201.
[25] Dreyer G, Hull S, Mathur R, Chesser A, Yaqoob MM. Progression of chronic kidney disease in a multi-ethnic community cohort of patients with diabetes mellitus. *Diabet*
[26] Ali O, Mohiuddin A, Mathur R, Dreyer G, Hull S, Yaqoob MM. A cohort study on the rate of progression of diabetic chronic kidney disease in different ethnic groups. *BMJ Open.* 2013; 3:e001855–e001855.
[27] Williams B, Poulter NR, Brown MJ, Davis M, McInnes GT, Potter JF, Sever PS, McG Thom S, British Hypertension Society. Guidelines for management of hypertension:

report of the fourth working party of the British Hypertension Society, 2004-BHS IV. J Hum Hypertens. 2004; 18:139–185.

[28] American Diabetes Association. Standards of medical care in diabetes. Diabetes Care. 2005; 28 Suppl 1:S4–S36.

[29] KDOQI Clinical Practice Guidelines and Clinical Practice Recommendations for Diabetes and Chronic Kidney Disease. *American Journal of Kidney Diseases*. 2007; 49:S12–S154.

[30] Effects of ramipril on cardiovascular and microvascular outcomes in people with diabetes mellitus: results of the HOPE study and MICRO-HOPE substudy. Heart Outcomes Prevention Evaluation Study Investigators. *Lancet*. 2000; 355:253–259.

[31] Lewis EJ, Hunsicker LG, Bain RP, Rohde RD. The effect of angiotensin-converting-enzyme inhibition on diabetic nephropathy. The Collaborative Study Group. *N. Engl. J. Med.* 1993; 329:1456–1462.

[32] Lewis EJ, Hunsicker LG, Clarke WR, Berl T, Pohl MA, Lewis JB, Ritz E, Atkins RC, Rohde R, Raz I, Collaborative Study Group. Renoprotective effect of the angiotensin-receptor antagonist irbesartan in patients with nephropathy due to type 2 diabetes. *N. Engl. J. Med.* 2001; 345:851–860.

[33] Fox KM, EURopean trial On reduction of cardiac events with Perindopril in stable coronary Artery disease Investigators. Efficacy of perindopril in reduction of cardiovascular events among patients with stable coronary artery disease: randomised, double-blind, placebo-controlled, multicentre trial (the EUROPA study). *Lancet*. 2003; 362:782–788.

[34] Yusuf S, Sleight P, Pogue J, Bosch J, Davies R, Dagenais G. Effects of an angiotensin-converting-enzyme inhibitor, ramipril, on cardiovascular events in high-risk patients. The Heart Outcomes Prevention Evaluation Study Investigators. *N. Engl. J. Med.* 2000; 342:145–153.

[35] Randomised trial of a perindopril-based blood-pressure-lowering regimen among 6105 individuals with previous stroke or transient ischaemic attack. Commentary. *Lancet*. 2001; 358:1033–1041.

[36] Weber MA, Julius S, Kjeldsen SE, Brunner HR, Ekman S, Hansson L, Hua T, Laragh JH, McInnes GT, Mitchell L, Plat F, Schork MA, Smith B, Zanchetti A. Blood pressure dependent and independent effects of antihypertensive treatment on clinical events in the VALUE Trial. *Lancet*. 2004; 363:2049–2051.

[37] Turnbull F, Blood Pressure Lowering Treatment Trialists' Collaboration. Effects of different blood-pressure-lowering regimens on major cardiovascular events: results of prospectively-designed overviews of randomised trials. *Lancet*. 2003; 362:1527–1535.

[38] GISSI-AF Investigators, Disertori M, Latini R, Barlera S, Franzosi MG, Staszewsky L, Maggioni AP, Lucci D, Di Pasquale G, Tognoni G. Valsartan for prevention of recurrent atrial fibrillation. *N. Engl. J. Med.* 2009; 360:1606–1617.

[39] ACTIVE I Investigators, Yusuf S, Healey JS, Pogue J, Chrolavicius S, Flather M, Hart RG, Hohnloser SH, Joyner CD, Pfeffer MA, Connolly SJ. Irbesartan in patients with atrial fibrillation. *N. Engl. J. Med.* 2011; 364:928–938.

[40] Goette A, Schön N, Kirchhof P, Breithardt G, Fetsch T, Häusler KG, Klein HU, Steinbeck G, Wegscheider K, Meinertz T. Angiotensin II-antagonist in paroxysmal atrial fibrillation (ANTIPAF) trial. *Circulation: Arrhythmia and Electrophysiology*. 2012; 5:43–51.

[41] Goette A. The vanishing story of angiotensin II receptor blockers in the treatment of atrial fibrillation. *Europace*. 2011; 13:451–452.

[42] Jafar TH, Schmid CH, Landa M, Giatras I, Toto R, Remuzzi G, Maschio G, Brenner BM, Kamper A, Zucchelli P, Becker G, Himmelmann A, Bannister K, Landais P, Shahinfar S, de Jong PE, de Zeeuw D, Lau J, Levey AS. Angiotensin-converting enzyme inhibitors and progression of nondiabetic renal disease. A meta-analysis of patient-level data. *Ann Intern Med*. 2001; 135:73–87.

[43] Giatras I, Lau J, Levey AS. Effect of angiotensin-converting enzyme inhibitors on the progression of nondiabetic renal disease: a meta-analysis of randomized trials. Angiotensin-Converting-Enzyme Inhibition and Progressive Renal Disease Study Group. *Ann Intern Med*. 1997; 127:337–345.

[44] Strippoli GFM, Craig M, Deeks JJ, Schena FP, Craig JC. Effects of angiotensin converting enzyme inhibitors and angiotensin II receptor antagonists on mortality and renal outcomes in diabetic nephropathy: systematic review. *BMJ*. 2004; 329:828.

[45] Casas JP, Chua W, Loukogeorgakis S, Vallance P, Smeeth L, Hingorani AD, MacAllister RJ. Effect of inhibitors of the renin-angiotensin system and other antihypertensive drugs on renal outcomes: systematic review and meta-analysis. *Lancet*. 2005; 366:2026–2033.

[46] Rahman M, Pressel S, Davis BR, Nwachuku C, Wright JT, Whelton PK, Barzilay J, Batuman V, Eckfeldt JH, Farber M, Henriquez M, Kopyt N, Louis GT, Saklayen M, Stanford C, Walworth C, Ward H, Wiegmann T. Renal outcomes in high-risk hypertensive patients treated with an angiotensin-converting enzyme inhibitor or a calcium channel blocker vs a diuretic: a report from the Antihypertensive and Lipid-Lowering Treatment to Prevent Heart Attack Trial (ALLHAT). *Arch Intern Med*. 2005; 165:936–946.

[47] Suissa S, Hutchinson T, Brophy JM, Kezouh A. ACE-inhibitor use and the long-term risk of renal failure in diabetes. *Kidney Int*. 2006; 69:913–919.

[48] Onuigbo MAC, Onuigbo NTC. Late-onset renal failure from angiotensin blockade (LORFFAB) in 100 CKD patients. *Int Urol Nephrol*. 2008; 40:233–239.

[49] Mauer M, Zinman B, Gardiner R, Suissa S, Sinaiko A, Strand T, Drummond K, Donnelly S, Goodyer P, Gubler MC, Klein R. Renal and retinal effects of enalapril and losartan in type 1 diabetes. *N. Engl. J. Med*. 2009; 361:40–51.

[50] Haller H, Ito S, Izzo JL Jr, Januszewicz A, Katayama S, et al.. Olmesartan for the delay or prevention of microalbuminuria in type 2 diabetes. N Engl J Med. 2011 Mar 10;364(10):907-17. doi: 10.1056/NEJMoa1007994.

[51] Mann JFE, Schmieder RE, Dyal L, McQueen MJ, Schumacher H, Pogue J, Wang X, Probstfield JL, Avezum A, Cardona-Munoz E, Dagenais GR, Diaz R, Fodor G, Maillon JM, Rydén L, Yu CM, Teo KK, Yusuf S, TRANSCEND (Telmisartan Randomised Assessment Study in ACE Intolerant Subjects with Cardiovascular Disease) Investigators. Effect of telmisartan on renal outcomes: a randomized trial. *Ann Intern Med*. 2009; 151:1–10– W1–2.

[52] Mann J, Schmieder RE, McQueen M, Dyal L. Renal outcomes with telmisartan, ramipril, or both, in people at high vascular risk (the ONTARGET study): a multicentre, randomised, double-blind, controlled trial. *The Lancet*. 2008.

[53] Parving H-H, Brenner BM, McMurray JJV, de Zeeuw D, Haffner SM, Solomon SD, Chaturvedi N, Persson F, Desai AS, Nicolaides M, Richard A, Xiang Z, Brunel P, Pfeffer MA, ALTITUDE Investigators. Cardiorenal end points in a trial of aliskiren for type 2 diabetes. *N. Engl. J. Med.* 2012; 367:2204–2213.

In: ACE Inhibitors. Volume 2
Editor: Macaulay Amechi Onuigbo
ISBN: 978-1-62948-422-8

Chapter 15

USE OF ACE-INHIBITORS AND ANGIOTENSIN-2 RECEPTOR BLOCKERS IN THE MANAGEMENT OF THE CARDIO-RENAL SYNDROME

Chike Nathan Okechukwu,[*] MD[1,2] and Muhammad Tahseen, MD[1]
[1]Department of Medicine, Crozer-Chester Medical Center, Upland, PA, US
[2]Department of Medicine, Temple University, Philadelphia, PA, US

ABSTRACT

Acute decompensated heart failure (ADHF) is one of the leading causes of initial hospitalizations and readmissions in the United States. 25% of patients hospitalized for acute decompensated heart failure also have significant worsening of renal function, which is associated with worse outcomes. The cardio-renal syndrome (CRS) can be defined as the coexistence of cardiac and renal dysfunctions, each of varying degrees, in which the acute or chronic dysfunction of either organ causes and/or accelerates the acute or chronic dysfunction of the other.

Patients with cardiac failure have a higher mortality when there is the coexistence of renal failure as measured by decrease in the Glomerular Filtration Rate (GFR). Mortality is increased in patients with heart failure (HF) who have a reduced GFR.

Patients with chronic kidney disease have an increased risk of both atherosclerotic cardiovascular disease and heart failure, and cardiovascular disease is responsible for up to 50 percent of deaths in patients with renal failure. Renal dysfunction in the setting of ADHF can happen as new-onset injury in the setting of previously normal kidney function or against the backdrop of chronic kidney disease. Zhou Q et al have shown that in the setting of ADHF, patients with acute-on-chronic kidney injury compared with those with AKI, had higher risk for in-hospital mortality, long hospital stay, and failure in renal function recovery.

The pathophysiology of CRS is poorly understood but likely involves interrelated hemodynamic and neurohormonal mechanisms including activation of the renin-angiotensin aldosterone system (RAAS), inflammation, disturbed bioavailability of nitric oxide, dysregulation of the sympathetic nervous system.

[*] Corresponding author: Chike Nathan Okechukwu MD: Email: chikeo66@gmail.com.

Chronic Kidney Disease (CKD) is associated with increased sympathetic activity and activation of the RAAS. These induce chronic inflammation and oxidative stress. In patients with mild to moderate renal disease, angiotensin-converting enzyme inhibitors (ACEIs) have been shown to improve cardiovascular survival independent of the severity of myocardial disease. Their positive effects on neurohormonal activation, hemodynamics, and ventricular remodeling may explain their positive effect on arrhythmic events in dialysis patients. Pun et al. noted that the use of ACEIs or angiotensin receptor blockers (ARBs) were associated with significant improvement in survival in ESRD patients who suffer cardiac arrest. Additionally ARBs have been shown to reduce oxidative stress and inflammation, suppress the RAAS, and decrease cardiovascular events in hypertensive patients.

In this chapter we will explore the effect and role of the RAAS in the cardio-renal syndrome and evaluate the utility of manipulating the RAAS as part of the overall therapeutic strategy for the management of the cardio-renal syndrome.

INTRODUCTION

The Cardio-Renal syndromes (CRS) are a group of disorders in which there is the coexistence of cardiac and renal dysfunctions, each of varying degrees, in which the acute or chronic dysfunction of either organ causes and/or accelerates the acute or chronic dysfunction of the other. Others have chosen to describe the syndrome as "a state in which therapy to relieve CHF symptoms is limited by further worsening renal function." [22].

There has been, for some time now, the recognition of the coexistence of cardiac and renal dysfunction. There has also been the recognition that patients with heart failure have an increase in mortality risk if there is coexistent renal dysfunction measured as a reduction in glomerular filtration rate [2-8]. Additionally, patients with end stage kidney disease have an increased risk of atherosclerotic cardiovascular disease and heart failure, and cardiovascular disease is responsible for 169 deaths per 1000 lives in 2009 [2-8, 11].

Mahan NG et al demonstrated in a sub-analysis of the Digitalis Investigation Group (DIG) trial that in ambulatory patients with congestive heart failure, the coexistence of kidney disease, as estimated by creatinine clearance, predicted all-cause mortality independent of other prognostic variables [4]. Equally poignantly, they noted that this risk was linear with worsening mortality risk as renal function declined.

There is also clear evidence demonstrating the progressive increase in cardiovascular disease with advanced chronic kidney disease (CKD) stage and age. Compared to non-CKD population, in which only about 3.6 percent of patients age 66–69, and 15 percent of those aged 85 and older have CHF, CHF occurs in 34% and 48% respectively in patients with Stage 4–5 CKD. [4-6] Additionally, Zhou Q et al [12], showed that in the setting of ADHF, patients with acute-on-chronic kidney injury compared with those with AKI, had higher risk for in-hospital mortality, long hospital stay, and failure in renal function recovery.

Finally although renal dysfunction as often described in terms of serum creatinine, creatinine clearance or GFR [4], the Blood Urea Nitrogen (BUN), has also emerged as an equally potent independent predictor of outcomes indeed a powerful predictor of ADHF [5,7,10, 17].

CLASSIFICATION AND NOMENCLATURE

Ronco et al [13], at a consensus conference organized under the auspices of the Acute Dialysis Quality Initiative (ADQI) in Venice, Italy proposed a classification system. This system is based on the recognition of the variety of heart-kidney interactions, the time frame of disease onset (acute versus chronic) and the definition of the presumed primary organ dysfunction (renal versus cardiac).

The consensus conference classified CRS into five groups:

Type 1 Acute cardio-renal syndrome:

This represents a group in which primary acute heart failure or acute coronary syndrome results in acute kidney injury or renal dysfunction.

Type 2 Chronic cardio-renal syndrome

Here chronic cardiac dysfunction leads to kidney injury or dysfunction.

Type 3 Acute reno-cardiac syndrome

These patients have primary acute worsening of kidney function leading to cardiac injury and/or dysfunction. For example reno-vascular disease causing acute heart failure

Type 4 Chronic reno-cardiac syndrome

This category includes patients in whom chronic kidney disease (CKD) leads to heart injury, disease, and/or dysfunction.

Type 5 Secondary cardio-renal syndromes

A systemic condition such as diabetes, hypertension leads to simultaneous injury and/or dysfunction of heart and kidney.

The appreciation for this bidirectional relationship, has led some authors to attempt to use these different terms to better depict the organ in which the primary dysfunction arose (and thus the provocatuer of the secondary dysfunction in the other organ) e.g., cardiorenal versus reno-cardiac syndrome. In this chapter we will use the terms cardiorenal syndrome or cardiorenal syndromes to describe this bidirectional coexistence of renal and cardiac dysfunction regardless of which organ is affected first.

EPIDEMIOLOGY

The prevalence, incidence and timing of coexistent renal dysfunction in patients hospitalized with decompensated heart failure vary depending on definition.

Heart disease and strokes statistics update from the American Heart Association estimates that in the United States, there are about 5.8 million people living with heart failure [20, 21]. This prevalence rises with age, and is higher in African-American patients.

At admission with ADHF the occurrence of acute renal dysfunction happens early [17,18]. However the definition of baseline creatinine, which in some series is taken as the admission creatinine, could miss renal dysfunction that begun prior to admission [17]. An analysis of the ADHERE database by Heywood JT et al showed that at admission, only 10,660 of 118,465 patients (9.0%) had normal renal function defined as GFR > or = 90 mL/min/1.73m2. [14]. In the same analysis only 33.4% of men and 27.3% of women were diagnosed with renal insufficiency. A retrospective analysis of 200 consecutive patients admitted to the coronary unit of Hospital Italiano de Buenos Aires with acute decompensated heart failure (ADHF) from January 1, 2006 to March 31, 2007, showed that fully 82 % of subjects had renal dysfunction. In the same series the factors predictive of intra-hospital progression/worsening of renal function were: age older than 80, renal dysfunction on presentation and systolic blood pressure <90 mm Hg on admission [15].

It is equally important to understand that the cardiorenal syndrome occurs also in patients with preserved ejection fraction [18,19]. This is especially common in older female patients with hypertension and/or diabetes. The presumed pathophysiologic mechanisms are thought to be from increased intra-abdominal and central venous pressure and also activation of the renin-angiotensin-Aldosterone system [17-19].

Certain factors/patient characteristics have been associated with the cardiorenal syndrome Table 1. [17-19]. The most significant of these considerations appears to be baseline renal dysfunction.

Table 1.

FACTORS ASSOCIATED WITH THE CARDIO-RENAL SYNDROME
Older age
Pre-existing renal dysfunction
Diabetes Mellitus
Hypertension
Hypotension
Right ventricular dysfucntion
Anemia
Severe diastolic dysfunction

PATHOPHYSIOLOGY

Heart failure leads to a variety of hemodynamic derangements, including decreased cardiac output, reduced stroke volume, raised atrial filling pressures, elevated atrial pressures, sodium and water retention and venous congestion [22].

A complex interplay of various factors has been implicated in ADHF and in the pathophysiology and pathogenesis of the Cardiorenal syndromes. The putative mechanisms include various neurohormonal adaptations including activation of the renin-angiotensin-aldosterone system, decreased cardiac output with resultant impaired renal perfusion, increased renal venous pressure, cytokine release and oxidative stress and right ventricular dysfunction and venous hypertension [22-25].

I. Reduced Cardiac Output, Decreased Renal Perfusion and Renal Venous Congestion

Cardiac Output and Renal Blood Flow

Renal blood flow appears to be the chief determinant of GFR in patients with cardiac dysfunction [26]. Worsening of renal function in the setting of ADHF is often thought to be secondary to decreased renal perfusion secondary to poor cardiac output and reduced effective circulatory volume. However this simplistic view of CRS has been challenged by different studies [26-31]. Nohria et al [31] in an analysis using the ESCAPE (Evaluation Study of Congestive Heart Failure and Pulmonary Artery Catheterization Effectiveness) database demonstrated no correlation between baseline hemodynamics or change in hemodynamics and the occurrence of renal dysfunction. They also showed that compared to clinical assessment alone, guiding therapy using pulmonary artery catheter-derived measurements did not decrease the incidence of renal failure during hospitalization or affect renal function after discharge relative to clinical assessment alone.

Also there is evidence that patients often have renal dysfunction on admission, a time when they are symptomatically hypervolemic. In the study by Gottlieb *et al.* significant numbers of patients admitted with decompensated heart failure had worsening renal function in the first 3 days of hospitalization, a time also when patients would be expected to be still hypervolemic [32].

Although renal dysfunction does occur from impaired perfusion as can be seen in the setting of catastrophic drops in cardiac output as in cardiogenic shock, ADHF-associated renal failure in renal blood flow (RBF) is well maintained by a significant increase in filtration fraction until the cardiac index falls below 1.5 l/m^2 [33].

The above observations suggest that the cardiorenal syndrome is not easily explained by the thesis of general has not been tightly correlated with poor perfusion.

Venous Congestion

Several studies have shown an association between right –sided failure with venous congestion measured by elevated central venous pressure (CVP) on the one hand and decrease in GFR with sodium and water retention on the other [27, 28, 34,35). This concept argues that the oliguria, azotemia, and reduced glomerular filtration rate happen as a result of the transmission of the elevated CVP back to the renal veins and thus the kidneys with resulting renal congestion and raised renal venous pressure. This model is not new and was demonstrated by Winton who observed that urine formation by isolated canine kidney was markedly reduced as renal venous pressures (RVP) rose above 20 mm Hg. He noted that rising RVP limited renal blood flow and urine production far more steeply than decrease in renal arterial pressure [38].

The elevated pressure within the kidney, which is encapsulated in a near-rigid capsule, results in sharp rise in intracapsular pressure, which leads to increased kidney interstitial pressure. This pressure rise causes a compression of the tubules, increases tubular fluid pressure, with reduced GFR due to an increase in hydrostatic pressure in the Bowman's capsule [36]. Also increased interstitial pressure may promote tubular inflammation and fibrosis, affect tubuloglomerular feedback and activate neurohormonal systems.

II. Neurohormonal Maladaptations and the Role of the Renin-Angiotensin-Aldosterone System

The hemodynamic abnormalities in ADHF provoke an assortment of neurohormonal compensatory mechanisms. These include the activation of the renin-angiotensin-aldosterone system (RAAS), the sympathetic nervous system and the release of vasoconstricting and sodium-retaining hormones like endothelin-1, angiotensin -2, norepinephrine, arginine vasopressin and adenosine. [36,37-39]

In early asymptomatic stages of ventricular dysfunction the counterbalancing effects of vasodilatory and natriuretic hormones such as natriuretic peptides, nitric oxide, prostaglandins (PGE2, PGI2), bradykinin act to maintain renal perfusion, support hemodynamic equilibrium and avoid fluid retention. As the cardiac dysfunction worsens, however, the vasodilatory/natriuretic mechanisms are overwhelmed by the vasoconstriction/sodium retention mechanisms, an imbalance that favors the worsening of renal function and sodium retention seen in the cardiorenal syndrome [17,23,25,36,37].

Therefore, efforts aimed at correcting these neurohormonal abnormalities in patients with heart failure would be expected to ameliorate symptoms, decrease hospitalizations and possibly, decrease mortality risk At the present time, amongst the potential pharmacological interventions acting on NHS in CHF, the blockade of the RAA system with ACE-inhibitors is generally accepted as the most feasible, the safest and the most effective therapeutic tool.

The Sympathetic System

Adaptive activation of the sympathetic nervous system in heart failure leads to increased release of Norepinephrine. This SNS activation results in increased myocardial contractility, vasoconstriction. The vasoconstriction involves systemic, renal and pulmonary blood vessels all geared towards maintaining cardiac output, blood pressure, renal perfusion and filtration fraction. This increased in Norepinephrine concentration and has been shown to be a prognostic indicator of outcome in heart failure [40, 41].

Adenosine

Adenosine is a precursor to ATP and binds to surface receptors found in various organs including the kidneys, brain and lungs. In the kidneys, receptors to adenosine exist in afferent arterioles, the proximal tubule and juxtaglomerular cells. Via its binding to Adenosine-1-receptor (A1R), adenosine inhibits renin release and mediates activated tubulo-glomerular feedback (TGF), which can decrease GFR [42]. With the effect on TGF and rennin, Levels of adenosine are elevated in patients with heart failure. Elevated adenosine in HF could decrease GFR by vasodilatation of postglomerular capillaries and/or provoke vasoconstriction of afferent arterioles. In theory at least one would expect to improve the GFR and urine output, and thus renal function,by antagonizing the effects of adenosine. However data from the PROTECT study using Rolofylline an A1R-antagonist failed to demonstrate any favorable effect with respect to the end points of post-treatment development of persistent renal impairment and the 60-day rate of death or readmission for cardiovascular or renal causes [43].

The Renin-Angiotensin-Aldosterone Axis

Decreased delivery of chloride to the macula densa, reduced stretch of the glomerular afferent arteriole, and the increased beta-1 adrenergic activity all incite increased renin secretion from the juxtaglomerular apparatus of the afferent arteriole [44].

This increased renin secretion leads ultimately to an increase n production of angiotensin-2 (A-2) which in turn promotes sodium avidity, stimulates thirst, and acts as a potent systemic vasoconstrictor by direct effect and also by stimulating the sympathetic nervous system.

The sodium avidity is mediated via effect of Angiotensin II-induced aldosterone production and release. Aldosterone also increases the myocardial fibrosis of the failing human heart.

Diagnosis

Renal dysfunction is defined by the worsening of GFR measred by a rise in serum creatinine. As implied by the Ronco classification model, renal dysfunction in the setting of ADHF can happen acutely or chronically. Patients admitted for ADHF who have renal dysfunction could have background chronic kidney disease with superimposed acute renal worsening.

Management Strategies for CRS and the Role of RAAS Disruption

Although there are guidelines for managing HF and CKD, there are no consensus guidelines on the management of patients with cardio-renal syndromes.

The clinical strategies for the management of CRS should include: fluid removal, avoidance of further renal impairment, avoidance of hypotension, avoidance of electrolyte imbalance, and management of diuretic resistance. [24]

Current therapeutic options include use of diuretics, use of RAAS blockers (ace-inhibitors, angiotensin-II receptor blockers, and anti-aldosterone agents), and use of beta-blockers. Also inotropes and natriuretic hormones have been used, as well as aquaretics (vasopressin antagonists), and vasodilators. There are also investigational therapies such as adenosine A1 receptor antagonists, ultrafiltration, and calcium sensitizers (levosimendan).

Fluid Removal

In acute decompensated hospitalized HF patients, use of diuretics remains the first line of fluid removal. The loop diuretics including Furosemide, Torsemide, Bumetanide, because of their class potency, have remained the preferred diuretic choice.

However thiazide diuretics and thiazide-like diuretics can be added to intensify diuresis and overcome diuretic resistance.

Loop diuretics use particularly in high doses is associated with worsening of renal function and higher mortality is associated with use of higher loop diuretic dosages

[24,39,49,50]. The increase in mortality could be related to the activation of the RAAS with possible resultant cardiac fibrosis, and the significant electrolyte abnormality, (e.g., hypokalemia, hypomagnesemia) which might lead to significant arrhythmias [51].

In the ADHF veno-venous extracorporeal ultrafiltration may be useful in settings of diuretic resistance. In a randomized study comparing the safety and efficacy of ultrafiltration versus standard intravenous diuretic therapy for hypervolemic heart failure (HF) patients, the UNLOAD investigators [52] found that ultrafiltration safely produced greater fluid removal than intravenous diuretics. They also found significantly lower 90-day rehospitalizations and hospital days per patient.

Inotropes

Use of inotropes has been shown to improve cardiac index and renal blood flow post cardiac surgery. However there are conflicting conclusions about effects on glomerular filtration rate (GFR), effective renal plasma flow, and diuresis [45-47].

Additionally a retrospective analysis of 949 patients from the Outcomes of a Prospective Trial of Intravenous Milrinone for Exacerbations of Chronic Heart Failure (OPTIME-CHF) showed that Milrinone use in these patients did not improve outcomes despite modest improvements in the renal function [48].

In the new 2013 ACC/AHA heart failure guidelines, low-dose short term continuous inotropic infusion is added as a Class IIb recommendation as adjunct to diuretic therapy in patients with severe systolic dysfunction, low blood and significantly depressed cardiac output. [50]

ACE-Inhibitors/Angiotensin-2 Receptor Blockade

Activation of the RAAS axis results in the elaboration of angiotensin II (AT-II) which upregulates Transforming growth factor-β (TGF-β), tumor necrosis factor-α (TNFα), nuclear factor-κB, (nf κB), interleukin-6 and it also stimulates fibroblasts. These cytokines promote cell growth, inflammation, and fibrotic damage in the renal parenchyma [56]. This results in direct cell injury in the heart, kidney and vascular endothelium.

The use of angiotensin-converting enzyme (ACE) inhibitors/angiotensin-receptor blockers (ARBs), beta-blockers, remain a Class I recommendation in the new 2013 ACCF/AHA Heart Failure guidelines [50] for the treatment of class1-4 heart failure patients. The guidelines recommend that absent contraindications (e.g., pregnancy, angioedema), ACE inhibitors should be prescribed to all patients with HF with reduced EF. The writers however advised use of Ace-inhibitors with caution in the settings of "very low systemic blood pressures (systolic blood pressure <80 mm Hg), markedly increased serum levels of creatinine (>3 mg/dL), bilateral renal artery stenosis, or elevated levels of serum potassium (>5.0 mEq/L)".

The reluctance to use ACE-inhibitors often comes from the fact that Angiotensin converting enzyme inhibitor and ARB therapies may cause or contribute to the worsening of renal function.

Testani JM et al, in 2011, analyzed data on 6337 subjects from the Studies Of Left Ventricular Dysfunction (SOLVD) trial. They showed that early worsening renal function defined as a decrease in estimated GFR ≥20 percent at 14 days) was not associated with increased mortality in the ACE-inhibitor group. However when the analysis was restricted to the placebo group they found a 40% increase in adjusted mortality (P=0.004). Consequently significant survival advantage was seen in patients who stayed on the Enalapril notwithstanding initial worsening renal function.

Drop in eGFR and Increases in serum creatinine can therefore occur after initiation of ACE inhibitor/ARB therapy, especially when patients are receiving concomitant diuretic treatment. However this temporary worsening of renal function in response to an ACE inhibitor does not necessarily indicate long-term mortality risk intolerance to angiotensin inhibition, but should prompt evaluation of the diuretic regimen and other possible causes of worsening renal function.

It is vital to note that in many heart failure studies, the percentage of patients with high serum creatinines has been modest ranging between10%-35%. Also the degree of renal insufficiency has been relatively mild, for instance, in the SOLVD trial, in which patients with serum creatinine> 2.0 mg/dL were excluded [52, 53,55].

The Cooperative North Scandinavian Enalapril Survival Study (CONSENSUS) in patients with severe heart failure, included patients albeit a minority with more significant renal impairment (up to creatinines of 3.4mg/dL). In a subgroup analysis of CONSENSUS patients with creatinines above 2.0mg/dL, there was evidence of improved outcomes when treated with ACE inhibitors. The authors also demonstrated that patients with severe heart failure had >30% rise in their serum creatinines, independent of baseline creatinines, when ACE-inhibitor therapy was added to their regime. Most patients were able to continue on the ACE-inhibitor, while those from whom the drug was withdrawn returned back to baseline creatinines. [54, 55]

Anti-Aldosterone Therapy

Aldosterone Blockade with spironolactone, in patients with left ventricular ejection fraction of 35% or less, was shown to decrease mortality by 30% and hospitalizations by 35% when compared with placebo [58].

However, the addition of these drugs to a therapeutic regimen that already contains ACE-inhibitors or ARBs has raised concerns of hyperkalemia. It should be noted that the RALES study excluded patients with a creatinine >2.5 mg/dL, and that the vast majority (95%) of patients had creatinines ≤1.7 mg/dL. [50,58]. Massoud et al [60] studied the adoption of spironolactone therapy, after publication of the RALES study, in national cohorts of older patients hospitalized for heart failure. They found that spironolactone prescription increased from 3% (pre-RALES publication) to 21.3% post-RALES, a seven-fold increase. Additionally, their study noted that 30.9% patients not meeting RALES enrollment criteria received spironolactone prescription. This included 22.8% of patients with a serum potassium >5meq/L, and 14.1% with a serum creatinine value > 2.5 mg/dL.

It is therefore crucial to prescribe anti-aldosterone drugs in a carefully selected population of patients with decreased left ventricular ejection fraction excluding those with significant

CKD serum creatinine ≥2.5 mg/dL or with potassium level >5.0 mEq/L, which were exclusion criteria in RALES.

Non-Pharmocological Therapies

Cardiac re-synchronization therapy is recommended for symptomatic CHF patients (NYHA III–IV) with poor left ventricular ejection fraction (LVEF) and QRS prolongation,

Also implantable cardiac defibrillators have been used for both survivors of cardiac arrest and those with symptomatic low EF heart failure. In selected patients who do not respond to treatment, MCS is beneficial in carefully selected patients [50].

Finally mechanical device management may be used as a bridge to cardiac transplantation.

Conclusion

Despite the clearly high prevalence of renal dysfunction in the setting of heart failure [9-10], the recognition remains suboptimal. In the analysis of the ADHERE database only 33.4% of men and 27.3% of women were diagnosed with renal insufficiency [9]. Although the pathophysiology of the cardiorenal syndromes involve the complex interplay of various systems including maladaptive neurohormonal pathways, the renin-angiotensin-aldosterone system plays a central role in the pathogenesis and pathophysiology of the cardiorenal syndromes.

The exclusion of patients with significant renal dysfunction in heart failure outcomes studies has caused a dearth of robust information on the place and roles of ACE-inhibitors and angiotensin 2 blockers in the management of CRS.

Despite this, continued judicious use of these drugs even in the decompensated heart failure patient remains reasonable. Special consideration should be given to patients at high risk for renal decline such as bilateral renal artery stenosis and dehydration. Also patients should be started on the lowest dose of ACE inhibitor/ARB and the dose slowly uptitrated. Non-steroidal anti-inflammatory drugs should be avoided if possible, and close watch on these patients should be kept for the possible development of hyperkalemia.

ACE inhibitors and angiotensin receptor blockers use should be continued in many patients despite a rise in creatinine, as long as renal dysfunction does not progressively worsen and/or significant hyperkalemia does not develop. Initiation of ACE-I/ARB should be followed by gradual dose increments if lower doses have been well tolerated. Renal function and serum potassium should be assessed within 1 week of initiation of therapy and periodically thereafter [50].

In patient with severe deterioration of renal function post-initiation of ACE-inhibitors/ARB, consideration should be made towards excluding renal artery stenosis [50, 57]. Careful selection of patients and avoidance of hypotension and NSAIDS would go some way in averting renal dysfunction in ACE-inhibitor treated patient with ADHF [60].

REFERENCES

[1] Heywood JT. The cardiorenal syndrome: lessons from the ADHERE database and treatment options. *Heart Fail Rev.* 2004;9:195–201.

[2] United States Renal Data System: 2012 Annual Data Report.

[3] Dries DL, Exner DV, Domanski MJ, Greenberg B, Stevenson LW. The prognostic implications of renal insufficiency in asymptomatic and symptomatic patients with left ventricular systolic dysfunction. *J Am Coll Cardiol.* 2000; 35: 681–689.

[4] Mahan NG, Blackstone EH, Francis GS, Starling RC III, Young JB, Lauer MS. The prognostic value of estimated creatinine clearance alongside functional capacity in patients with chronic congestive heart failure. *J Am Coll Cardiol.* 2002; 18;40(6):1106-13.

[5] Aronson D, Hammerman H, Beyar R et al. Serum blood urea nitrogen and long-term mortality in acute ST-elevation myocardial infarction. *Int. J. Cardiol.* 127, 380–385 (2008).

[6] Schrier R Role of diminished renal function in cardiovascular mortality: marker or pathogenetic factor? *J Am Coll Cardiol* 47: 1–8, 2006.

[7] Fonarow GC, Adams KF Jr, Abraham WT, Yancy CW, Boscardin WJ. Risk stratification for in-hospital mortality in acutely decompensated heart failure: classification and regression tree analysis. *JAMA* 293, 572–580 (2005).

[8] Go AS, Chertow GM, Fan D, McCulloch CE, Hsu CY Chronic kidney disease and the risks of death, cardiovascular events, and hospitalization. *N Engl* Med351: 1296–1305, 2004.

[9] Kazory A. Emergence of blood urea nitrogen as a biomarker of neurohormonal activation in heart failure. *Am. J. Cardiol.* 106, 694–700 (2010).

[10] Aronson D, Mittleman MA, Burger AJ. Elevated blood urea nitrogen level as a predictor of mortality in patients admitted for decompensated heart failure. *Am. J. Med.* 116, 466–473 (2004).

[11] Damman K, Masson S, Hillege HL et al. Clinical outcome of renal tubular damage in chronic heart failure. *Eur. Heart J.* 32(21), 2705–2712 (2011).

[12] Zhou Q, Zhao C, Xie D, Xu D, Bin J, Chen P, Liang M, Zhang X, Hou F Acute and acute-on-chronic kidney injury of patients with decompensated heart failure: impact

[13] Ronco et al Cardio-renal syndromes: report from the consensus conference of the Acute Dialysis Quality Initiative. *Eur Heart J.* 2010; 31(6): 703–711.

[14] Heywood JT, Fonarow GC, Costanzo MR, Mathur VS, Wigneswaran JR, Wynne J; ADHERE Scientific Advisory Committee and Investigators. High prevalence of renal dysfunction and its impact on outcome in 118,465 patients hospitalized with acute decompensated heart failure: a report from the ADHERE database. *J Card Fail.* 2007;13(6):422-30.

[15] César A. Belzitia, Rodrigo Bagnatia, Paola Ledesmaa, Norberto Vulcanoa, Sandra Fernández Worsening Renal Function in Patients Admitted With Acute Decompensated Heart Failure: Incidence, Risk Factors and Prognostic Implications. *Rev Esp Cardiol.* 2010;63:294-302.

[16] Shamseddin MK, Parfrey PS. Mechanisms of the Cardiorenal syndromes. *Nat Rev Nephrol* 2009; 5:641.

[17] Aronson Doron Cardiorenal Syndrome in Acute Decompensated Heart Failure Expert *Rev Cardiovasc Ther.* 2012;10(2):177-189.

[18] Forman DE, Butler J, Wang Y, Abraham WT, O'Connor CM, Gottlieb SS, Loh E, Massie BM, Rich MW, Stevenson LW, Young JB, Krumholz HM Incidence, predictors at admission, and impact of worsening renal function among patients hospitalized with heart failure. *J Am Coll Cardiol.* 2004;43(1):61.

[19] Chiara Lazzeri,1 Serafina Valente,1 Roberto Tarquini,2 and Gian Franco Gensin Cardiorenal Syndrome Caused by Heart Failure with Preserved Ejection Fraction International Journal of NephrologyVolume 2011 (2011), Article ID 634903.

[20] Lloyd-Jones D, Adams RJ, Brown TM, Carnethon M, Dai S, De Simone G, Ferguson TB, Ford E, Furie K, Gillespie C, Go A, Greenlund K, Haase N, Hailpern S, Ho PM, Howard V, Kissela B, Kittner S, Lackland D, Lisabeth L, Marelli A, McDermott MM, Meigs J, Mozaffarian D, Mussolino M, Nichol G, Roger VL, Rosamond W, Sacco R, Sorlie P, Roger VL, Stafford R, Thom T, Wasserthiel-Smoller S, Wong ND, Wylie-Rosett J, American Heart Association Statistics Committee and Stroke Statistics Subcommittee. Heart disease and stroke statistics--2010 update: a report from the American Heart Association. *Circulation.* 2010;121(7):e46.

[21] Cadnapaphornchai MA, Gurevich AK, Weinberger HD, Schrier RW Pathophysiology of sodium and water retention in heart failure. *Cardiology.* 2001;96(3-4):122.

[22] NHLBI Working Group: Cardio-Renal Connections in Heart Failure and Cardiovascular Disease. August 2004. Available at http://www.nhlbi.nih.gov/meetings /workshops/cardiorenal-hf-hd.htm.

[23] Schrier RW, Abraham WT Hormones and hemodynamics in heart failure. *N Engl J Med.* 1999;341(8):577.

[24] Sarraf, Mohammed, Masoumi Amirali, Schrier Robert W. Cardiorenal Syndrome in Acute Decompensated Heart failure CJASN 20091;2(4):2013-2026.

[25] Kiernan MS, Udelson JE, Sarnak M, Konstam M. Cardiorenal syndrome: Definition, prevalence, diagnosis, and pathophysiology In: UpToDate, Basow, DS (Ed), UpToDate, Waltham, MA, 2013.

[26] Ljungman S., Laragh J.H., Cody R.J. Role of the kidney in congestive heart-failure — relationship of cardiac index to kidney-function. *Drugs* 1990;39:10-21.

[27] Damman K, Navis G, Smilde TD, et al. Decreased cardiac output, venous congestion and the association with renal impairment in patients with cardiac dysfunction. *Eur J Heart Fail.* 2007;9(9):872–878.

[28] Mullens W, Abrahams Z, Skouri HN, et al. Elevated intra-abdominal pressure in acute decompensated heart failure: a potential contributor to worsening renal function? *J Am Coll Cardiol.* 2008;51(3):300–306

[29] Tang WH, Mullens W. Cardiorenal syndrome in decompensated heart failure. *Heart.* 2010; 96(4): 255–260.

[30] Hatamizadeh P, Fonarow GC, Budoff MJ, Darabian S, Kovesdy CP, Kalantar-Zadeh K. Cardiorenal syndrome: pathophysiology and potential targets for clinical management. *Nat Rev Nephrol.* 2013 Feb;9(2):99-111.

[31] Nohria A, Hasselblad V, Stebbins A, Pauly DF, Fonarow GC, Shah M, Yancy CW, Califf RM, Stevenson LW, Hill JA. Cardiorenal interactions: insights from the ESCAPE trial. *J Am Coll Cardiol.* 2008 Apr 1;51(13):1268-74.

[32] Gottlieb SS, Abraham W, Butler J, Forman DE, Loh E, Massie BM, O'Connor CM, Rich MW, Stevenson LW, Young J, Krumholz HM: The prognostic importance of different definitions of worsening renal function in congestive heart failure. *Card Fail* 2002;8: 136–141.

[33] Ljungman S, Laragh JH, Cody RJ. Role of the kidney in congestive heart failure. Relationship of cardiac index to kidney function. *Drugs* 1990;39 Suppl 4:10–21; discussion 22–14.

[34] Wencker D Acute cardio-renal syndrome: progression from congestive heart failure to congestive kidney failure. *Curr Heart Fail Rep.* 2007;4(3):134.

[35] Firth JD, Raine AE, Ledingham JG. Raised venous pressure: a direct cause of renal sodium retention in oedema? *Lancet.* 1988;1(8593):1033-5.

[36] Fiksen-Olsen M.J., Strick D.M., Hawley H., Romero J.C. Renal effects of angiotensin II inhibition during increases in renal venous pressure. *Hypertension* 1992;19:137-141.

[37] Blair JE, Manuchery A, Chana A, Rossi, J, Schrier RW, Burnett JC, Gheorghiade M. Prognostic markers in heart failure--congestion, neurohormones, and the cardiorenal syndrome. *Acute Card Care.* 2007;9(4):207-13.

[38] Winton FR. The influence of venous pressure on the isolated mammalian kidney. *J Physiol.* 1931; 72: 49–61.

[39] Bock, Jeremy, Gottlieb SS. Cardiorenal Syndrome New Perspectives. *Circulation.* 2010; 121: 2592-2600.

[40] Cohn JN, Levine TB, Olivari MT, Garberg V, Lura D, Francis GS, Simon AB, Rector T. Plasma norepinephrine as a guide to prognosis in patients with chronic congestive heart failure. *N Engl J Med.* 1984;311(13):819.

[41] Colucci WS. Pathophysiology of heart failure: Neurohumoral adaptations. In: UpToDate, Basow, DS (Ed), UpToDate, Waltham, MA, 2013.

[42] Vallon V, Miracle, C, Thomson S. Adenosine and kidney function: Potential implications in patients with heart failure. *Eur J Heart Fail.* 2008;10 (2):176-187.

[43] Massie BM, O'Connor CM, Metra M, Ponikowski P, Teerlink JR, Cotter G, Weatherley BD, Cleland JG, Givertz MM, Voors A, DeLucca P, Mansoor GA, Salerno CM, Bloomfield DM, Dittrich HC, PROTECT Investigators and Committees;. Rolofylline, an adenosine A1-receptor antagonist, in acute heart failure. *N Engl J Med.* 2010;363(15):1419-28.

[44] Harrison-Bernard LM. The renal renin-angiotensin system *Adv Physiol Educ.* 2009; 33(4): 270-274.

[45] Drexler H, Höing S, Faude F, Wollschläger H, Just H. Central and regional vascular hemodynamics following intravenous milrinone in the conscious rat: comparison with dobutamine. *J Cardiovasc Pharmacol.* 1987; 9: 563–569.

[46] Sato Y, Matsuzawa H, Eguchi S. Comparative study of effects of adrenaline, dobutamine and dopamine on systemic hemodynamics and renal blood flow in patients following open heart surgery. *Jpn Circ J.* 1982; 46: 1059–1072.

[47] Wang DJ, Dowling TC, Meadows D, Ayala T, Marshall J, Minshall S, Greenberg N, Thattassery E, Fisher ML, Rao K, Gottlieb SS. Nesiritide does not improve renal function in patients with chronic heart failure and worsening serum creatinine. *Circulation.* 2004; 110: 1620–1625.

[48] Klein L, Massie BM, Leimberger JD, O'Connor CM, Piña IL, Adams KF Jr, Califf RM, Gheorghiade M, for the OPTIME-CHF Investigators. Admission or changes in renal

function during hospitalization for worsening heart failure predict postdischarge survival: results from the Outcomes of a Prospective Trial of Intravenous Milrinone for Exacerbations of Chronic Heart Failure (OPTIME-CHF). *Circ Heart Fail.* 2008; 1:25–33.

[49] Stampfer M, Epstein SE, Beiser GD, Braunwald E. Hemodynamic effects of diuresis at rest and during intense upright exercise in patients with impaired cardiac function. *Circulation.* 1968;37(6):900.

[50] Yancy CW, Jessup M, Bozkurt B, Butler J, Casey DE Jr, Drazner MH, Fonarow GC, Geraci SA, Horwich T, Januzzi JL, Johnson MR, Kasper EK, Levy WC, Masoudi FA, McBride PE, McMurray JJV, Mitchell JE, Peterson PN, Riegel B, Sam F, Stevenson LW, Tang WHW, Tsai EJ, Wilkoff BL. 2013 ACCF/AHA guideline for the management of heart failure: a report of the American College of Cardiology Foundation/American Heart Association Task Force on Practice Guidelines. *Circulation.* 2013: published online before print June 5, 2013, 10.1161/CIR.0b013e31829e8776.

[51] Brater DC: Diuretic therapy. *N Engl J Med* 339: 387–395, 1998.

[52] Testani JM, Kimmel SE, Dries DL, Coca SG. Prognostic importance of early worsening renal function after initiation of angiotensin-converting enzyme inhibitor therapy in patients with cardiac dysfunction. *Circ Heart Fail.* 2011;4(6):685-91. Epub 2011 Sep 8.

[53] The SOLVD Investigators.Effect of enalapril on survival in patients with reduced left ventricular ejection fractions and congestive heart failure. *N Engl J Med* 1992; 325:293–302.

[54] Ljungman S, Kjekshus J, Swedberg K.Renal function in severe congestive heart failure during treatment with enalapril (the Cooperative North Scandinavian Enalapril Survival Study Trial). *Am J Cardiol* 1992; 70:479–487.

[55] Geisberg C, Butler J. Addressing the challenges of cardiorenal syndrome. Cleveland Clinic *Journal of Medicine* 2006;73(5) : 485-491.

[56] Ruiz-Ortega M, Ruperez M, Lorenzo O, Esteban V, Blanco J, Mezzano S, Egido J. Angiotensin II regulates the synthesis of proinflammatory cytokines and chemokines in the kidney. *Kidney Int.* 2002; 82: S12–S22.

[57] Shlipak MG, Massie BM. The clinical challenge of cardiorenal syndrome. *Circulation* 110, 1514–1517 (2004).

[58] Pitt B, Zannad F, Remme WJ, Cody R, Castaigne A, Perez A, Palensky J, Wittes J: The effect of spironolactone on morbidity and mortality in patients with severe heart failure. *N Engl J Med* 341: 709, 1999.

[59] Pitt B, Bakris G, Ruilope LM, Dicarlo L, Mukherjee R,. Eplerenone Post-Acute Myocardial Infarction Heart Failure Efficacy and Survival Study Investigators:Serum potassium and clinical outcomes in the Eplerenone Post-Acute Myocardial Infarction Heart Failure Efficacy and Survival Study (EPHESUS). *Circ.* 2008;118:1643–1650.

[60] Masoudi FA, Gross CP, Wang Y, et al. Adoption of spironolactone therapy for older patients with heart failure and left ventricular systolic dysfunction in the United States, 1998-2001. *Circulation* 2005;112(1):39-47. Epub 2005 Jun 27.

In: ACE Inhibitors. Volume 2
Editor: Macaulay Amechi Onuigbo

ISBN: 978-1-62948-422-8

Chapter 16

A THREE-YEAR CLINICAL EXPERIENCE WITH ACE INHIBITORS AT NNAMDI AZIKIWE UNIVERSITY TEACHING HOSPITAL, NNEWI, NIGERIA, DEPARTMENT OF PEDIATRICS, 2010-2012

Ebele Francesca Ugochukwu**, BSc MBBS FWACP[Ped]
Department of Pediatrics, Nnamdi Azikiwe University Teaching Hospital, Nnewi, Nigeria

ABSTRACT

Objective: To determine the frequency of use and indications for ACE Inhibitors (ACEI) among pediatric patients at Nnamdi Azikiwe University Teaching Hospital, Nnewi, Nigeria.

Design: A retrospective analysis of data from 151 children treated with ACEI, in the Pediatric clinics and wards over a three-year period [January 2010 to December 2012], was conducted.

Results: There were 98 boys (64.9%) and 53 girls (35.1%). Age at commencement of therapy ranged from 2 months to 17 years. Patients were categorized into primary clinical diagnoses and indications for ACEI therapy. The clinical diagnoses were ventricular septal defect (31.1%), nephrotic syndrome (23.9%), rheumatic heart disease (11.3%), acute post-streptococcal glomerulonephritis (7.9%), chronic kidney disease (6.0%), posterior urethral valves (3.3%), HIV associated nephropathy (3.3%), acute renal failure (2.6%), chronic renal failure (2.0%), cardiomyopathy (2.0%), HIV-associated congestive cardiac failure (2.0%), transposition of the great arteries (1.3%), sickle cell nephropathy (1.3%), congenital hydronephrosis (1.3%), and patent ductus arteriosus (0.7%). Indications for therapy were heart failure (48.3%), renoprotective effect (37.8%), and hypertension (13.9%). The ACEI used were lisinopril (88.0%), enalapril (9.3%), and ramipril (2.7%). Lisinopril and enalapril were dosed at 0.1mg/kg/day, while ramipril was given in a dose range of 2.5–5mg/day. Hypotension (4.6%) and dizziness (3.0%) were documented adverse effects. Serum electrolytes in cardiac patients remained unaffected,

*Ebelechuku Ugochukwu BSc MBBS FWACP [Ped]; Email: efugochukwu@gmail.com

while the underlying pathology in renal patients made it difficult to attribute any change in serum biochemistry to the use of ACEIs.

Conclusion: ACEIs are efficacious and well tolerated in children.

INTRODUCTION

The renin-angiotensin system (RAS), in addition to maintaining cardiovascular homeostasis, regulates renal cell survival and cell death, and development of the kidneys. In fact, an intact RAS is a prerequisite for normal renal development [1]. Adverse events on the developing kidney have been reported with use of ACEIs in pregnancy and in neonates [2-5]. These include oligohydramnios, pulmonary hypoplasia, neonatal renal failure, bony deformities and an increased incidence of perinatal mortality. The postulated mechanism of insult in late pregnancy is related to fetal hypotension and a prolonged decrease in glomerular filtration secondary to the inhibition of ACE [5]. Neonates are far more sensitive than older children to the hypotensive actions of these agents hence doses must be markedly reduced to avoid precipitating oliguria [6].

Beyond the neonatal age the effects of ACEIs on the renin-angiotensin-aldosterone (RAA) system in pediatric patients are similar to those in adults; hence they are indicated in kidney disease, hypertension and heart failure.

METHODS AND PATIENTS

The Nnamdi Azikiwe Teaching Hospital, Nnewi is located in south east Nigeria and serves as a tertiary referral center for Anambra state and other surrounding states. The Pediatric department runs daily general out-patient and specialty clinics. It also has a neonatal unit, children emergency unit and two pediatric wards. The pediatric population spans from birth to age 17 years. The patients included in this review were recruited from the cardiac, renal, and infectious diseases clinics.

A retrospective analysis of data from clinical records of 151 children treated with ACEIs, in the Pediatric clinics and wards over a three-year period [January 2010 to December 2012], was conducted. These children constitute 0.27% of all patients seen in the pediatric department during the study period.

RESULTS

Clinical charts of 151 children, 98 boys (64.9%) and 53 girls (35.1%) were scrutinized. Age at commencement of therapy ranged from 2 months to 17 years with a mean of 7.48 (6.04) years. Table 1 outlines the age and sex distribution of the subjects.

Table 1. Age and Sex distribution of subjects

Age (years)	Males (%)	Females (%)	Total (%)
< 1	23 (15.2)	10 (6.6)	33 (21.8)
1 – 5	22 (14.6)	11(7.3)	33 (21.9)
6 – 13	25 (16.6)	23 (15.2)	48 (31.8)
13 – 17	28 (18.5)	9 (6.0)	37 (24.5)
Total	98 (64.9)	53 (35.1)	151 (100.0)

Patients were categorized into primary clinical diagnoses and indications for ACEI therapy. The clinical diagnoses were ventricular septal defect (31.1%), nephrotic syndrome (23.9%), rheumatic heart disease (11.3%), acute post-streptococcal glomerulonephritis (7.9%), chronic kidney disease (6.0%), posterior urethral valves (3.3%), HIV associated nephropathy (3.3%), acute renal failure (2.6%), chronic renal failure (2.0%), cardiomyopathy (2.0%), HIV-associated congestive cardiac failure (2.0%), transposition of the great arteries (1.3%), sickle cell nephropathy (1.3%), congenital hydronephrosis (1.3%), and patent ductus arteriosus (0.7%).

Indications for therapy and ACEI used are given in Table 2.

Table 2. ACE inhibitors used and their indications

Indication	ACE Inhibitor		
	Lisinopril N [%]	Enalapril N [%]	Ramipril N [%]
Heart failure	64 [42.4]	8 [5.3]	0
Hypertension	14 [9.3]	3 [2.0]	4 [2.6]
Renoprotective effect	55 [36.4]	3 [2.0]	0
Total	133 [88.1]	14 [9.3]	4 [2.6] 151 [100.0]

Lisinopril and enalapril were dosed at 0.1mg/kg/day, while ramipril was given in a dose range of 2.5 – 5mg/day. Hypotension (4.6%) and dizziness (3.0%) were documented adverse effects. Serum electrolytes in cardiac patients remained unaffected, while the underlying pathology in renal patients made it difficult to attribute any change in serum biochemistry to the use of ACEI.

DISCUSSION

The commonest indication for ACEIs was cardiac failure. In children, the causes of cardiac failure differ appreciably from what obtains in adults. Congenital malformations, such as left-to-right shunts, commonly ventricular septal defects [VSD] are seen in younger children, while rheumatic heart disease and cardiomyopathy are commoner in older children.

The rational for use of ACEIs in cardiac failure is that they reduce the effects that result from the activation of the RAS which occurs in heart failure [7-9]. The beneficial effects of ACEIs in heart failure may therefore include:

- reduced angiotensin II mediated vasoconstriction
- reduced angiotensin II mediated potentiation of sympathetic nervous system activity
- reduced angiotensin II mediated aldosterone release and therefore
    - reduced sodium and water retention
    - reduced myocardial fibrosis
    - reduced inhibition of nitric oxide release
- reduced breakdown of vasodilatory bradykinin

The principal action through which ACEIs improve survival and reduce symptoms derives from their ability to target raised filling pressures, reduced cardiac output and increased systemic vascular resistance through vasodilatation and after-load reduction [10].

A number of ACEIs have been studied in large randomized trials in the management of cardiac failure in adults, with generally consistent findings of reduced symptoms, morbidity and mortality, however, there is no data directly comparing the different ACEIs on which any conclusions about the superiority of one over another can be drawn [7]. Effects of ACEIs on the RAS in pediatric patients are similar to those in adults [11]. ACEIs lower aortic pressure and systemic vascular resistance, do not affect pulmonary vascular resistance significantly, and lower left atrial and right atrial pressures in pediatric patients with heart failure [11]. In infants with a large VSD and pulmonary hypertension, ACEIs decrease left-to-right shunt in those infants with elevated systemic vascular resistance. Enalapril and captopril have been more widely used in pediatric cardiology than other ACEIs, even though in this center lisinopril and enalapril have been more popularly prescribed.

Transforming growth factor-β (TGF-β) and nitric oxide are important mediators of renal disease progression. TGF-β is a fibrinogenic cytokine involved in normal wound healing and pathological fibrosis [12]. Glomerular scarring enhances intrarenal production of TGF-β. Nitric oxide is a short-acting signaling molecule that is involved in the regulation of glomerular hemodynamics, mesangial proliferation, and net mesangial matrix production [13]. Diminished renal production in chronic renal disease may contribute to kidney fibrosis [14].

Both proteinuria [15, 16] and hypertension [17] are considered among the most significant nonimmunologic causes of progression of renal damage [18]. Therefore, their treatment is considered the most effective strategy to preserve renal function [19].

Angiotensin II is recognized presently as one of the most important mediators of progressive renal failure. It is responsible for several hemodynamic effects such as vasoconstriction, proteinuria (secondary to glomerular hyperfiltration attributable to increased intraglomerular pressure), and structural changes to the glomeruli caused by proinflammatory mediators, fibroblast proliferation, and production of superoxide free radicals [20]. The administration of ACEIs reduces the progression of renal damage from varying causes, by blocking the RAS and therefore lowering proteinuria and/or arterial blood pressure.

Treatment with ACEIs is renoprotective in virtually all proteinuric forms of kidney disease [21]. By reducing intraglomerular hypertension, ACEIs prevent glomerular hyperfiltration. However, because angiotensin II is a potent inducer of TGF-β release, ACEIs may also diminish renal fibrosis by a non-hemodynamic mechanism [22]. Both ACEIs and nitric oxide retard the progression to kidney failure and their renoprotective effects correlate with suppression of TGF-β [23].

Angiotensin blockade has been put to the most use among our renal patients with nephrotic syndrome of the steroid-dependent and steroid-resistant varieties. Chander et al [24] retrospectively analyzed data from 146 children treated with ACEIs as sole agents for non-diabetic proteinuria and observed effective control of proteinuria and stabilization of kidney function in the children. Likewise Milliner and Morgenstern reported the treatment of six children with steroid-resistant nephrotic syndrome with enalapril resulting in a significant decrease in proteinuria and fall in urine protein/creatinine ratio [25].

Chronic glomerulonephritis resulting in substantial renal damage is frequently characterized by relentless progression to end-stage renal disease. Renal angiotensin II, the production of which is enhanced in chronic glomerulonephritis can elevate intraglomerular pressure, increase glomerular cell hypertrophy, and augment extracellular matrix accumulation [26, 27]. ACEIs were also used as part of treatment regimen in children with acute postinfectious glomerulonephritis (APGN) and their blood pressure reduction was better than with the use of alpha methyl dopa, amlodipne and propranolol. A study in Lithuania [28] also recorded superior antihypertensive effect with enalapril-treated patients with APGN. This could be explained by the fact that ACEIs alter the balance between the vasoconstrictive, salt-retentive, and cardiac hypertrophic properties of angiotensin II and the vasodilatory and natriuretic properties of bradykinin; they also alter the metabolism of other vasoactive substances [29].

Two patients with sickle cell nephropathy treated with lisinopril for 10 – 12 weeks also showed good blood pressure control and regression of proteinuria, even though their serum biochemistry remained unaltered. Falk et al [30] did report a good response to enalapril in their patients with sickle cell nephropathy.

Kidney disease is an important complication of the human immunodeficiency virus (HIV) infection, kidney function being abnormal in up to 30% of HIV-infected patients [31]. AIDS-related kidney disease has become a relatively common cause of end-stage renal disease requiring dialysis, and kidney disease may be associated with progression to AIDS and death [32, 33]. Five patients with HIV associated nephropathy were treated with HAART and lisinopril for varied periods of time. The outcome was not favorable probably due to late presentation and consequent late onset of therapy.

Adverse effects of ACEIs may be classified into four main types, 1) effects due to interfering with the activity of the RAS in the maintenance of blood pressure and serum potassium, 2) effects due to interfering with the activity of other enzymes and receptors, 3) allergic reactions; and 4) effects on the fetus. Hypotension, early decrease in glomerular filtration rate, and hyperkalemia are dose-related adverse effects related to the mechanism of reduced angiotensin II levels through inhibition of ACE. Dose decreases and slow dose titration were used to manage hypotension in the patients. The dizziness waned off with bed rest and continued therapy.

Even though renal failure incident on use of ACEIs has been reported [34, 35], it was not observed in these patients.

In spite of the fact that the use of ACEIs in pediatric patients at the Nnamdi Azikiwe University Teaching Hospital has not been quite robust, they have proved reasonably efficacious in the various clinical entities they have been used to treat cardiac failure, proteinuria and hypertension. ACEIs have also been well tolerated with minimal side effects.

ACKNOWLEDGMENTS

The assistance of Staff of Medical Records Department and Dr. Ifeanyi Nwaeju in assembling the clinical records of the patients is acknowledged. The kind permission of Dr. John Chukwuka and Dr. Joy Ebenebe to include their patients in this review is also acknowledged.

DISCLOSURES

The author declares no conflicts of interests

REFERENCES

[1] Guron G, Friberg P. An intact rennin-angiotensin system is a prerequisite for normal renal development. *J Hypertens* 2000; 18: 123 – 37.

[2] Shotan A, Widerhorn J, Hurst A. Risk of angiotensin-converting enzyme inhibition during pregnancy: experimental and clinical evidence, potential mechanisms, and recommendations for use. *Am J Med* 1994; 96: 451 – 6.

[3] Schubiger G, Flury G. Enalapril for pregnancy-induced hypertension; acute renal failure in a neonate. *Ann Intern Med* 1988; 108: 215 – 16.

[4] Cunniff C, Jones KL, Phillipson J. Oligohydramnios sequence and renal tubular malformation associated with maternal enalapril use. *Am J Obstet Gynecol* 1990; 162: 187 – 9.

[5] Filler G, Wong H, Condello AS, Charbonneau C, Sinclair B, Kovesi T, Hutchison J. Early dialysis in a neonate with intrauterine lisinopril exposure. *Arch Dis Child Fetal Neonatal Ed* 2003; 88: F154 – F156.

[6] Chevalier RL. Mechanisms of fetal and neonatal renal impairment by pharmacologic inhibition of angiotensin. *Curr Med Chem* 2012; 19(27): 4572 – 80.

[7] Beggs S, Thompson A, Nash R, Tompson A, Peterson G. Cardiac failure in children. 17th Expert Committee on the Selection and Use of Essential Medicines. Geneva, March 2009.

[8] Scammell AM, Diver MJ. Plasma rennin activity in infants with congenital heart disease. *Arch Dis Child* 1987; 62: 1136 – 1138.

[9] Dutertre JP, Billand EM, Autret E, Chantepie A, Oliver I, Langier J. Inhibition of angiotensin converting enzyme with enalapril maleate in infants with congestive heart failure. *Br J Clin Pharmac* 1993; 35: 528 – 530.

[10] Fenton M, Burch M. Understanding chronic heart failure. *Arch Dis Child* 2007; 92: 812 – 16.

[11] Momma K. ACE inhibitors in pediatric patients with heart failure. *Paediatr Drugs* 2006; 8(1): 55 – 69.

[12] Border WA, Noble NA. Transforming growth factor-β in tissue fibrosis. *N Engl J Med* 1994; 331: 1286 – 92.

[13] Haynes WG, Hand MF, Dockrell MEC, Eadington DW, Lee MR, Hussein Z, Benjamin N, Webb DJ. Physiological role of nitric oxide in regulation of renal function in humans. *Am J Physiol* 1997; 272: F364 – F371.

[14] Schmidt RJ, Baylis C. Total nitric oxide production is low in patients with chronic renal disease. *Kidney Int* 2000; 58: 1261 – 66.

[15] Burton MB, Harris KGP. The role of proteinuria in the progression of chronic renal disease. *Am J Kidney Dis* 1996; 27: 765 – 75.

[16] Remuzzi G, Bertani T. Pathophysiology of progressive nephropathies. *N Engl J Med* 1998; 339: 1448 – 56.

[17] Soeergel M, Schaefer F. Effect of hypertension on the progression of chronic renal failure in children. *Am J Hypertens* 2002; 15 (suppl 1): 53 – 6.

[18] Klahr S,Schreiner G, Ichikawa I. The progression of renal disease. *N Engl J Med* 1998; 318: 1657 – 66.

[19] Wolf G, Ritz E. Combination therapy with ACE inhibitors and angiotensin II receptor blockers to halt progression of chronic renal disease: pathophysiology and indications. *Kidney Int* 2005; 67: 799 – 812.

[20] Wolf G, Butzmann U, Wenzel UO. The rennin-angiotensin system and progression of renal disease: from hemodynamics to cell biology. *Nephron Physiol* 2003; 93: P3 – P13.

[21] Taal MW, Brenner BM. Renoprotective benefits of RAS inhibition: from ACEI to angiotensin II antagonists. *Kidney Int* 2000; 57: 1803 – 17.

[22] Shin GT, Kim SJ, Ma KA, Kim HS, Kim D. ACE inhibitors attenuate expression of renal transforming growth factor-β in humans. *Am J Kidney Dis* 2000; 36: 894 – 902.

[23] Ketteler M, Border WA, Noble NA. Cytokines and L-arginine in renal injury and repair. *Am J Physiol* 1994; 267: F197 – F207.

[24] Chandar J, Abitbol C, Montane B, Zilleruelo G. Angiotensin blockade as sole treatment for proteinuric kidney disease in children. *Nephrol Dial Transplant* 2007; 22: 1332 – 1337. Doi:10.1093/ndt/gf1839.

[25] Milliner DS, Morgenstern BZ. Angiotensin converting enzyme inhibitors for reduction of proteinuria in children with steroid-resistant nephrotic syndrome. *Pediatr Nephrol* 1991; 5: 587 – 90.

[26] Kohan DE. Angiotensin II and endothelin in chronic glomerulonephritis. *Kidney International* 1998; 54(2): 646 – 7.

[27] Urushihara M, Kobori H. Angiotensinogen expression is enhanced in the progression of glomerular disease. *International Journal of Clinical Medicine* 2011; 2(4): 378 – 87.

[28] Jankauskiene A, Cerniauskiene V, Jakutovic M, Malikenas A. Enalapril influence on blood pressure and echocardiographic parameters in children with acute postinfectious glomerulonephritis. *Medicina (Kaunas)* 2005; 41 (12): 1019 – 1025.

[29] Brown NJ, Vaughan DE. Angiotensin-converting enyme inhibitors. *Circulation* 1998; 97: 1411 – 20.

[30] Faulk RJ, Scheinman J, Phillips G, Orringer E, Johnson A, Jennette JC. Prevalence and pathologic features of sickle cell nephropathy and response to inhibition of angiotensin-converting enzyme. *N Engl J Med* 1992; 326: 910 – 915.

[31] Gupta SK, Eustace JA, Winston JA, Boydstun II, Ahuja TS, Rodriguez RA, Tashima KT, Roland M, Franceschini N, Palella FJ, Lennox JL, Klotman PE, Nachman SA, Hall

SD, Szczech LA. Guidelines for management of chronic kidney disease in HIV/AIDS. CID 2005: 40 (1 June): 1559 – 1585.

[32] Gupta SK, Mamlin BW, Johnson CS, Dollins MD, Topf JM, Dube MP. Prevalence of proteinuria and development of chronic kidney disease in HIV-infected patients. *Clin Nephrol* 2004; 61: 1 – 6.

[33] Ademola AD, Asinobi OO, Oladokun RE, Ogunkunle OO, Okoloz CA, Ogbole GE. Kidney disease in hospitalized HIV positive children in Ibadan, southwest Nigeria. *Afr J Med Med Sci* 2012; 41(2): 221 – 230.

[34] Olowu WA, Adenowo OA, Elusiyan JBE. Reversible renal failure in hypertensive idiopathic nephrotics treated with captopril. *Saudi J Kidney Dis Transplant* 2006; 17(2): 216 – 21.

[35] Leversha AM, Wilson NJ, Clarkson PM, Calder AL, Ramage MC, Neutze JM. Efficacy and dosage of enalapril in congenital and acquired heart disease. *Arch Dis Child* 1994; 70: 35 – 39.

In: ACE Inhibitors. Volume 2
Editor: Macaulay Amechi Onuigbo
ISBN: 978-1-62948-422-8

Chapter 17

Is There a Role for ACEIs in the ICU?

Pascale Khairallah, MD[1] and Kianoush Kashani, MD[2,3]*
[1]Division of Internal Medicine,
American University of Beirut Medical Center, Beirut, Lebanon
[2]Division of Nephrology and Hypertension, Mayo Clinic, Rochester, MN, US
[3]Division of Pulmonary and Critical care, Mayo Clinic, Rochester, MN, US

Abstract

Renin-angiotensin-aldosterone system (RAAS) exerts a range of physiologic effects on the cardiovascular and renal system through various mechanisms leading to increased afterload and intraglomerular trans-membrane pressure. Its effects also include cardiac and vascular wall remodeling. The role of angiotensin II blockers such as angiotensin-converting enzyme inhibitors (ACEI) and angiotensin receptor blockers (ARB) in enhancing survival in patients with heart failure, diabetes, hypertension and post myocardial infarction has been proven through various studies. In the critically ill patient, however, the role of ACEI/ARBs is still unclear. Therefore, the intensivists in surgical and medical intensive care units are often faced with the decision to discontinue them especially in the setting of acute kidney injury. It is well known that ACEI/ARBs decrease renal efferent arteriolar tone, intraglomerular pressure and GFR. This is beneficial in proteinuric kidney disease. Critically ill patients commonly have a decrease in effective circulating volume. This will lead to decreased renal function. In these patients, withholding ACEI/ARBs will prevent further decline in GFR and kidney damage. On the other hand ACEI/ARBs provide benefit to patients who are admitted to ICU for hypertensive crisis secondary to enhanced Renin-Angiotensin-Aldosterone system (RAAS) activation or patients with scleroderma renal crisis and thrombotic microangiopathy. In these patients blocking RAAS will not only reduce in blood pressure but also mitigates vascular endothelial damage. An area in which the decision to continue an ACEI/ARB presents a particular challenge is that of chronic heart failure. The favorable effects of ACEI/ARBs in patients with heart failure include, but are not limited to, a decrease in afterload and an increase in cardiac output. Due to the documented survival benefit, chronic heart failure patients are often on these medications. In acute decompensation, angiotensin II becomes a main contributor maintaining the systemic

* Corresponding author: Kianoush Kashani MD; Email: Kashani.Kianoush@mayo.edu.

vascular resistance and renal perfusion. In the same setting, ACEI/ARBs lead to afterload reduction which in turn improves cardiac function and renal perfusion. So the decision to keep the patient on ACEI/ARB would depend on where the cardiac and renal function lies with respect to each other. In cases of low blood pressure, rise in serum creatinine, or the development of hyperkalemia, ACEI/ARBs can be temporarily withheld and replaced by other afterload reducing agents.

INTRODUCTION

The intensive care unit (ICU) mortality rate remains high particularly among elderly patients [1]. The mean age of patients who are admitted to the ICU is about 62 years old and within the last decade admission of patients older than 85 years old showed the fastest growth [2]. As patients age, they are more likely to have more complex diseases. Therefore, polypharmacy in elderly is a common finding and the reported incidence has been reported as 13-92% [3]. Angiotensin converting enzyme inhibitors (ACEIs) is a common medication that is used particularly by old patients. Protective effects of ACEI on multiple organs have been shown in several studies [4]. However, in the critical care setting, due to hemodynamic changes, ACEI could have some unintended consequences and side effects [5]. These considerations would generally in turn influence clinicians' decisions to therefore not use ACEIs in the ICUs liberally. Many patients in the ICU have multiple organ dysfunction; therefore, the decision to initiate, withhold or continue ACEIs becomes dependent on a risk and benefit assessment.

The following chapter looks at the role of ACEIs in the critical care setting according to the primary organ system dysfunction.

THE ROLE OF ANGIOTENSIN II IN HEMODYNAMICS

The renin-angiotensin-aldosterone system (RAAS) plays a crucial role in maintaining hemodynamic stability in the body. Renin, angiotensinogen, angiotensin I and angiotensin II are the main components of the RAAS [6]. Increasing knowledge about the RAAS consistently portrays angiotensin II as being a key player [7,8]. Angiotensin II has multiple origins; circulating, paracrine and neuronal [7,9,10].

The neuronal recently described source of angiotensin II, as determined by immunocytology, is likely to be an independent modulator of salt and water homeostasis [9]. Moreover, the components of the RAAS can all be locally found in the proximal tubules where they are produced [8]. This guarantees angiotensin II as a physiologic moderator independent of the systemic activity of RAAS.

Angiotensin II affects blood pressure through both direct systemic vasoconstriction and renal salt and water excretion. Intrarenally, angiotensin II binds to the angiotensin II receptor type 1 (AT1 receptor) and constricts the afferent and efferent arterioles. This effect is more pronounced on the efferent arterioles [11]. This in turn leads to an increase in the glomerular filtration rate (GFR) [12,13]. The increase in GFR consequently increases the filtration fraction leading to increased tubular flow. This, in turn, translates into increased proximal sodium and water reabsorption [11].

The hemodynamic contributions of angiotensin II are not limited to its effect on GFR but also on direct tubular actions. More specifically, angiotensin II acts on the proximal tubules, distal tubules, and collecting ducts via binding to the AT1 receptor. In the proximal tubules, the main action of angiotensin II is to promote sodium bicarbonate and water reabsorption. At the molecular level, this is achieved by altering the membrane properties of the proximal tubule through activation of apical Sodium/Proton (Na/H) exchanger, basolateral Sodium/Bicarbonate (Na-HCO3) cotransporter, and basolateral Sodium/Potassium Adenosine Triphosphatase (Na/K-ATPase) as well as via insertion of Proton Adenosine Triphosphatase (H-ATPase) into the apical membrane [8]. At the level of the distal tubules, angiotensin II activates both Na/H exchangers and H-ATPase enzymes, which further enhances the reabsorptive process that was initiated at the proximal tubules [14]. Finally, in the collecting ducts, angiotensin II exerts its effects via two distinct mechanisms. The first mechanism is aldosterone dependent and acts by up-regulating sodium reabsorption and potassium secretion via their luminal channels and the basolateral Na/K-ATPase [15]. The second mechanism is aldosterone independent; angiotensin II directly stimulates the luminal epithelial sodium channels (ENaC) which increases sodium reabsorption [16].

Patients in critical care units commonly suffer from Congestive Heart Failure (CHF) exacerbation, sepsis, or other conditions that result in decreased effective intravascular volume and vascular tone. This leads to decreased perfusion pressure to the various organs, including the kidneys. The normal physiological activity of angiotensin II described above is usually altered in the patient population admitted to the critical care units. Specifically, the activity of angiotensin II is further amplified to maintain effective intravascular volume and end organ perfusion [17]. Any interference with the action of angiotensin II renders this compensatory response suboptimal, and becomes potentially deleterious to renal function.

ACEIs by blocking the enzymatic conversion of angiotensin I to angiotensin II, prevent this effort at maintaining an adequate effective perfusion, and can therefore lead to organ injury or failure.

ACEI in the ICU

Renal Considerations

Acute Kidney Injury (AKI)

AKI complicates 5-7% of hospital admissions [18], and two thirds of admissions to the intensive care unit [19]. The etiology of AKI is multifactorial with acute tubular necrosis, being the greatest contributor. In states of hypoperfusion or volume depletion, angiotensin II becomes essential for the maintenance of GFR [5]. Using ACEI would block the compensatory angiotensin II mediated vasoconstriction, and renal perfusion would further decline. Decline in the renal perfusion in the setting of heart failure, volume depletion and bilateral renal artery stenosis are the risk factors of development of AKI [20]. Moreover, ACEIs were found to be independent predictors of AKI in patients admitted to the ICU [19]. For example, Arora and colleagues reported pre-operative use of ACEI was associated with significant increase in the Post-Operative risk for AKI [21]. In the chronic setting, a rise in the baseline serum creatinine of up to 30% is well tolerated and reversible; however, in the ICU where hemodynamic status is changed and many other risk factors for the AKI exist, the general recommendation is to withhold or withdraw ACEI whenever effective blood volume has decreased.

One instance where the use of ACEIs is justified in AKI is in systemic sclerosis renal crisis [22-25]. AKI complicates scleroderma and is characterized by new onset malignant hypertension, kidney dysfunction, and microangiopathic hemolytic anemia [26]. ACEIs have improved renal outcome and are now considered one of the mainstays of therapy. Captopril is the most studied ACEI in this scenario; however, enalapril was found to be effective in patients who did not tolerate captopril [27]. Generally ACEIs in the setting of scleroderma hypertension crisis need to be continued even in the case of worsening kidney function and the goal remains as decline in blood pressure. ACEI are to be given continuously until reaching consistently values below 120 mmHg for Systolic Blood Pressure (SBP) and below 80 mmHg for Diastolic Blood Pressure (DBP) [28].

Cardiovascular Considerations

Acute Heart Failure

Despite being on optimal medical management, patients with left ventricular dysfunction often suffer acute exacerbations and require frequent admissions in the hospitals or critical care settings [29]. ACEIs have become one of the main treatments for chronic heart failure [30,31]. The mechanism of cardioprotective effects of ACEIs is mainly due to afterload reduction, prevention of abnormal remodeling of myocardium after an infarct and therefore prevention of cardiac hypertrophy, reduction of myocardial infarct size, reduction of sympathetic activity and improvement in arterial compliance [32-36]. Decline in cardiac output would result systemic hypoperfusion and decrease in renal blood flow, congestion of the kidneys and hence impaired kidney function [37]. Particularly in the patients with cardiorenal syndrome type I, when acute decompensated heart failure causes acute deterioration of kidney function, kidney vasculature becomes dependent on angiotensin II and the sympathetic nervous system to maintain the glomerular filtration pressure [38]. Thus blocking the RAAS could be deleterious in these patients and create a more severe state of hypoperfusion. On the other hand, due to the significant importance of ACEIs in the treatment of heart failure, discontinuation of this medications are not recommended unless they are associated with progressive kidney dysfunction, hypotension or hyperkalemia [39] Therefore, if patients have been on ACEI at home, are not hypotensive or hyperkalemic and are not suffering from acute kidney injury, then keeping them on ACEI can be justified. Caution arises with patients presenting with acute heart failure and who have never been on ACEI [39]. The decision to start an ACEI would then depend on blood pressure and kidney function status. It is recommended to use short acting afterload reducers in the setting of acute decompensated heart failure particularly in patients who have borderline hypotension and switch them to ACEI as soon as they can tolerate [40].

Myocardial Infarction (MI)

Patients having suffered an ST segment elevation MI have been shown to benefit from ACEI. The role of ACEI after MI has been corroborated in multiple trials. In the acute setting, patients who require admission to a critical care setting show a 30-day survival advantage over those who are not started on ACEI. In the first day post-MI, the ACEI group showed an average of 30% survival advantage [41,42]. This effect is more proven in patients who were not revascularized [43]. Following revascularization, although some studies showed improvement in mortality, some other studies failed to show such results [44,45]. Early and late initiation of ACEIs is both associated with improvement in mortality. In addition other studies have proven the effect of ACEI on reduction in sudden death, recurrent MI, myocardial remodeling and progression to congestive heart failure [46]. As an important precaution, when starting this class of medication, is to start from a low dose, and up-titrate to reach a maximum tolerable dose. The main benefit of such an approach is to prevent hypotension and hyperkalemia, known complications of ACEI therapy [47]. The only group where ACEI did not show a clear survival advantage was in patients older than 75 years as this group is most commonly affected by ACEI-induced hypotension [46].

Thus, in non-hypotensive post MI patients, it is recommended to start ACEI. This is arguable in individuals above 75, whose risk from ACEI induced hypotension outweighs the benefits.

Cardiogenic Shock

Cardiogenic shock is a state of end-organ hypoperfusion due to cardiac failure. The diagnosis is based on altered hemodynamic parameters and clinical signs such as cool extremities, decreased urine output or altered mental status [48]. ACE inhibitors are vasodilators that act on the arterial tree to decrease afterload. Afterload reduction is important in cardiogenic shock because it decreases myocardial strain and oxygen consumption [49]. In one small retrospective study amongst patients with multi-organ dysfunction with cardiogenic shock, mortality was significantly lower on patients who were on ACEI during their ICU stay [50]. Larger trials are however needed to explore whether the mortality benefit clearly compensates for the risk of ACEI induced hypotension and renal failure.

Septic Shock

Septic shock is defined by both IV fluid refractory hypotension and a source of infection. The RAAS has been shown to be implicated in both elements comprising this definition. In septic hypotension, RAAS is activated and Angiotensin II is released to maintain vascular tone and organ perfusion. Nevertheless, this same vasoconstriction can become unregulated from increased angiotensin II release and can lead to further end organ hypoperfusion. Using ACEI was found to be associated with increased risk of acute kidney injury in the setting of sepsis [51].

On the other hand, Angiotensin II has also been found to have proinflammatory and procoagulant effects that exacerbate tissue and vascular damage and potentiate the state of sepsis. ACEI is protective of endothelial cell when these cells are damaged during sepsis [52]. Therefore, the spectrum at which the septic patient is presenting is important to determine whether ACEI might be advantageous.

In early sepsis, before hypotension has completely ensued, the use of ACE inhibition was shown to limit organ failure through both decreasing endothelial damage and exerting anti-inflammatory effects. In late shock, however, ACEI use leads to refractory hypotension as vascular tone becomes angiotensin II dependent [53].

Neurologic Considerations

Encephalopathy

Hypertension alters the blood brain barrier physiology by modulating the cerebral microvasculature. Even though the pathophysiology of these changes is poorly understood, a positive feedback loop stimulating the release of vasoactive mediators seems to be implicated. Activation of this feedback loop causes a continuous increase in blood pressure and end organ damage leading to encephalopathy [54,55]. Hypertension resulting in encephalopathy is a hypertensive emergency. Hypertensive emergency is thought to be induced by a multitude of factors, including mechanical shear stress from blood flow, endothelial dysfunction and oxidative damage [55]. Endothelial injury then causes release of cytokines, prostaglandins and nitric oxide which alter the blood brain barrier. The RAAS was found to be critical in the initiation and maintenance of hypertensive emergencies and in target organ damage. Interestingly, inhibition of the AT_1 receptor blocks the hypertension-related enhanced cell permeability and cerebral edema. These effects suggest an important role for Angiotensin II blockade in modulating BBB function to reduce brain damage [56].

Respiratory Considerations

Acute Respiratory Distress Syndrome (ARDS)

The involvement of the RAAS in the pathogenesis and evolution of inflammatory responses has received considerable attention lately. Various experimental studies have shown RAAS as a key inflammatory mediator [57]. Recent studies suggest a role for the RAAS in pulmonary disease as ACE levels were found to be elevated in bronchoalveolar lavage fluid from subjects with acute respiratory distress syndrome (ARDS) [58]. Moreover, mortality from ARDS is positively correlated with genetic polymorphisms of ACE. ACE_2, an ACE homolog which is found mostly in the endothelial cells of heart and kidney, decreases levels of angiotensin II and provides protection from acute lung injury [59]. These observations suggest that ACE activity, angiotensin II and its receptor may play as important modulators of inflammation in ARDS [60]. Recent studies on animal models have shown that enalapril can down-regulate angiotensin II and suppress cytokine levels in serum, thus preventing acute lung injury [60]. Further studies need to be undertaken to evaluate the effectiveness of ACEI in humans, but results seem promising and we might be using ACEI to treat ARDS in ICU patients in the future.

CONCLUSION

In many clinical scenarios in ICU, the role of ACEIs is not very well defined. On the other hand, based on the current data, there is a potential role for ACEIs in cell and organ protection. This class of medications potentially can cause hypotension, hyperkalemia and acute kidney injury, if they are used in high risk patients. Their usage in many ICU-related clinical syndromes has been tested with some degree of success. Therefore, we suggest prescribing these medications based on the individual cases after balancing the risks and benefits associated with them. There is a great interest in the academic medicine to investigate the effect of these drugs in the treatment and/or prevention of ICU-related clinical syndromes. These studies will determine the role of ACEIs in ICU with more clarity in the future.

REFERENCES

[1] Conti M, Merlani P, Ricou B. Prognosis and quality of life of elderly patients after intensive care. *Swiss Med. Wkly* 2012;142:w13671.

[2] Mullins PM, Goyal M, Pines JM. National Growth in Intensive Care Unit Admissions From Emergency Departments in the United States from 2002 to 2009. *Academic Emergency Medicine* 2013;20:479-86.

[3] Lees J, Chan A. Polypharmacy in elderly patients with cancer: clinical implications and management. *The Lancet Oncology* 2011;12:1249-57.

[4] Stojiljkovic L, Behnia R. Role of renin angiotensin system inhibitors in cardiovascular and renal protection: a lesson from clinical trials. *Curr. Pharm. Des.* 2007;13:1335-45.

[5] Schoolwerth AC SD, Ballermann BJ, Wilcox CS, Association. CotKiCDatCfHBPRotAH. Renal considerations in angiotensin converting enzyme inhibitor therapy: a statement for healthcare professionals from the Council on the Kidney in Cardiovascular Disease and the Council for High Blood Pressure Research of the American Heart Association. *Circulation* 2001:1985-91.

[6] Brewster UC SJ, Perazella MA. The renin-angiotensin-aldosterone system: cardiorenal effects and implications for renal and cardiovascular disease states. *The American journal of the medical sciences* 2003:15-24.

[7] Carey RM SH. Newly recognized components of the renin-angiotensin system: potential roles in cardiovascular and renal regulation. Endocrine reviews 2003:261-71.

[8] Kobori H NM, Navar LG, Nishiyama A. The intrarenal renin-angiotensin system: from physiology to the pathobiology of hypertension and kidney disease. *Pharmacological reviews* 2007:251-87.

[9] Bohlender J NJ, Imboden H. Angiotensinergic innervation of the kidney: present knowledge and its significance. *Current hypertension reports* 2013:10-6.

[10] Zhuo JL LX. New insights and perspectives on intrarenal reninangiotensin system: Focus on intracrine/intracellular angiotensin II. *Peptides* 2011:1551-65.

[11] Navar LG H-BL, Imig JD, Wang CT, Cervenka L, Mitchell KD. Intrarenal angiotensin II generation and renal effects of AT1 receptor blockade. *Journal of the American Society of nephrology* 1999:266-72.

[12] Hilal-Dandan R. Renin and Angiotensin. Goodman & Gilman's The Pharmacological Basis of Therapeutics New York: McGraw-Hill 2011.

[13] Kobori H, Nangaku M, Navar LG, Nishiyama A. The Intrarenal Renin-Angiotensin System: From Physiology to the Pathobiology of Hypertension and Kidney Disease. *Pharmacological Reviews* 2007;59:251-87.

[14] Barreto-Chaves ML M-AM. Effect of luminal angiotensin II and ANP on early and late cortical distal tubule HCO3- reabsorption. *The American journal of physiology* 1996:977-84.

[15] David Pearce VB, John W. Funder, John B. Stokes. Aldosterone Regulation of Ion Transport. In: Brenner & Rector's The Kidney, Ninth Edition: Saunders; 2012:202- 25.
[16] Peti-Peterdi J WD, Bell PD. Angiotensin II directly stimulates ENaC activity in the cortical collecting duct via AT(1) receptors. *Journal of the American society of nephrology* 2002:1131-5.
[17] Sladen RN. Renal Physiology. In: Miller's Anesthesia, Seventh Edition: Churchill Livingstone; 2010:441-76.
[18] Langenberg C WL, Egi M, May CN, Bellomo R. Renal blood flow in experimental septic acute renal failure. *Kidney international* 2006:1996-2002.
[19] Plataki M KK, Cabello-Garza J, Maldonado F, Kashyap R, Kor DJ, Gajic O, Cartin-Ceba R. Predictors of acute kidney injury in septic shock patients: an observational cohort study. *Clinical journal of the American Society of Nephrology* 2011:1744-51.
[20] Bentley ML, Corwin HL, Dasta J. Drug-induced acute kidney injury in the critically ill adult: Recognition and prevention strategies. *Critical Care Medicine* 2010;38:S169-S74 10.1097/CCM.0b013e3181de0c60.
[21] Arora P, Rajagopalam S, Ranjan R, et al. Preoperative use of angiotensin-converting enzyme inhibitors/angiotensin receptor blockers is associated with increased risk for acute kidney injury after cardiovascular surgery. *Clin. J. Am. Soc. Nephrol.* 2008;3:1266-73.
[22] Beckett VL, Donadio JV, Jr., Brennan LA, Jr., et al. Use of captopril as early therapy for renal scleroderma: a prospective study. *Mayo Clin. Proc.* 1985;60:763-71.
[23] Penn H, Howie AJ, Kingdon EJ, et al. Scleroderma renal crisis: patient characteristics and long-term outcomes. *QJM* 2007;100:485-94.
[24] Steen VD, Costantino JP, Shapiro AP, Medsger TA, Jr. Outcome of renal crisis in systemic sclerosis: relation to availability of angiotensin converting enzyme (ACE) inhibitors. *Ann. Intern. Med.* 1990;113:352-7.
[25] Bussone G, Bérezné A, Pestre V, Guillevin L, Mouthon L. The Scleroderma Kidney: Progress in Risk Factors, Therapy, and Prevention. *Curr. Rheumatol. Rep.* 2011;13: 37-43.
[26] Yang Y ZL, Tang Y, Zhao Y, Su B, Fu P. Systemic sclerosis with thrombotic thrombocytopenia purpura and malignant hypertension. *Renal. failure* 2012:1170-2.
[27] Smith CD, Smith RD, Korn JH. Hypertensive crisis in systemic sclerosis: treatment with the new oral angiotensin converting enzyme inhibitor MK, 421 (Enalapril) in captopril-intolerant patients. *Arthritis Rheum.* 1984;27:826-8.
[28] Harrison W. Farber RWSaRL. Analytic Review: Care of Patients With Scleroderma in the Intensive Care Setting. *Journal of Intensive Care Medicine* 2010:247-58.
[29] Coffey RM, Misra A, Barrett M, Andrews RM, Mutter R, Moy E. Congestive Heart Failure: Who Is Likely to Be Readmitted? *Medical Care Research and Review* 2012;69:602-16.
[30] Effect of enalapril on survival in patients with reduced left ventricular ejection fractions and congestive heart failure. The SOLVD Investigators. *N. Engl. J. Med.* 1991;325:293-302.
[31] Cohn JN, Johnson G, Ziesche S, et al. A comparison of enalapril with hydralazine-isosorbide dinitrate in the treatment of chronic congestive heart failure. *N. Engl. J. Med.* 1991;325:303-10.

[32] Stauss HM, Zhu YC, Redlich T, et al. Angiotensin-converting enzyme inhibition in infarct-induced heart failure in rats: bradykinin versus angiotensin II. *J. Cardiovasc. Risk* 1994;1:255-62.

[33] Scholkens BA, Linz W. Cardioprotective effects of ACE inhibitors: experimental proof and clinical perspectives. *Clin. Physiol. Biochem.* 1990;8 Suppl 1:33-43.

[34] Giannattasio C, Achilli F, Failla M, et al. Radial, carotid and aortic distensibility in congestive heart failure: effects of high-dose angiotensin-converting enzyme inhibitor or low-dose association with angiotensin type 1 receptor blockade. *J. Am. Coll. Cardiol.* 2002;39:1275-82.

[35] Grassi G, Cattaneo BM, Seravalle G, et al. Effects of chronic ACE inhibition on sympathetic nerve traffic and baroreflex control of circulation in heart failure. *Circulation* 1997;96:1173-9.

[36] Dibner-Dunlap ME, Smith ML, Kinugawa T, Thames MD. Enalaprilat augments arterial and cardiopulmonary baroreflex control of sympathetic nerve activity in patients with heart failure. *J. Am. Coll. Cardiol.* 1996;27:358-64.

[37] Ronco C, Haapio M, House AA, Anavekar N, Bellomo R. Cardiorenal Syndrome. *J. Am. Coll. Cardiol.* 2008;52:1527-39.

[38] McCullough P.A. KJA, Mehta R.L., Murray P.T., Ronco C. ADQI Consensus on AKI Biomarkers and Cardiorenal Syndromes: Karger; 2013.

[39] Hollenberg SM. Vasodilators in acute heart failure. *Heart Failure Reviews* 2007:143-7.

[40] Allen LA, O'Connor CM. Management of acute decompensated heart failure. *Canadian Medical Association Journal* 2007;176:797-805.

[41] ISIS-4: a randomised factorial trial assessing early oral captopril, oral mononitrate, and intravenous magnesium sulphate in 58,050 patients with suspected acute myocardial infarction. ISIS-4 (Fourth International Study of Infarct Survival) Collaborative Group. *Lancet* 1995;345:669-85.

[42] GISSI-3: effects of lisinopril and transdermal glyceryl trinitrate singly and together on 6-week mortality and ventricular function after acute myocardial infarction. Gruppo Italiano per lo Studio della Sopravvivenza nell'infarto Miocardico. *Lancet* 1994;343:1115-22.

[43] Ambrosioni E, Borghi C, Magnani B. The effect of the angiotensin-converting-enzyme inhibitor zofenopril on mortality and morbidity after anterior myocardial infarction. The Survival of Myocardial Infarction Long-Term Evaluation (SMILE) Study Investigators. *N Engl J Med* 1995;332:80-5.

[44] Borghi C, Marino P, Zardini P, Magnani B, Collatina S, Ambrosioni E. Short- and long-term effects of early fosinopril administration in patients with acute anterior myocardial infarction undergoing intravenous thrombolysis: results from the Fosinopril in Acute Myocardial Infarction Study. FAMIS Working Party. *Am. Heart J.* 1998;136:213-25.

[45] Baur LH, Schipperheyn JJ, van der Wall EE, et al. Beneficial effect of enalapril on left ventricular remodelling in patients with a severe residual stenosis after acute anterior wall infarction. *Eur. Heart J.* 1997;18:1313-21.

[46] Group AIMIC. Indications for ACE Inhibitors in the Early Treatment of Acute Myocardial Infarction. *Circulation* 1998:2202-12.

[47] Spinar J VJ, Pluhacek L, Spinarova L, Fischerova B, Toman J. First dose hypotension after angiotensin converting enzyme inhibitor captopril and angiotensin II blocker

losartan in patients with acute myocardial infarction. *International Jouranl of Cardiology* 2000:197-204.
[48] Robert M. Califf aJRB. Cardiogenic Shock. *N. Engl. J. Med.* 1994:1724-30.
[49] Ng R YY. Post myocardial infarction cardiogenic shock: a review of current therapies. *Journal of intensive care medicine* 2013:151-65.
[50] Schmidt H, Hoyer D, Rauchhaus M, et al. ACE-inhibitor therapy and survival among patients with multiorgan dysfunction syndrome (MODS) of cardiac and non-cardiac origin. *International Journal of Cardiology* 2010;140:296-303.
[51] Plataki M, Kashani K, Cabello-Garza J, et al. Predictors of Acute Kidney Injury in Septic Shock Patients: An Observational Cohort Study. *Clinical Journal of the American Society of Nephrology* 2011;6:1744-51.
[52] Boldt J, Papsdorf M, Kumle B, Piper S, Hempelmann G. Influence of angiotensin-converting enzyme inhibitor enalaprilat on endothelial-derived substances in the critically ill. *Critical Care Medicine* 1998;26:1663-70.
[53] Diamantino Ribeiro Salgado JRR, Eliezer Silva, Jean-Louis Vincent. Modulation of the renin-angiotensin-aldosterone system in sepsis: a new therapeutic approach? *Expert opinion on therapeutic targets* 2010:11-20.
[54] Catherine Lamy J-LM. Hypertensive Encephalopathy. In: Stroke: Pathophysiology, Diagnosis, and Management, Fifth Edition: Saunders; 2011:734-40.
[55] Andrew R. Haas PEM. CRITICAL CARE ISSUES FOR THE NEPHROLOGIST: Current Diagnosis and Management of Hypertensive Emergency. *Seminars in Dialysis* 2006:502-12.
[56] Ito H TK, Kawai J, Suzuki T. AT1 receptor antagonist prevents brain edema without lowering blood pressure. *Acta neurochirurgica Supplement* 2000:141-5.
[57] Marshall RP, Webb S, Bellingan GJ, et al. Angiotensin Converting Enzyme Insertion/Deletion Polymorphism Is Associated with Susceptibility and Outcome in Acute Respiratory Distress Syndrome. *American Journal of Respiratory and Critical Care Medicine* 2002;166:646-50.
[58] Wösten-van Asperen RM LR, Specht PA, Moll GN, van Woensel JB, van der Loos CM, van Goor H, Kamilic J, Florquin S, Bos AP. Acute respiratory distress syndrome leads to reduced ratio of ACE/ACE2 activities and is prevented by angiotensin-(1–7) or an angiotensin II receptor antagonist. *Journal of Pathology* 2011:618-27.
[59] Imai Y KK, Rao S, Huan Y, Guo F, Guan B, Yang P, Sarao R, Wada T, Leong-Poi H, Crackower MA, Fukamizu A, Hui CC, Hein L, Uhlig S, Slutsky AS, Jiang C, Penninger JM. Angiotensin-converting enzyme 2 protects from severe acute lung failure. *Nature* 2005:112-6.
[60] Hagiwara S IH, Matumoto S, Hidaka S, Noguchi T. Effects of an angiotensin-converting enzyme inhibitor on the inflammatory response in in vivo and in vitro models. *Critical care medicine* 2009:626-33.

In: ACE Inhibitors. Volume 2
Editor: Macaulay Amechi Onuigbo

ISBN: 978-1-62948-422-8

Chapter 18

THE IMPACT OF ACE INHIBITION IN THE MANAGEMENT OF SICKLE CELL DISEASE IN NIGERIAN ADULTS

Ademola Aderibigbe,* MBBS FMCP FWACP[1], Fatiu Abiola Arogundade, MBBS FMCP FWACP[2] and Timothy Olanrewaju, MBBS FMCP[3]

[1]University of Ilorin Teaching Hospital, Ilorin, & AB Consultant Medical Centre Nigeria
[2]Obafemi Awolowo University / Teaching Hospitals Complex, Ile-Ife, Nigeria
[3]University of Ilorin Teaching Hospital, Ilorin, Nigeria

ABSTRACT

Sickle Cell Disease (SCD) is a constellation of various disorders resulting from changes consequent on gene mutation on the 6th codon of chromosome 11. The resultant abnormality alters the physiochemical property of the haemoglobin hence the red blood corpuscle changes into sickle form with hypoxia. SCD includes sickle cell anaemia, Hemoglobin SC disease, Hemoglobin CC-Disease, sickle cell trait and various forms of sickle–thalassemia syndromes. The pathological basis of the manifestations and complications of SCD is mainly the vaso-occlusive phenomenon due to the rigid and tactoid hemoglobin which occurs on exposure of sickle hemoglobin to hypoxic or an acidotic environment. The consequences of this occlusion include stasis and subsequently, vascular endothelial damage and the generation of proinflammatory and restorative cytokines. These actions and reactions result in the pathological features which include acute chest syndrome, various cardiovascular conditions including stroke, glomerular hypertrophy, interstitial fibrosis tubular atrophy and various forms of glomerular diseases among others. The renal manifestations in adults range from increased glomerular filtration rate, enlarged kidneys, microalbuminria, macroalbuminuria, nephrotic syndrome, and Chronic Kidney Disease (CKD) progressing to ESRD. Renal failure accounted for 40% of SCD patients that died in a large follow-up cohort study by Platt et al. The risk of developing renal disease in SCD has been shown

* Corresponding author: Ademola Aderibigbe MBBS FMCP FWACP; Email: academolanan@yahoo.com.

to be enhanced by the presence of a non-muscle myosin heavy chain 9 (MYH9) and Apolipoprotein 1 (APOL1) genes (haplotype) located on chromosome 22q13. This might have contributed to the high prevalence of renal complications in Africans with SCD. Angiotensin II has been implicated in the renal vaso-occlusion in SCD. Thus ACE inhibition is particularly indicated in SCD for managing some of these complications and manifestations particularly the glomerular hypertension, microalbuminria, relative hypertension and chronic kidney disease in addition to the use of Hydroxyurea, stem cell treatment, and Dipyridamole, among others. More recently, there has been increasing use of ACEIs in SCD in Africa including Nigeria; however the literature is limited on this paradigm. Some researchers in Africa have reported significant reduction of proteinuria with the use of ACE inhibition in adult SCD patients. The pathophysiological basis of the complications of SCD and the property of ACEIs and its success story in various cardiovascular conditions recommend the use of ACEIs in SCD. The ACEI has value-added effect in the management of SCD as it is cardio-protective, lowers the glomerular hypertension, is effective in treating the relative hypertension and proteinuria, and also slows down the progression to end stage renal failure and development of glomerulosclerosis in SCD. However it requires intense work and further clarifications of its safety in order to enhance confidence in its usage in adult SCD in Nigeria. It's high cost and the perceived complications also influence its usage for adult SCD with proteinuria in Africa and particularly in Nigeria.

INTRODUCTION

What is Sickle Cell Disease

Sickle cell disease remains the commonest genetic disorder with significant geographical and racial predilection principally affecting blacks. It results from a single base-pair DNA mutation in the globin gene. This leads to the formation of an abnormal haemoglobin tetramer, haemoglobin S. This inheritance could be in double form termed homozygous or in various combinations with normal haemoglobin termed sickle cell trait or with other abnormal globin chains. The various combination of these mutations result in various hemoglobinopathies with variegated presentations and clinical outcomes [1,2]. The abnormality in the synthesis of the α and β chains quantitatively of the haemoglobin gene could combine with various sickled haemoglobins to produce various forms of the diseases. When inherited with HbS, it results in HBS-thalassemia which could be major or minor depending on the quantity or quality of the α and β chains produced [1,3].

The abnormal sickled haemoglobin and allied qualitative and quantitative changes in the globin chains alter the physiochemical property of the haemoglobin with resultant variable presentations and complications of SCD. The combination of all these inheritable haemoglobin disorders is termed Sickle Cell Disease. The commonest and most devastating of them is called Sickle Cell Anaemia (SCA) which has double SS Haemoglobin (HbSS) inheritance [1,3].

EPIDEMIOLOGY, PRESENTATIONS AND COMPLICATIONS OF SICKLE CELL DISEASE

Sickle Cell Disease is one of the commonest inherited disorders all over the world affecting over 200 million people. The occurrences of the abnormal gene and its polymorphism have been shown to relate to migration pressure with its origin in Africa [4]. Sickle cell disease has been recognized in Africa and described in West Africa by various local names [5,6], centuries before it was discovered in 1904 and reported by Dr Herrick in 1910 [7]. It was called Äbiku"and "Ogbanje" respectively by the Yorubas and Igbos in Nigeria. In Ghana, the Ga called it Chwechechue, Ahotuitui in Twi, Nuidudui by the Ewe and Anniwi by the Fante tribes (Kotoney.Ahulu) [2].

Most countries do not have exact figures for SCD prevalence, but estimates suggests that there are 12,000 persons with SCD in United Kingdom [8], and about 72,000 in the United States [9].

In the USA, one out of 600 black Americans has HBSS disease and 8% of the same population are carriers [5]. It is also present in other European countries such as France, Greece, Turkey, Cyprus and Italy. Other countries where SCD have been reported in sizeable proportion are Sicily, Israel, Latin and South America, the Middle East, Riyadh and the South East part of India [1,2]. In Nigeria, 3% of the population have SCA, while 25% have the sickle cell disease trait [10]. This large pool of carriers provides the reservoir for the sustenance of the disease. The global spread of this chronic disease portends the impact of its global socio-economic burden [11].

The clinical presentations of SCD are protean and variable depending on the type of inheritance. In SCA which is the most studied, clinical presentations are age-specific and modulated by various factors including socio economic status, age and access to health care. In childhood, presentations could take various forms which include polyuria, dactylitis (termed hand and foot syndrome), chronic anemia, failure to thrive, increased susceptibility to infections and acute splenic sequestration crisis [12-14]. In adults, the severity of these symptoms and signs are reduced but other complications in tandem with the chronicity of vaso-occlusive crisis occur such as increased GFR, acute pulmonary syndrome due to infarction at the pulmonary bed manifesting as chest pain, fever, cough and pulmonary infiltrates on chest radiograph, leg ulcer, stroke, nephrotic syndrome, chronic kidney disease leading to end stage renal failure (ESRF), skeletal abnormalities, infertility problems, relative hypertension which does not increase with age and other cardiovascular abnormalities [15-19].

The asplenic phenomenon in SCD leads to increased susceptibility to infection particularly encapsulated organisms like Streptococcus pneumonia and Salmonella species. A cohort study in Uganda showed that Staphylococcus Aureus was implicated in 60% of the cohorts studied and followed up as against 19% with streptococcus pneumonaie [20]. This finding queries the rationale for the general use of pneumococcal vaccine in African SCD patients. This also gives credence to the postulate that treatment of SCD would vary from area to area, even if within the same geographical expanse [21]. For example, in Nigeria, it has been shown that the presentations and responses to treatment by the Bini tribe in the South-South part of the country are different from the Yoruba tribe in the Western part of the same country [22]. The haplotype influences variability in manifestations and complications. There are three distinct haplotypes; the Senegalese haplotype mostly common in Atlantic West Africa, the Benin/Algeria haplotype which is domicile mainly among Arab and North Africans and the Bantu/Central Africa haplotype originating from the Central Africa [23]. Furthermore, Powars et al has shown that the Central African haplotype in African-Americans predisposes or has an enhanced risk of developing chronic renal failure [24]. The latter has been shown to influence renal complications in SCD [25-27].

The Renin Angiotensin Cascade

Renin-Angiotensin-Aldosterone-System (RAAS) consists of a cascade of proteolytic events leading to the formation of angiotensin II (Ang II). Hypoperfusion and hypoxia stimulate the release of renin, an enzyme produced by the macula densa cells in juxta glomerular apparatus that cleaves Angiotensinogen present in circulation into Angiotensin I which lacks biological activity [28]. Angiotensin converting enzyme has two isotypes, ACE1 and ACE2. The ACE1 isotype does the final conversion of Angiotensin I to Angiotensin II, a pro-fibrotic molecule with strong vasoconstrictor properties. ACE inhibition therefore reduces Angiotensin II activity and therefore protects against Angiotensin II receptor–mediated effects such as vasoconstriction, cell growth and proliferation and inflammation [29].

The ACE1 is the enzyme involved in the cleavage of Angiotensin I to Angiotensin II. It is the larger somatic form which has two metalloproteinase terminals; the C and N terminals. The C terminal domain is important for blood pressure regulation. Angiotensin II binds to AT1 receptor to invoke vasoconstriction of the smooth muscle. In the kidneys it binds to AT1 receptor to influence sodium ion reabsorption leading to water retention and increase in blood pressure [30,31]. The effective inhibition of this powerful vasoconstrictor would definitely have profound effects in reducing blood pressure. In addition to this, it affects the glomerular permeability.

Moreover, Angiotensin II has direct effects on vascular tone by stimulating vascular smooth muscle contraction, thus increasing both systemic and intraglomerular pressures. It also stimulates the release of aldosterone, a strong mineralocorticoid secreted from zona glomerulosa of adrenal cortex and causing avid sodium reabsorption from distal convoluted tubules and collecting ducts [32]. It is also a pro-fibrotic cytokine that encourages the stimulation of growth factors leading to laying down of collagen with consequent fibrosis [29,30].

Ang II also has significant effects on intrarenal haemodynamics leading to increase in the filtration of protein and trafficking of macromolecules across the glomeruli. It also stimulates cell growth leading to fibrosis [30]. Thus, the activation of the RAAS plays a major role in the relentless progression of kidney diseases to end stage renal disease (ESRD) [29]. This has been clearly demonstrated in hypertensive nephrosclerosis, diabetic nephropathy and various glomerulonephritides but less so defined in patients with SCD [28-32].

The discovery of angiotensin converting enzyme inhibitors (ACEIs), [28], and the findings of its salutary effects in the management of patients with hypertension, diabetes and glomerulopathies have opened a new frontier for its trials in SCD patients [31,32]. ACEIs are effective drugs in retarding progression of renal injury. This is achieved through the blockage of the conversion of Angiotensin I to Angiotensin II. This leads in part to better control of hypertension, reduction in secondary hyperaldosteronism with consequent regression or blockage of fibrotic changes [31,32]. Of note, vitamin D, which is naturally present in the skin of blacks and which occurs as vitamin D3 following exposure to sunlight, has been reported to reduce high blood pressure by interacting with Angiotensin II. It inhibits rennin hence interfering with the RAAS [33]. It would be of interest to investigate the impact of race vis a viz this mechanism, on the potentiation of ACEI effects in blacks and and in patients with SCD.

Pathophysiological Basis of the Use of ACEI in the Management of SCD

The physiochemical changes in the sickle haemoglobin into tactoid gelatinized structure on exposure to low oxygen state is the basis of the cascade of inflammatory events followed by responses and repairs with the consequential changes resulting in various complications of the disease. The normal haemoglobin HbA and sickle haemoglobin HbS have the same solubility under normal conditions. However when there is de-oxygenation, the solubility of haemoglobin S is altered, thereby blocking blood flow and causing stasis which further promotes hypoxia and acidosis [34].

In the process, there is vascular endothelial damage with resultant interplay of pro-inflammatory cytokines induction such as IL-1, Il-6, TNF-α, EGF, TGF and the response by the restorative cytokines like Insulin-like Growth Factor, Fibroblast Growth Factor (FBG), Transforming Growth Factor (TGF-β), Platelet derived Growth Factor (PDGF). Also involved in these interactions are the adhesion molecules with their surface receptors on leucocytes and endothelin which mediate transcellular signals [35]. This process does not spare the Angiotensin Aldosterone System which plays an active role in this cascade. The Angiotensin II (AII) up regulates TGF-β which leads to tissue fibrosis [35,36]. These actions and reactions are well elaborated in the lung, brain, kidney and skeletal tissues. In-spite of these processes, the role of ACEIs in SCD patients with hyperfiltration remains to be established.

In the kidney, the polymerization of sickled red blood corpuscles on exposure to low oxygen is enhanced at the renal medulla by its hypertonic environment. Vascular obstruction occurs with attendant stasis within the plexus. This leads to vascular injury via endothelial damage and adhesion. Some of the cytokines involved in this cascade are mitogenic to glomerular mesangial cells, including PDGF [37]. The cell free plasma haemoglobin which is released from the destroyed red blood cell in SCD contributes to the vascular resistance and resistance to blood flow by inhibiting NO in the vasculature of SCD. This dsyregulation of endothelium-derived vasodilator: vasoconstrictor system leads to vasoconstriction and proliferative vasculopathy in SCD [38].

The resolution of these reactions and interactions leads to various pathological manifestations including hyperfiltration (markedly increased GFR) which characterises the manifestation of kidney disease in children with SCD. However, renal plasma flow is elevated to an even greater extent than is GFR, so the filtration fraction is lower in patients with SCD than in healthy individuals [39,40]. One explanation for this discrepancy is that increased cortical blood flow, caused by prostanglandin-induced vasodilation decreases filtration by limiting effluent diffusion from rapidly flowing plasma. Hyperfiltration together with endothelial damage through vaso-occlusion by sickled cells might lead to endothelial hyperplasia and ultimately glomerular fibrosis [41].

Transgenic mice made sickled have been shown to induce nitric oxide synthase II in the glomerular and distal nephron. The concomitant increase of nitric oxide is postulated to be responsible for the intense vasodilatation and hyperfiltration that is observed in SCD [43]. Hyperfiltration leads to glomerular hypertrophy which could promote glomerulosclerosis under various conditions. This glomerular hyperfiltration mediates proteinuria. This has been confirmed by the reduction of proteinuria with angiotensin converting enzyme inhibitor [44]. The prevalence of hypertension is relatively low in Sickle Cell Disease, at about 2-6%, when compared with the prevalence of hypertension in blacks in the USA [17]. The prevalence of hypertension is also reported to be low in Nigerian SCD patients [45,46].

Management of Sickle Cell Disease Patients and the Role of ACE Inhibition

The approach to the management of SCD involves the management of the symptoms as well as managing the pathological consequences of SCD with its complications. The former includes prevention of crisis, treatment of pain, and increasing total body fluid by infusion of liberal fluids and blood transfusion. The latter encompasses the use of Erythropoietin (EPO) and Hydroxyurea [27]. There is a suggestion by Fitzhugh et al that combination therapy of ACEI and Hydroxyurea may be beneficial. They managed 3 patients with combination therapy including Enalapril and Hydroxyurea and found improvement in proteinuria to near normal levels [47].

Stem cell and gene therapy, and the inhibition of RAAS system with ACEIs have found various uses in patients with SCD even though some of the indications have not been extensively studied [48,49]. SCD patients have chronic anaemia and consequently exhibit a hyperdynamic circulation which imposes volume and pressure loads on the heart leading to increased myocardial contractility, chamber enlargement and wall hypertrophy with resulting increase in left ventricular mass. Left ventricular hypertrophy has been found to be a cardiovascular predictor of mortality. Another common cardiovascular disease in SCD patients is pulmonary hypertension [50,16].

Furthermore, sickle cell disease also adversely affects the kidneys with increasing age with children manifesting hyperfiltration while microalbuminria, overt proteinuria, reduction in glomerular filtration rate and end stage renal failure, set in later [51,52]. ACEIs have been found to be useful in reducing proteinuria and microalbuminuria as well as retardation of progression of chronic kidney disease in patients with SCD [53]. Proteinuria is common in SCD, and is present in up to 30-40% of adult patients [54]. The proportion of SCD patients with proteinuria and renal insufficiency increases with increasing age, though only about 3-5% of patients have nephrotic range proteinuria and about the same proportion have end stage renal disease. Nephrotic syndrome in SCD is a recognised predictor of progression to chronic renal failure [55].

ACEIs have been found to reduce the degree of proteinuria in SCD patients with nephropathy. In two non-randomized studies, Enalapril was found to reduce urinary albumin excretion in patients with sickle cell disease who have microalbuminuria or proteinuria. Falk and colleagues conducted a 2 week trial with Enalapril therapy in 10 SCD patients with mild nephropathy, showed that proteinuria decreased by 57%, but proteinuria returned to high levels after treatment withdrawal [56]. Similarly, Aoki et al observed a decline in overt albuminuria to normal in 75% of the patients studied [57]. However, these studies were not blinded, randomized or placebo-controlled [56,57]. Foucan et al in a randomized controlled trial reported a decrease in albuminuria and blood pressure in patients with sickle cell disease who had microalbuminuria after receiving Captopril over a period of 6 months [58]. These authors argued for a specific antiproteinuric effect of ACE inhibitors while others think that this effect cannot be dissociated from its effects on blood pressure [55-57].

Rosenberg has recently demonstrated in a 4 years prospective study, that ACEI treatment in hypertensives is associated with a 10% reduction in all-cause mortality [59]. The benefit of ACEIs is thought to be secondary to a decrease in activity of the renin-angiotensin system but systemic alterations in renin and/or Angiotensin II have been difficult to document in two chronic models of progressive glomerulosclerosis. Moreover, normal renin and aldosterone values are found in sickle cell anaemia both under standard and volume depleted conditions. This paradox could be explained by an intrarenal angiotensin axis separate from the systemic one, thereby reducing proteinuria without affecting blood pressure [60]. Also ACE inhibition has been found to reduce pain during sickle cell crisis [61].

Thus ACE inhibition is particularly indicated in SCD for reducing hyperfiltration, glomerular hypertension, treating relative arterial hypertension, reducing the incidence of stroke, treatment of pain and is indicated to modulate and limit the rate of sclerosis of tissue since Angiotensin II up-regulated Fibroblast Growth Factor. Furthermore, pathological evidence shows that interstitial fibrosis which leads to tubular atrophy can be attenuated by angiotensin converting enzyme inhibition [64].

Safety of ACEIs in SCD

ACEIs have various known adverse effects and the SCD patients are not excluded from these problems. However, of all the recognised adverse effects of ACEIs, only hyperkalemia has been found to limit its uses in a few anecdotal reports. Mckie et al observed that hyperkalemia developed in 4 of 9 patients treated with ACEIs, and resulted in discontinuation of treatment in 3 children [64]. Children with HbSS may be particularly at risk for hyperkalemia as they have preserved tubular function unlike adults with SCD. Higher serum potassium levels and lower fractional excretion of potassium have been documented in children with HbSS.

Conclusion

In spite of the fact that SCD is predominant and originated from Africa, the documented cases and literature on it were scanty until the late thirties and forties. Hence, it is not surprising that the use of adequate measures to prevent and treat the condition including ACEIs are not well documented in spite of its usefulness being both potentially renoprotective and cardio-protective in adult SCD patients. A little reduction in proteinuria and slowing of progression to ESRD translates in absolute terms to huge savings in cost when the huge population of prospective patients are considered. This is in addition to the resultant improvement in quality of life among millions of adults with SCD in Nigeria. The untoward effects of ACEIs particularly the chronic cough, angioedema and hyperkalaemia are issues to be considered in balancing the advantages of using ACEIs in adult SCD patients. The improvement in medical care of patients with SCD has yielded a significant adult population of SCD patients that would benefit from the advantage of using ACEIs in limiting the progression and complication of SCD in Africa. The risk of developing renal disease in SCD has been shown to be enhanced by the presence of a myosin heavy chain 9 non-muscle MYH9 and APOL1 genes (haplotype) located on chromosome 22q13 which have been shown to increase the risk of developing FSGS and HIVAN in Africans [65]. This might have contributed to the high prevalence of renal complications in Africans with SCD. These two genes had earlier been associated with the risk of developing nephropathy in black hypertensives.

REFERENCES

[1] Sickle Cell Disease. Serjeant G. 1985. *Oxford university Press* (epidemiology

[2] Kotoney – Ahulu FID The sickle cell from myths to molecules by Eldelstein Book review. *Tropical Diseases Bullentin.* 1986 85: 511 – 513

[3] Fairbanks VF: The 'common' hemoglobin variants. *Hemoglobinopathies and Thalassemia.* New York, Decker, 1980, pp 10–14.

[4] Serjeant GR (ed). Sickle Cell Disease. *Oxford University Press: Oxford,* 1992, pp 261–281.

[5] Angastiniotis M, Modell B. Global Epidemiology of Hemoglobin Disorders. *Annals of the New York Academy of Sciences* 1998;850:251-69.

[6] Kotoney – Ahulu FID. The spectrum of phenotypic expression of clinical hemoglobinopathies in West Africa. *New Istanbul contribution to clinical science* 12; 246 – 257

[7] Herrick JB: Peculiar elongated and sickle-shaped red blood corpuscles in a case of severe anemia. *Arch Intern Med* 1910;6:517–520.

[8] Streetly A, Maxwell K, Mejia A. 1997. Fair shares for London report. Sickle cell disorders in greater London: A needs assessment of screening and care services. London: United Medical and Dental Schools; Department of Public Health Medicine.

[9] Bonds DR. Three decades of innovation in the management of sickle cell disease: The road to understanding the sickle cell disease clinical phenotype. *Blood Reviews* 2005. 19:99-110.

[10] Serjeant GR, Serjeant BE. Sickle Cell Disease 3 rd ed. *Oxford University Press* 2001.

[11] Akinyanju O, Johnson AO. Acute illness in Nigerian children with Sickle Cell Anemia. *Ann. Trop. Paedir.* 1987;7: 181-186.

[12] Voskaridou E, Terpos E, Michail S, Hantzi E,Ananquostopoulos A, Margel A Simirloglou D Loukopolous D Papassortirou I. *Early markers of renal dysfunction in patients with Sickle/β-thallassemia. KI.* 2006;693: 2037 – 2042.

[13] Statius van Eps LW, Pinedo-Veels C, De Vries GH, De Koning J. Nature of concentrating defect in sickle cell nephropathy. Microradioangiographic studies. *Lancet* 1970; 1: 450–452.

[14] Steinberg MH. 2005. Predicting clinical severity in sickle cell anaemia. *British Journal of Haematology* 129:465-81.

[15] Aderibigbe A, Arije AS, Akinkugbe OO. Glomerular function in Sickle Cell Disease patients during crisis. *Afri J. Med Med Sci. 1994* 23: 153 – 160.

[16] Castro O, Brambilla DJ, Thorington B, et al. The acute chest syndrome in sickle cell disease: incidence and risk factors. The Cooperative *Study of Sickle Cell Disease. Blood* 1994;84:643-649.

[17] Pegelow CH, Colangelo L, Steinberg M, Wright EC, Smith J, Phillips G, Vichinsky E. 1997. Natural history of blood pressure in sickle cell disease: Risks for stroke and death associated with relative hypertension in sickle cell anemia. *American Journal of Medicine* 102:171-177.

[18] Sklar AH, Campbell H, Carnana BJ, Lightfoot BO, Gaier JG, Milroof. A population study of renal function in SCA. *Int J. Artif. Organs* 1990; 13,231 – 236.

[19] Allon M. Renal abnormalities in sickle cell disease. *Arch Intern Med* 1990; 150: 501–504.

[20] Ebah LM. Renal involvement in sickle cell Disease: an African perspective for an African condition. *CKJ.* 2013; 1: 6-7.

[21] Ayanniyi O. Musculoskeletal complications and general Health status of individual with SCD. *NJMR.* 2006, 11: 65-71

[22] Schnog JB, Duits AJ, Muskiet FA, Ten Cate H, Rojer RA, Brandjes DP. 2004. Sickle cell disease; a general overview. *Netherlands Journal of Medicine* 62:364-374.

[23] Styllianos EA, Stuart HO, Haig HK., Sabra CG, Corinne DB, Pamela GW, Julianne PS Harry O, Virgil FF, Aravinda C. Evidence for multiple origins of the β E-globin gene in South-East Asia. *Proc. Natl. Acad. Sci. USA.* 1982;79:6606-6611.

[24] Powars DR, Elliot-Mills DD, Chan L, Hisi AL, Opas LM, Johnson C. Chronic renal failure in sickle cell disease: Risk factors, clinical course and mortality. *Ann Intern Med* 1991;115:614-620.

[25] Steinberg MH. Management of sickle cell disease. *New England Journal of Medicine.* 1999. 340:1021-30.

[26] Abbott KC, Hypolite IO, Ogodoa LY. Sickle cell nephropathy at end stage renal disease in the United States: Patient characteristics and survival. *Clin Nephrol* 2002;58(1):9-15.

[27] Powars DR, Chan LS, Hiti A, Ramicone E, Johnson C. Outcome of sickle cell anemia: a 4-decade observational study of 1056 patients. *Medicine.* (Baltimore) 2005;85:363-76.

[28] Skeggs,LT, Dorer FE, Kahn JR, Lentz KE, Levin M. Experimental renal hypertension: the discovery of the Renin-Angiotensin system. *Biochemical Regulation of Blood Pressure.* 1981 Soffer, R eds. John Wiley & Sons Inc Hoboken. 3-38.

[29] Brew K. Structure of human ACE gives new insights into inhibitor binding and design. *Trends Pharmacol Sci.* 2003;24(8): 391 394.

[30] Natesh R, Schwager SL, Sturrock ED, Acharya KR. Crystal structure of the human Angiotensin –converting enzyme –lisinopril complex. *Nature.* 2003; 421(6922): 551 554.

[31] Weir MR. The Effects of renin-Angiotensin system inhibition on end-organ protection: can we do better?. *Clin Ther.* 2007;29(9):1803-1824.

[32] Van Vark LC, Bertrand M, Akkerhuis Km, et al. Angiotensin-converting enzyme inhibitors reduce mortality in hypertension: A meta-analysis of randomised clinical trials of rennin-Angiotensin-Aldosterone system inhibitors involving 158998 patients. *Eur. Herat J.* 2012: DOI:10, 1093-http://eurheartj.oxfordjournals.org.

[33] Eckle Holger Eltzschig. Sunlight protect heart attack by activating Period -2 protein *Nature medicine*. 2012. April 15.

[34] Poillon WN, Kim BC, Castro O. 1998. Intracellular hemoglobin S polymerization and the clinical severity of sickle cell anemia. *Blood* 91:1777-1783.

[35] Kaul KD, Fabry ME, Nagel RL. Microvascular sites and characteristics of sickle cell adhesion to vascular endothelium in shear flow conditions; pathophysiological implications. *Proc Nalt Acad Sci (USA)* 1989; 86:3356 – 3360.

[36] Mohtat R,Thomas Z,Du Z,Moulton T,Driscoll C,Woroniccki R, Urinary Tranforming Growth Factor β1 as a marker of renal dysfunction in sickle cell Di7ease. *Paedric Nephrol.* 2011;26: 275 -280.

[37] Floege J, Topley N, Hoppe J, Barrett TB, Resch K. Mitogenic effect of platelet-derived growth factor in human glomerular mesangial cells: modulation and/or suppression by inflammatory cytokines. *Clin Exp Immunol.* 1991;86(2):334-41.

[38] Reiter CD, Wang X, Tanus-Santos JE, et al. Cell- free hemoglobin limits nitric oxide bioavalability in sickle cell Disease. *Nat. Med.* 2002;8:1383-1389.

[39] de Jong PE and Statins van Eps. Sickle cell nephropathy: new insights into its pathophysiology. *Kidney Int.*1985;27:711-717.

[40] Allon M et al. Effects of nonsteroidal anti-inflammatory drugs on renal function in sickle cell anaemia. *Kidney Int.*1988; 34:500-506.

[41] Buckalew VM and Someren A. Renal manifestation of sickle cell disease. *Nephron.* 1974; 133:660-669.

[42] Kaul DK, Liu XD, Fabry ME, Nagel RL. Impaired nitric oxide mediated -vasodilatation in transgenic sickle mouse. *Am J. Physiol Heart Circ Physiol.* 2000;278: H1799 - H1806.

[43] Bank N, Aynedran HS, Qiu JH, Osei SY, Ahima RS, Fabry ME, Nagel RL: Renal nitric oxide synthases in transgenic sickle cell mice. *Kidney Int* 1996;50:184–189.

[44] Falk RJ, Scheinman J, Phillips G *et al.* Prevalence and pathologic features of sickle cell nephropathy and response to inhibition of angiotensin-converting enzyme. *N Engl J Med* 1992; 326: 910–915.

[45] Aderibigbe A, Omotoso AB, Awobusuyi JO, Akande TM. Arterial blood pressure in adult Nigerian sickle cell anaemia patients. *West Afr J Med.*1999; 18 (2):114-8.

[46] Arogundade FA, Sanusi A.A., Hassan M.O., Salawu L., Durosinmi M.A., Akinsola A. (2011) An Appraisal of Kidney Dysfunction and Its Risk Factors in Patients with Sickle Cell Disease. *Nephron Clin Pract.* 118: c225-c231 (DOI: 10.1159/000321138).

[47] Fitzhugh CD, Wigfall DR, Ware RE. Enalapril and Hydroxyurea therapy for children with sickle nephropathy. *Pediatr Blood Cancer.* 2005; 45:982-985.

[48] Ilesanmi OO. Sickle Cell Disease and Stem Cell: Implications for psychotherapy and Genetic counseling in Africa Medicine and Stem. *Cell Research " innovation in stem cell Book eds Demier T.T* (51) pp 978-953. Published CC BY.

[49] Lima CS, Ueti OM, Ueti AA, Francini KG, Costa FF, Saad ST. Enalapril therapy and cardiac remodelling in sickle cell disease patients. *Acta Cardiol.* 2008;63(5):599-602.

[50] Ristow B, Schiller NB. Pulmonary hypertension in Sickle Cell Disease. *New Engl J Med* 2011;365:1645-1649.

[51] Falk RJ, Jenettle JC: Sickle cell nephropathy. *Adv. Nephrol Necker Hosp.* 1994; 23: 133-147.

[52] Alvarez O, Lopez-Mitnik G, Zilleruelo G: Short-term follow-up of patients with sickle cell disease and albuminuria. *Pediatr Blood Cancer* 2008;50:1236–1239.

[53] Sasongko Th, Nagalla S. Balla SK. Angiotensin Converting Enzyme for proteinuria and microalbuminuria in people with sickle cell Disease. *Cochrane Database Sys. Rev.* 2013 3 CD009191.

[54] Bolarinwa RA, Akinlade KS, Kuti M, Olawale OO. Akiola NO. Renal Disease in Adult Nigerians with Sickle Cell Anaemia: A prevalence, clinical features and risk factors. *Saudi J. Kidney Dis* 2012;23:171 -175.

[55] Pardo V. Kramer H, Levi D, Strauss J. Glomerular change in patients with Sickle Cell Disease and Nephrotic Syndrome. *Am J.pathol* 1973, 70 49.

[56] Falk RJ, Scheinman J, Philip G, Orringer E, Johnson A, Jennetta C. Prevalence and pathological features of SCN and response to inhibition of ACE. *NEJM* 1992: 326, 347 – 351.

[57] Aoki RY, Saad ST. Enalapril reduces the albuminuria of patients with sickle cell disease. *Am J Med.*1995; 98:432-435.

[58] Foucan L, Bourhis V, Bangon J, et al. A randomized trial of captopril for microalbuminuria in normotensive adults with sickle cell disease. *Am J Med.* 1998; 104: 339-342.

[59] Rosenberg ME, Smith LJ, Correa-Rotter R, Hosteller TH. The paradox of the renin-angiotensin system in chronic renal disease. *Kidney Int.* 1994; 45:403-410.

[60] De Jong PE, Statins van Eps LW. Sickle cell nephropathy: new insight into its pathophysiology. *Kidney Int.* 1985; 27:711-717.

[61] Williams RM, Moskowitz DW. The prevention of pain from sickle cell disease by trandolapril. *J Natl Med Assoc.* 2007;99 (3): 276-278.

[62] De Jong LE, Landman H. Statius Van Eps L.W. Blood pressure in Sickle Cell Disease. *Arch intern Med.* 1982; 142: 1239 – 1240.

[63] Rodgers GP, Walker EC, Podgor MJ. Is "Relative" Hypertension a risk factor for vaso-occlusive complications in sickle cell disease? *American Journal of Medicine Science.* 1993. 305:150-156.

[64] Mckie KT, Hanevold VD, Hernandez C, et al. Prevalence, Prevention and treatment of microalbuminuria and proteinuria in children with sickle cell disease. *J Pediatr Hematol Oncol.* 2007; 29 (3): 140-144.

[65] Ashley-Koch AE, Okocha EC, Garrett ME, Soldano K, De Castro LM, Jonassaint JC. MYH9 and APOL1 are both associated with sickle cell nephropathy. *Br. J. Hematol.* 2011; 155(3): 386-394.

SECTION 3. NEW AND EMERGING INDICATIONS FOR ACE INHIBITORS AND ANGIOTENSIN RECEPTOR BLOCKERS

In: ACE Inhibitors. Volume 2
Editor: Macaulay Amechi Onuigbo
ISBN: 978-1-62948-422-8

Chapter 19

HYPERTENSION-MISATTRIBUTED KIDNEY DISEASE IN AFRICAN AMERICANS

Karl Skorecki, MD FRCP(C) FASN*[*1] and Walter G. Wasser, MD[2]

[1]Rappaport Faculty of Medicine and Research Institute, Technion - Israel Institute of Technology, Rambam Health Care Campus, Haifa, Israel

[2]Rambam Health Care Campus, Haifa, Israel

ABSTRACT

It has recently been demonstrated that African ancestry populations develop kidney disease previously misattributed to hypertension, but now more properly understood to be related to powerful kidney risk variants in the chromosome 22 region containing the gene for APOL1. The African American Study of Kidney Disease (AASK) trial and cohort follow-up studies resolved the "chicken and egg" conundrum of hypertension as a cause of secondary kidney disease or a consequence of primary kidney disease, but only at the therapeutic intervention level. The epidemiologic studies did not shed light on a potential solution to the failure of blood pressure control to effectively slow kidney injury. Addition of genetics to the AASK datasets has now provided an important clue. Analysis of genotypes at the newly appreciated APOL1 risk region for non-diabetic kidney disease, in the combined case-control cohorts of more than 1,200 individuals, provides further strong evidence that the expectation that effective blood pressure control in the major etiologic category of chronic kidney disease with hypertension designated in the past as "hypertensive nephrosclerosis" would slow progression, has been overly simplistic. Rather, many of these African-ancestry individuals should be designated instead under a new category of APOL1-genetic region associated chronic kidney disease with secondary hypertension. The clinical implications are enormous and mandate urgency in a multi-team and interdisciplinary effort to unravel the mechanisms whereby the genetic risk interacts with environmental triggers to cause progressive kidney disease accompanied by dangerous hypertension. Recent research postulates a role for intrarenal angiotensin converting enzyme (ACE) as a downstream target for APOL1. Furthermore, it raises the testable hypothesis that African ancestry individuals with hypertensive kidney disease without APOL1 risk allele variants may respond to hypertension treatment

* Correponding author: Karl Skorecki MD FRCP(C) FASN; Email: skorecki@tx.technion.ac.il.

paradigms that presently apply to non-Africans. For example, such individuals may manifest a favorable response to ACE-inhibition. This novel formulation raises the optimistic possibility that nephropathic viral triggers can be identified and treated, toprevent hypertension secondary to kidney disease in persons at genetic risk.

1. Hypertension in African Americans

Essential hypertension is not a single disorder but a collection of disorders that when untreated results in cardiovascular, cerebrovascular and kidney disease. Different pathogenesis and clinical characteristics have been observed in diverse population groups. Patients of African ancestry more commonly develop hypertension [1], at an earlier age that is more severe, more often "salt sensitive" with renin suppression, and manifesting a higher incidence and prevalence of target organ damage [2]. Pathophysiologic features include delayed excretion of a salt load, elevated red blood cell intracellular sodium concentration, reduced renal blood flow and increased catecholamine sensitivity [2]. Comparison with other population groups has consistently shown that treatment with renin-angiotensin blockers is generally less effective in African ancestry patients than calcium channel blockers and diuretics [3,4]. In resistant hypertension, aldosterone blockers may be useful as an additional agent and hyperaldosteronism may contribute to salt sensitive hypertension [5].

2. Hypertension and Chronic Kidney Disease in African Americans

Despite the fact that the hypertension of African Americans is more responsive to monotherapy with calcium channels blockers and diuretics than ACE-inhibitors, African Americans with chronic kidney disease (CKD) show clear benefit from ACE-inhibitors usually in combination with other anti-hypertensive agents. This was shown in the African American Study of Kidney Disease and Hypertension (AASK) [6].

An analysis of a total of 1094 patients with hypertension, otherwise unexplained chronic kidney disease and mild proteinuria (mean about 500-600 mg per day) indicates a histologic pattern compatible with hypertensive nephrosclerosis in this population [7]. The patients were treated with one of three drugs: ramipril, metoprolol, or amlodipine, while targeting one of two blood pressure goals, 125/75 or 140/90. The primary end point was the rate of change of GFR; the secondary endpoint was a secondary clinical composite of reduction in GFR of 50%, actual decrease in GFR of 25 mL/min per 1.73 m^2, onset of end-stage kidney failure, or death. At study end, the mean rate of change in GFR and secondary composite end point was similar with both blood pressure goals, suggesting that lower blood pressure would not further slow progression of kidney disease. There was however, a non-significant trend favoring lower blood pressure in patients with higher proteinuria at baseline. However, among the different anti-hypertensive agents, patients receiving ramapril had significantly decreased risk of secondary outcomes compared to patients treated with metoprolol or amlodipine [8]. As a result of the AASK finding, consensus recommendations were expanded to include the use of ACE inhibitors for proteinuric CKD to include kidney protection in African Americans with hypertensive nephrosclerosis [9].

3. High Rate of Subsequent ESKD in AASK Patients

Of the initial trial participants, 691 (90%) were followed for an additional cohort phase. During 11 years of follow up, the rate of ESKD (3.9/100 patient-years) was significantly higher than rates of total mortality (2.2/100 patient years) and CVD mortality (0.8/100 patient years). The incident rate of ESKD to CVD mortality was 5.0. This was despite the fact that 84% of AASK cohort patients received renin-angiotensin blockers [10]. This is consistent with the general observation of nephrologists in North America that African Americans with hypertension associated kidney disease display a poor long term kidney protective response to medications that effectively lower arterial blood pressure compared to non-Africans.

The AASK studies strongly suggest that an underlying factor(s) other than hypertension *per se* might be responsible for chronic kidney disease risk with hypertension as an accompaniment, at least among African-Americans. The epidemiologic inference is further strengthened by the strikingly different histopathology in the kidneys of African versus non-African ancestry individuals, clinically labeled with “hypertensive nephrosclerosis” [11]. The foregoing would not be expected if a single disease entity were present.

4. Population Genetics and the Discovery of the APOL1 Locus

The discovery of the APOL1 kidney disease locus really goes back to the initial studies of Ferguson R et al. [12], and Freedman BI et al. [13], regarding the familial clustering of CKD and the 4 to 5 fold increased risk for End-Stage Kidney Disease (ESKD) in African Americans over the general population [14]. This led Freedman to postulate the existence of overarching renal susceptibility genes [15].

How did we advance from the bold hypothesis of the existence of such an overarching genetic susceptibility locus in early 1990s to its discovery three years ago?. The answer to this question requires an understanding of certain principles of population genetics and evolutionary medicine. Reviews of the population genetics of the APOL1 discovery have been published recently [16,17].

In human genetics, a population is described as a group of people who share genome-wide or genetic locus specific ancestry as demonstrated by genetic variation markers which define “population genetic architecture” [18]. There are many categories of such markers. The choices and combinations utilized in a given study depend on the scientific question of interest [19]. SNVs are single nucleotide variants caused by a base pair substitution in the germ-line of an individual, which is then propagated in his other descendants [20]. For any given SNV, the combination of occurrence at a given nucleotide site and its propagation to a substantial number of descendants, has usually occurred only once in the short course of human evolutionary history. When an SNV has risen in frequency to a conventional global frequency cutoff of 1%, it is often designated as a Single Nucleotide Polymorphism (SNP). Globally there are ~18 million SNPs [20]. Any pair of individuals differs in only a subset, perhaps 3 million out of a total of ~3.2 billion nucleotides in the human genome [20]. Most of these different SNVs/SNPs do not have any phenotypic effects. Their allele frequencies in different parts of the world are influenced by demographic history. However, even without phenotypic effects, these SNP differences can be used to infer demographic history and as signposts in disease gene mapping. A small percentage of SNVs do encode health and disease phenotypes [21]. In such cases, population frequency may be influenced by adaptive selection in response to environmental challenges: nutritional, climactic and by far most powerfully, by microbial pathogens. In terms of disease gene mapping, SNVs and other markers have been used successfully in positional cloning and identifying causal mutations using family based linkage approaches now in combination with, or supplanted by whole exome mapping [22]. At the population level, the results of many hundreds of genome-wide association studies (GWAS), performed based on linkage disequilibrium (LD), have been somewhat disappointing, since most loci have yielded low odds ratios and the problem of so-called "missing heritability" [23]. The APOL1 discovery, on the other hand, has been a notable exception due to the power of admixture mapping studies in revealing high effect variants that appear to have risen to high frequency in a given large population under the influence of adaptive selection [22].

When performing a GWAS, a tagging SNV/SNP may be near a causal variant, but meiotic recombination breaks down linkage disequilibrium (LD) and genetic association into smaller and smaller regions making identifying these variants more challenging. Admixture restores this LD genetic association to a wider region and confers to a genome wide approach the power of family based linkage mapping by identifying a large genomic region which is nearly certain to contain a large effect variant [24]. In order for the admixture mapping to succeed, an admixed population is required, as well as disparity in disease frequency between the admixing parental populations, and a causal risk variant that has risen to a high frequency in the at risk parental population. The African American population represents an admixed population between African (~80%) and European (~20%) ancestry [25], with a disease disparity of FSGS and CKD, and contains a causal risk variant. The "overarching genetic risk" hypothesis posited the existence of a "common variant-common disease" model with a large effect size.

Kopp et al, and Kao et al in two simultaneous landmark publications used admixture mapping to discover a region of interest in chromosome 22q [26,27]. In the case of Kopp et al., the disease phenotype of interest for the discovery cohort was FSGS, and included often chronic kidney disease phenotypes, including what was designated as hypertensive nephrosclerosis [26]. In Kao et al., the discovery set disease phenotype included multiple etiologies of non-diabetic ESKD [27]. The initial association was with MYH9, containing at the time the most highly associated tag SNPs and haplotypes (E1 and S1) [28]. However, deep sequencing showed no candidate functional variants within the MYH9 gene itself [28]. *In silico* resequencing more widely within the region, but outside of MYH9, by means of data-mining of the 1000 Genomes Project showed that the MYH9 gene anchored and tagged even more highly associated functional variants in the adjacent gene, APOL1 missense haplotype, Ser342Gly and Ile384MeT (designated as G1) and a truncation deletion del.N388/Y389 (designated as G2) [29,30]. These APOL1 variants explain more strongly the disease phenotypes, than the variants in MYH9. When conditioned against MYH9, APOL1 completely explains the previously observed MYH9 associations [29]. This APOL1 association both explains a population level discrepancy and illustrates a crucial principle of evolutionary medicine [22].

What is the population level discrepancy? We reported many years ago that HIV infected Ethiopian Jews living in Israel exhibit an absence of HIVAN and a low prevalence of chronic kidney disease in general [31]. We also found this to be true among Ethiopians living in Ethiopia [32]. Of interest, the MYH9 tag SNPs, both E1 and S1 exhibit an allele frequency of 0.35 in Ethiopia, making the absence of HIVAN there even more intriguing [33]. However, the APOL1 G1 and G2 risk alleles were absent in Ethiopia just like HIVAN was absent in Ethiopia [32]. An evolutionary selection pressure has held MYH9 tagging SNPs in strong LD with APOL1 G1 and G2 which have risen to high frequency in sub-Saharan Africa but not north-East Africa [33].

What is the principle of evolutionary medicine alluded to above? The presence of high risk allele frequency in West Africans is due to the apparent adaptive advantage provided by even a single parental G1 or G2 parental allele against the pathogenicity of *Trypanosoma brucei rhodesiense.* Pays E and Raper J and colleagues, have shown that *Trypanosoma brucei rhodesiense* evades the trypanolytic effect of most forms of circulating apolipoprotein L1, by generating a serum-resistance associated protein, SRA, that binds, sequesters, and confers resistance to trypanolysis [34,35]. APOL1 G1 and G2 variants modify protein structures to overcome the invasion by the SRA of *Trypanosoma Brucei Rhodesiense.* Bioinformatics models predict the G1 and G2 variants to exert a disruptive effect on the SRA binding domain of APOL1 molecule [30]. Furthermore, experiments by Genovese et al. show *in-vitro* killing of *Trypanosoma Brucei Rhodesiense* by APOL1 G1 and G2 variants [29]. The same APOL1 variants in the two allele risk state are associated with and presumably responsible for the development of kidney disease in later life. Additionally, we see the hitchhiking of tag markers in the neighboring genes, including of MYH9. It is this evolutionary force which was conducive to a high odds ratio for a “common variant-common disease”. When one looks at the relationship of allele frequency and effect sizes, rare recent variants tend to be associated with a high risk for disease and are demonstrated in family cloning or whole exome studies, whereas common, ancient variants tend to be associated with low risk for disease and disappointingly low odds ratio (OR) in hundreds of GWAS [24]. The example of APOL1, however, appears to be an exception to this rule, showing a high frequency allele with a high odds ratio as a result of the powerful selection pressure.

5. Hypertension-Misattributed Kidney Disease

Further resolution to the understanding of hypertension-attributed kidney disease in African Americans at the molecular epidemiologic level has been obtained, by relating the AASK findings to the rapidly evolving story of powerful kidney disease risk variants at a chromosome 22q genomic region containing the genes MYH9 and APOL1 [36]. These studies report the G1 and G2 allelic state (as well as genotypes of several other sites in the region and at genome-wide ancestry informative markers) in 675 AASK cases and 618 non-nephropathy controls. The cases were African Americans recruited throughout the United States, between the ages 18 to 70 years of age with diastolic blood pressures >95 mmHg and a measured iothalamate GFR between 20 and 65 ml/min/1.78 m2, indicative CKD. Since non-nephropathy controls were not part of the AASK study cohort, these African American subjects were recruited at Wake Forest School of Medicine and fulfilled the enrollment criteria of serum creatinine concentrations < 1.5 mg/dl in men or < 1.3 mg/dl in women.

Case-control analysis showed a highly significant association of the G1 genotype and the AASK label of "hypertensive nephropathy" under a recessive inheritance model. While ORs are higher in HIVAN and FSGS as noted above, the finding of an OR of 2.57 (1.85-3.55 95% CI), with a p=1.4E^{8} despite the low sample size, can be considered a vindication of the currently much maligned "common disease common variant" formulation. The clinical phenotype of hypertension with chronic kidney disease affects millions worldwide and the associated G1 allele frequencies is well into the "common" range in the population of interest (51% of African Americans carry at least one risk allele) [33]. The association of APOL1 G1 was stronger still with more advanced kidney disease at AASK baseline (UPCR >0.6 g/g), [OR 6.29 (3.92-10.11); p=2.6E-^{14}], or with serum creatinine >3mg/dL during follow up [OR 4.61 (3.14-6.76); p=5.6E-^{15}]. As in previous studies, associations with the lower frequency G2 risk allele were more difficult to prove – perhaps for statistical or possibly biological reasons [37,38].

The authors also analyzed the treatment arms of the original AASK intervention trial 2X3 factorial design to examine the effects of medication class (calcium blocker, angiotensin converting enzyme inhibitor, and beta-blocker), and of intensity of blood pressure control ("usual" – Mean Arterial Pressure (MAP) < 102-107 mmHg versus "low" – MAP < 92). There was no observable influence of APOL1 genotype on achieved blood pressure in the usual or low intensity arms. Disappointingly perhaps, multiple analyses including a general linear model, did not demonstrate a significant interaction of age and gender adjusted medication class group, nor of intensity of blood pressure control arm, with the APOL1 allelic state, under a recessive model. In other words, in contrast to conclusions from recent kidney graft survival studies [39], African ancestry individuals with no APOL1 risk variants cannot yet be approached with treatment paradigms that seem to apply to non-African ancestry counterparts. Although the benefit reported for ACE inhibitors in the original non-genotyped AASK trial and cohort studies for proteinuric (PCR >0.22 gm/gm) subjects was not replicated in the current study, it still may be the case that APOL1 genotyping may be useful in guiding antihypertensive medication choice and usage in African ancestry populations.

6. Role of the "Second Hit"

A key consistent observation has been that only a small subset of individuals with 2 APOL1 risk alleles actually develops kidney disease [40]. This observation together with family studies lead to a central hypothesis - that an identifiable and modifiable requisite "second hit" is necessary to trigger disease expression in genetically susceptible individuals (Figure 1).

The prototype for such a viral, nephrotropic second hit is HIV. The lifetime risk of kidney disease in patients with two APOL1 alleles risk has been shown to rise from <10% to >50% in the presence of untreated or undertreated HIV infection [38]. Successful anti-retroviral therapy, which reduces the rate of GFR decline per year, is probably one of the most important pieces of evidence that HIV represents an important, pathogenic factor [41]. In contrast, as noted in our study of the Ethiopian population, HIV infection is not associated with HIVAN in populations with a zero G1 or G2 allele frequencies [32]. More than a decade of biologic work has been done on the pathogenesis of HIVAN beginning with the initial finding of the podocyte as a possible reservoir for the HIV virus [42-44], and expression of HIV viral proteins Nef and Vpr. Many models were developed long before the description of APOL1. However, importantly, the murine experimental models lack APOL1 and the direct introduction of Nef into murine or human podocytes, was performed under conditions where APOL1 was not present or induced, respectively. This leads to the necessity to develop kidney disease models to replicate the interaction of "second hits" with APOL1. If we presume a recessive inheritance model where non-risk APOL1 is protective, then a viral nephrotropic second hit could induce APOL1 through a cytokine. We could then suggest having at least one APOL1 non-risk allele would protect the podocyte, but in the absence of a non-risk APOL1 allele, the podocyte may be vulnerable to the second hit. In the case of an additive inheritance model, gain of injury and a viral second hit, IFNγ induction of two APOL1 risk alleles exceeds a threshold for podocyte injury, perhaps interacting with interferon or viral protein. Zero or 1 APOL1 risk alleles would, in this case, be below the threshold level for podocyte injury.

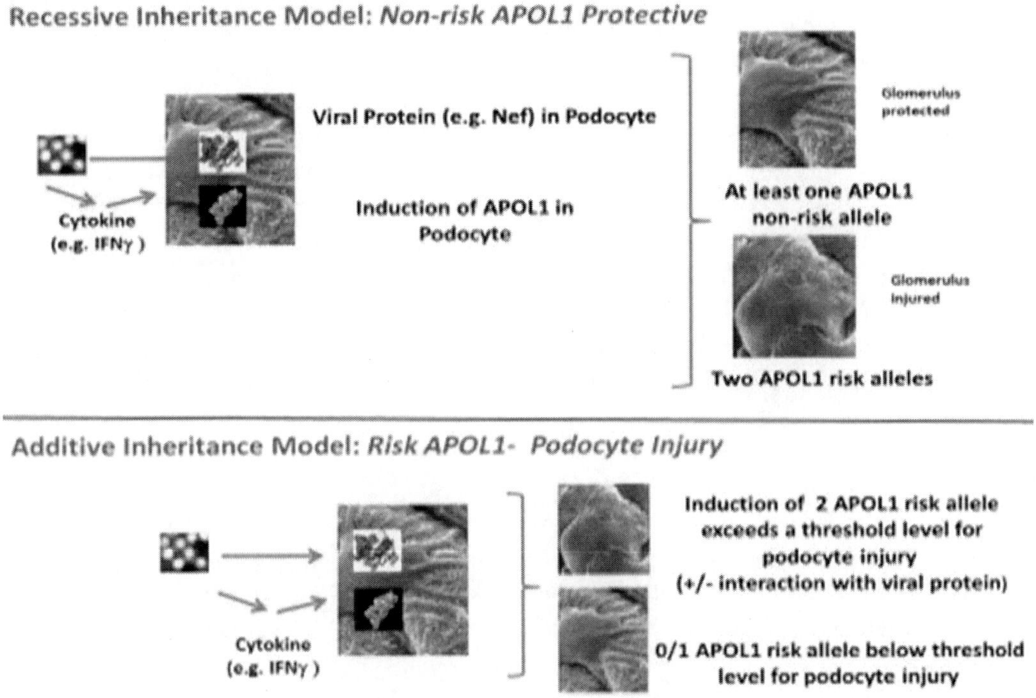

Figure 1. Alternative Proposed Mechanisms for APOL1 Injury based on Genetic Epidemiologic Clues.

Besides HIV, are there other additional human viral nephrotropic second hits? Parvovirus B19 is another attractive but as yet possible candidate. Parvovirus B19 was detected over 10 years ago in kidney tissue from patients with collapsing FSGS [45,46]. In-situ hybridization studies confirmed the presence of Parvovirus B19 with viral genome detected in kidney biopsies from patients with collapsing FSGS. Most of these subjects were African-American. Of course, these biopsy slides were not genotyped for APOL1 at that time. In light of the APOL1 discovery, this type of investigation would appear to be highly relevant. The recent demonstration that urine JC polyoma virus (JCV) confers protection to African Americans at risk for CKD as a result of two APOL1 risk variants and postulated inhibition of JCV-mediated inhibition of urinary tract replication by other more nephropathic viruses or modulation of gene expression profiles that alter susceptibility to CKD [47].

7. Role of APOL1 in Patients with Hypertension without CKD

The Lipkowitz et al. study also attempts to address the crucial question of whether or not hypertension, in the absence of clinically overt kidney disease, may also be associated with the APOL1 kidney disease risk region [36]. The investigators were able to query 409 of the 618 controls, and among these 171 (41.7%) recalled having been told of hypertension by their health care professionals or reported using anti-hypertensive medication. In particular, comparing subsets of controls phenotyped in this manner for hypertension status, showed no relation to APOL1 genotype. This provides a tentative suggestion that hypertension in the absence of chronic kidney disease in African-Americans may not be related to a clinical entity of subclinical APOL1 risk kidney disease. However, an important caveat is the possibility that in the absence of kidney biopsy, large numbers of individuals with subclinical forms of APOL1-associated primary kidney disease with hypertension as a first clinical manifestation might be present. Since it is unlikely that kidney biopsies would be performed, an appropriate clinical study should be designed to address this question. This new study should include large numbers of participants with careful and objective determination of blood pressure status, no other evidence of kidney disease at enrollment, and long-term follow-up with tailored examination of the benefit of the antihypertensive therapy conditioned to APOL1 genotype in the African ancestry population. Perhaps the most appropriate venue for such a study is the African continent, where recognition of hypertension accompanied by life-threatening complications is growing, and progressive CKD without recourse to kidney replacement therapy is the rule. Keeping in mind the need to effectively treat hypertension to prevent non-renal complications as well, in such a setting it becomes mandatory to have a comprehensive understanding of the possible kidney origin of hypertension (including APOL1 risk allele nephropathy), and the relationship between preferred modalities of treatment for hypertension and preservation of kidney integrity. Moreover, the genetic epidemiology should be more straightforward in the absence of the variable degree of non-Sub-Saharan African admixture seen in other study venues. Recently released guidelines of the British Hypertension Society, provide directives which inappropriately generalize African ancestry subjects together as a homogeneous group in terms of recommending calcium blockers as the preferred initial antihypertensive modality (http://www.bhsoc.org/Latest_BHS_management_Guidelines.stm.) In this regard, it will be important to know whether APOL1 or genotypes of relevance should be an additional guiding factor in making the antihypertensive choice which is most appropriate for a given individual.

8. Hypertension-Attributed CKD in Continental Africa

CKD affects an estimated 50 million people in continental Africa although these data may even underestimate the problem since they are mostly extrapolated from small population surveys [48]. Few patients have access to any form of dialysis and kidney transplantation is not widely available. In addition to those patients with CKD that progress to ESKD, significant numbers of people with CKD succumb to cardiovascular and cerebrovascular disease before reaching ESKD [49]. Small observational studies of hypertensive patients from Ghana and Nigeria document a high percentage of CKD and anecdotal reports from these areas indicate that the CKD prevalence is high [50]. Africa is also experiencing an increasing incidence of hypertension with an estimated prevalence of 75 million persons in 2008 expected to increase to 125 million persons by 2025 [51]. The areas of high distribution of APOL1 allelic risk variation seem to be associated with high prevalence rates of hypertension [51]. The Yoruba and Igbo populations of Nigeria are two examples of populations that exhibit high allelic variation in risk variants and show high levels of hypertension-attributed CKD [52,53]. These two populations are both major ancestral populations of modern African Americans [25].

9. The Role of Intrarenal ACE in Hypertension

Recent data allow one to postulate a role for intrarenal ACE in promoting hypertension as a potential downstream target for APOL1 [54]. The role of the kidney as a critical hypertension locus was initially suggested when kidneys transplants of hypertensive rats into control rats with normal blood pressures developed hypertension in the recipients; however the exact mechanism was not clarified at that time [55]. Recent studies have allowed the experiment to be refined and indicate that the kidney attributed hypertension is associated with local kidney activation of the renin-angiotensin system (RAS) [56]. In the activation of the systemic renal angiotensin system (RAS), angiotensinogen from the liver is cleaved by renin from the kidney to form angiotensin I. ACE present on endothelial cells surfaces throughout the body then utilize this to generate angiotensin II. The angiotensin II receptor type I (AT1R) is the receptor subtype that increases blood pressure and blood volume through vasoconstriction and adrenal gland stimulation of aldosterone secretion and kidney sodium retention. However, the systemic RAS as detected by plasma renin activity is not uniformly elevated in hypertension [57].

In a recent publication, Gonzalez-Villalobos, et al. demonstrated the potential role of local kidney intrarenal angiotensin activation associated with hypertension independent of the systemic RAS activation [56]. Conversely, inhibiting intrarenal angiotension II formation protects against hypertension. The model utilized in this study comprised mice specifically lacking kidney ACE. Since complete ACE removal causes severe developmental defects, the investigators generated ACE knockout mice expressing ACE either in hepatocytes (ACE 3/3 mice) or in myelomonocytic cells (ACE 10/10 mice). In these animals devoid of intrarenal ACE, the authors showed a blunted hypertensive response to ACE infusion and nitric oxide inhibition. The study further demonstrated a kidney response to high serum angiotensin 2 in wild type mice to cause intrarenal angiotensin II accumulation, sodium and water retention, activation of ion transporters in the loop of Henle (NKCC2) and distal nephron (NCC, ENaC, and pendrin) as well as the transporter kinases SPAK and OSR1 II which enhance sodium and water reabsorption throughout the nephron. These were effectively prevented in mice lacking ACE. The possibility of additional downstream targets for APOL1 in addition to intrarenal ACE is suggested by the only partial response to ACE inhibition in preventing hypertension and chronic kidney disease exhibited in the AASK study [10].

CONCLUSION

Based on these models, there is reason for optimism. Declining rates of HIVAN with the use of highly active anti-retroviral therapy (HAART) prove the treatment of a viral trigger can prevent kidney disease in those at genetic risk. In this regard, HAART can be considered as a novel treatment for CKD. In contrast, the conventional therapies (blood pressure control and ACE-inhibitors) in which the viral trigger has not yet been identified and treated, fail to reliably halt other forms of APOL1-associated kidney disease as we have seen with the large number of patients with hypertension-misattributed nephropathy in the AASK trial. It thus becomes imperative to determine if individuals with no APOL1 risk alleles might more effectively respond to ACE inhibition and to identify the inciting viral triggers, and their mechanisms of interaction with APOL1 risk moieties in the kidney and the immune system. These approaches will hopefully open up new avenues of thinking about hypertension and other common non-communicable diseases.

REFERENCES

[1] Keenan NL, Rosendorf KA. *Prevalence of hypertension and controlled hypertension -* United States, 2005-2008. MMWR Surveill Summ 2011;60 Suppl:94-7.

[2] Freedman BI, Divers J, Palmer ND. Population Ancestry and Genetic Risk for Diabetes and Kidney, Cardiovascular, and Bone Disease: Modifiable Environmental Factors May Produce the Cures. *Am J Kidney Dis.* 2013. pii: S0272-6386(13)00979-7. doi: 10.1053/j.ajkd.2013.05.024. [Epub ahead of print].

[3] Weir MR, Gray JM, Paster R, Saunders E. Differing mechanisms of action of angiotensin-converting enzyme inhibition in black and white hypertensive patients. The Trandolapril Multicenter Study Group. *Hypertension* 1995;26:124-30.

[4] Materson BJ, Reda DJ, Cushman WC, et al. Single-drug therapy for hypertension in men. A comparison of six antihypertensive agents with placebo. The Department of Veterans Affairs Cooperative Study Group on Antihypertensive Agents. *N Engl J Med* 1993;328:914-21.

[5] Saha C, Eckert GJ, Ambrosius WT, et al. Improvement in blood pressure with inhibition of the epithelial sodium channel in blacks with hypertension. *Hypertension* 2005;46:481-7.

[6] Agodoa LY, Appel L, Bakris GL, et al. Effect of ramipril vs amlodipine on renal outcomes in hypertensive nephrosclerosis: a randomized controlled trial. *JAMA* 2001;285:2719-28.

[7] Fogo A, Breyer JA, Smith MC, et al. Accuracy of the diagnosis of hypertensive nephrosclerosis in African Americans: a report from the African American Study of Kidney Disease (AASK) Trial. AASK Pilot Study Investigators. *Kidney Int* 1997;51:244-52.

[8] Wright JT, Jr., Bakris G, Greene T, et al. Effect of blood pressure lowering and antihypertensive drug class on progression of hypertensive kidney disease: results from the AASK trial. *JAMA* 2002;288:2421-31.

[9] Chobanian AV, Bakris GL, Black HR, et al. The Seventh Report of the Joint National Committee on Prevention, Detection, Evaluation, and Treatment of High Blood Pressure: the JNC 7 report. *JAMA* 2003;289:2560-72.

[10] Alves TP, Wang X, Wright JT, Jr., et al. Rate of ESRD exceeds mortality among African Americans with hypertensive nephrosclerosis. *J Am Soc Nephrol* 2010;21:1361-9.

[11] Marcantoni C, Ma LJ, Federspiel C, Fogo AB. Hypertensive nephrosclerosis in African Americans versus Caucasians. *Kidney Int* 2002;62:172-80.

[12] Ferguson R, Grim CE, Opgenorth TJ. A familial risk of chronic renal failure among blacks on dialysis? *J Clin Epidemiol* 1988;41:1189-96.

[13] Freedman BI, Spray BJ, Tuttle AB, Buckalew VM, Jr. The familial risk of end-stage renal disease in African Americans. *Am J Kidney Dis* 1993;21:387-93.

[14] USRDS. 2011 Annual Data Report:. *Atlas of End-Stage Renal Disease in the United States Bethesda, MD*: National Institutes of Heath, National Institute of Diabetes & Digestive & Kidney Diseases 2012.

[15] Freedman BI, Iskandar SS, Appel RG. The link between hypertension and nephrosclerosis. *Am J Kidney Dis* 1995;25:207-21.

[16] Pollak MR, Genovese G, Friedman DJ. APOL1 and kidney disease. *Curr Opin Nephrol Hypertens* 2012;21:179-82.

[17] Freedman BI, Kopp JB, Langefeld CD, et al. The apolipoprotein L1 (APOL1) gene and nondiabetic nephropathy in African Americans. *J Am Soc Nephrol* 2010;21:1422-6.

[18] Behar DM, Yunusbayev B, Metspalu M, et al. The genome-wide structure of the Jewish people. *Nature* 2010;466:238-42.

[19] Weiner MPGS SJ. *Genetic Variation: A laboratory Manual.* Cold Spring Harbor, NY, USA: Cold Spring Harbor Press; 2007.

[20] Feero WG, Guttmacher AE, Collins FS. Genomic medicine--an updated primer. *N Engl J Med* 2010;362:2001-11.

[21] Goldstein DB. Common genetic variation and human traits. *N Engl J Med* 2009;360:1696-8.

[22] Wasser WG, Tzur S, Wolday D, et al. Population genetics of chronic kidney disease: the evolving story of APOL1. *J Nephrol* 2012;25:603-18.

[23] McCarthy MI, Hirschhorn JN. Genome-wide association studies: potential next steps on a genetic journey. *Hum Mol Genet* 2008;17:R156-65.

[24] Winkler CA, Nelson GW, Smith MW. Admixture mapping comes of age. *Annu Rev Genomics Hum Genet* 2010;11:65-89.

[25] Tishkoff SA, Reed FA, Friedlaender FR, et al. The genetic structure and history of Africans and African Americans. *Science* 2009;324:1035-44.

[26] Kopp JB, Smith MW, Nelson GW, et al. MYH9 is a major-effect risk gene for focal segmental glomerulosclerosis. *Nat Genet* 2008;40:1175-84.

[27] Kao WH, Klag MJ, Meoni LA, et al. MYH9 is associated with nondiabetic end-stage renal disease in African Americans. *Nat Genet* 2008;40:1185-92.

[28] Nelson GW, Freedman BI, Bowden DW, et al. Dense mapping of MYH9 localizes the strongest kidney disease associations to the region of introns 13 to 15. Hum Mol Genet 2010;19:1805-15.

[29] Genovese G, Friedman DJ, Ross MD, et al. Association of trypanolytic ApoL1 variants with kidney disease in African Americans. *Science* 2010;329:841-5.

[30] Tzur S, Rosset S, Shemer R, et al. Missense mutations in the APOL1 gene are highly associated with end stage kidney disease risk previously attributed to the MYH9 gene. *Hum Genet* 2010;128:345-50.

[31] Behar DM, Shlush LI, Maor C, Lorber M, Skorecki K. Absence of HIV-associated nephropathy in Ethiopians. *Am J Kidney Dis* 2006;47:88-94.

[32] Behar DM, Kedem E, Rosset S, et al. Absence of APOL1 risk variants protects against HIV-associated nephropathy in the Ethiopian population. *Am J Nephrol* 2011;34:452-9.

[33] Rosset S, Tzur S, Behar DM, Wasser WG, Skorecki K. The population genetics of chronic kidney disease: insights from the MYH9-APOL1 locus. *Nat Rev Nephrol* 2011;7:313-26.

[34] Vanhamme L, Paturiaux-Hanocq F, Poelvoorde P, et al. Apolipoprotein L-I is the trypanosome lytic factor of human serum. *Nature* 2003;422:83-7.

[35] Molina-Portela MP, Samanovic M, Raper J. Distinct roles of apolipoprotein components within the trypanosome lytic factor complex revealed in a novel transgenic mouse model. *J Exp Med* 2008;205:1721-8.

[36] Lipkowitz MS, Freedman BI, Langefeld CD, et al. APOL1 variants associate with hypertension-attributed nephropathy and rate of kidney function decline in African-American Study of Kidney Disease and Hypertension. *Kidney Int* 2013; 83(1):114-20.

[37] Kanji Z, Powe CE, Wenger JB, et al. Genetic variation in APOL1 associates with younger age at hemodialysis initiation. *J Am Soc Nephrol* 2011;22:2091-7.

[38] Kopp JB, Nelson GW, Sampath K, et al. APOL1 genetic variants in focal segmental glomerulosclerosis and HIV-associated nephropathy. *J Am Soc Nephrol* 2011;22:2129-37.

[39] Reeves-Daniel AM, DePalma JA, Bleyer AJ, et al. The APOL1 gene and allograft survival after kidney transplantation. *Am J Transplant* 2011;11:1025-30.

[40] Freedman BI, Langefeld CD, Turner J, et al. Association of APOL1 variants with mild kidney disease in the first-degree relatives of African American patients with non-diabetic end-stage renal disease. *Kidney Int* 2012;82:805-11.

[41] Kalayjian RC, Lau B, Mechekano RN, et al. Risk factors for chronic kidney disease in a large cohort of HIV-1 infected individuals initiating antiretroviral therapy in routine care. *AIDS* 2012;26:1907-15.

[42] Winston JA, Bruggeman LA, Ross MD, et al. Nephropathy and establishment of a renal reservoir of HIV type 1 during primary infection. *N Engl J Med* 2001;344:1979-84.

[43] Wyatt CM, Meliambro K, Klotman PE. Recent progress in HIV-associated nephropathy. *Annu Rev Med* 2012;63:147-59.

[44] Bruggeman LA, Ross MD, Tanji N, et al. Renal epithelium is a previously unrecognized site of HIV-1 infection. *J Am Soc Nephrol* 2000;11:2079-87.

[45] Tanawattanacharoen S, Falk RJ, Jennette JC, Kopp JB. Parvovirus B19 DNA in kidney tissue of patients with focal segmental glomerulosclerosis. *Am J Kidney Dis* 2000;35:1166-74.

[46] Moudgil A, Nast CC, Bagga A, et al. Association of parvovirus B19 infection with idiopathic collapsing glomerulopathy. *Kidney Int* 2001;59:2126-33.

[47] Divers J, Nunez M, High KP, et al. JC polyoma virus interacts with APOL1 in African Americans with nondiabetic nephropathy. *Kidney Int* 2013 May 15. doi: 10.1038/ki.2013.173. [Epub ahead of print].

[48] Sumaili EK, Cohen EP, Zinga CV, Krzesinski JM, Pakasa NM, Nseka NM. High prevalence of undiagnosed chronic kidney disease among at-risk population in Kinshasa, the Democratic Republic of Congo. *BMC Nephrol* 2009;10:18.

[49] Odubanjo MO, Okolo CA, Oluwasola AO, Arije A. End-stage renal disease in Nigeria: an overview of the epidemiology and the pathogenetic mechanisms. *Saudi J Kidney Dis Transpl* 2011;22:1064-71.

[50] Ulasi, II, Arodiwe EB, Ijoma CK. Left ventricular hypertrophy in African Black patients with chronic renal failure at first evaluation. *Ethn Dis* 2006;16:859-64.

[51] Twagirumukiza M, De Bacquer D, Kips JG, de Backer G, Stichele RV, Van Bortel LM. Current and projected prevalence of arterial hypertension in sub-Saharan Africa by sex, age and habitat: an estimate from population studies. *J Hypertens* 2011;29:1243-52.

[52] Tayo BO, Kramer H, Salako BL, et al. Genetic variation in APOL1 and MYH9 genes is associated with chronic kidney disease among Nigerians. *Int Urol Nephrol* 2013;45:485-94.

[53] Ulasi II TS, Wasser WG, et al. High Population Frequencies of APOL1 Risk Variants Are Associated with Increased Prevalence of Non-Diabetic Chronic kidney Disease in the Igbo People from South-Eastern Nigeria. *Nephron Clin Pract 2013*; 123(1-2):123-8.

[54] Reudelhuber TL. Where hypertension happens. *J Clin Invest* 2013;123:1934-6.

[55] Grisk O, Kloting I, Exner J, et al. Long-term arterial pressure in spontaneously hypertensive rats is set by the kidney. *J Hypertens* 2002;20:131-8.

[56] Gonzalez-Villalobos RA, Janjoulia T, Fletcher NK, et al. The absence of intrarenal ACE protects against hypertension. *J Clin Invest* 2013;123:2011-23.

[57] Alderman MH, Cohen HW, Sealey JE, Laragh JH. Plasma renin activity levels in hypertensive persons: their wide range and lack of suppression in diabetic and in most elderly patients. *Am J Hypertens* 2004;17:1-7.

In: ACE Inhibitors. Volume 2
Editor: Macaulay Amechi Onuigbo
ISBN: 978-1-62948-422-8

Chapter 20

TREATMENT OF INFANTILE HEMANGIOMA WITH AN ACE INHIBITOR: A PARADIGM SHIFT

Tinte Itinteang, MBBS PhD[1], Paul F. Davis, PhD[1] and Swee T. Tan, MBBS FRACS PhD*[1-3]
[1]Gillies McIndoe Research Institute, New Zealand
[2]Centre for the Study & Treatment of Vascular Birthmarks, Hutt Hospital, New Zealand
[3]University of Otago, Wellington, New Zealand

ABSTRACT

Traditionally the use of angiotensin converting enzyme inhibitors (ACEi) has focused on their role in blocking angiotensin converting enzyme (ACE), and the downstream production of the vasoactive peptide, angiotensin II, typically in the setting of hypertension treatment. Earlier studies have demonstrated the lungs as the major site of ACE production, and therefore the predominant site of ACE inhibition. More recently the expression of ACE has been shown on hemangiongioblasts, the stem cell precursors of both endothelial and hematopoietic cells. The *in vivo* equivalent of hemangioblasts has been proposed to be the hemogenic endothelium, a developmentally primitive phenotypic endothelium, with the capacity for hematopoietic differentiation. This hemogenic endothelium constitutively expresses both primitive endothelial (CD34 and VEGFR-2) and hematopoietic (Tal-1, GATA-2, and Runx-1) associated markers. The novel finding of the expression of ACE on a phenotypic hemogenic endothelium has recently been reported on the endothelium of the microvessels of proliferating infantile hemangioma (IH), the most common tumour of infancy. IH which predominantly affects females, premature and white infants typically undergoes an initial rapid proliferation followed by spontaneous involution, often leaving a fibrofatty residuum. β-blockers, particularly propranolol, are now the preferred treatment for proliferating IH. The expression of ACE and the role of the angiotensin II peptide in regulating cellular proliferation via the angiotensin II receptor 2 has been proposed to account for the programmed biologic behavior of IH and its accelerated involution induced by β-blockers. Our recent clinical trial showing the efficacy of captopril, an ACEi, on IH confirms the crucial role of the renin-angiotensin system in the regulation of the hemogenic endothelium. This concept

* Corresponding author: Swee T Tan MBBS FRACS PhD; Email: Swee.Tan@huttvalleydhb.org.nz.

underscores the paradigm shift in the understanding and implications of ACE inhibition in human development, IH and other tumors.

INTRODUCTION

Angiotensin converting enzyme (ACE) was discovered by Skeggs and his colleagues at the Cleveland Veterans Administration Hospital in the 1950s [1]. This discovery of an enzyme that converts angiotensin I (ATI) to the vasoactive peptide, angiotensin II (ATII), later led to its isolation and purification [2]. Further work by Erdos *et al* demonstrated that ACE also inactivates bradykinin [3,4]. However, it was not until the pioneering work of Laragh and his team in the 1970s that suppression of ATII by the inhibition of ACE forms the basis of effective treatment for hypertension and cardiac failure [5,6]. This led to the discovery of captopril, the first orally active ACE inhibitor (ACEi) [7], followed by the pro-drugs such as enalapril and ramipril [8].

ACE inhibition now forms an important cornerstone in the management of hypertension with recent data showing a potential reduction in all-cause mortality by ACE inhibition [9].

ANGIOTENSIN CONVERTING ENZYME INHIBITORS

Since the discoveries of the mid to late 1950s, ACE has been the enzyme critically associated with the maintenance of the concentration of ATII, by the cleavage of the ATI, with its predominant effects on the cardiovascular system. The most profound of these is its effect on vasoconstriction of blood vessels and on cardiac muscle hypertrophy [10]. Since the introduction of ACE inhibitor (ACEi) in 1981 there have been multiple clinical indications for ACEi in reducing mortality from hypertension, congestive cardiac failure, myocardial infarction, diabetes mellitus, chronic renal insufficiency and atherosclerotic cardiovascular disease [11].

THE RENIN-ANGIOTENSIN SYSTEM

The renin-angiotensin system (RAS) is the endocrine system in which ATII is derived. Physiologically, renin is predominantly secreted from the juxtaglomerular cells of the kidney and this is primarily regulated by the macula densa in response to urine osmolality [12], and also by the stimulation of β-adrenergic receptors on the juxtaglomerular cells through the formation of the second messenger, cAMP [13]. Renin which is responsible for cleaving circulating angiotensinogen, is produced primarily in the liver and white adipose fat [14], to form the decapeptide, ATI, which is subsequently cleaved by ACE to form the vasoactive octapeptide, ATII [15]. The actions of ATII are predominantly mediated via its two receptors, angiotensin II receptor1 (ATIIR1) and angiotensin II receptor 2 (ATIIR2) [15].

HEMANGIOBLASTS AND HEMOGENIC ENDOTHELIUM

Hemangioblasts, primitive cells derived from the extra-embryonic mesoderm [16], which are regarded as the common precursor cells for both endothelial and hematopoietic cells were first demonstrated *in vitro* by Eichmann *et al,* in 1997 [17]. This was based on the expression of vascular endothelial growth factor receptor 2 (VEGFR-2) on cells derived from chicken embryos, and their differential response to the administration of VEGF [17]. This revealed the dual plasticity for a VEGFR-2 cellular signature that enabled the cells to undergo either hematopoietic or endothelial differentiation. Using cells derived from mice embryos, Sugiyama *et al*, subsequently generated hematopoietic cells through an endothelial intermediate [18]. However, it was not until 2009, using live cell imaging that two independent research groups confirmed the ability for hematopoietic differentiation from hemangioblasts to occur through a hemogenic endothelium intermediate (Figure 1) [19,20]. Although these studies have, for the most part, managed to generate hemangioblasts, the identification of an *in vivo* equivalent of the hemogenic endothelium currently remains elusive [21].

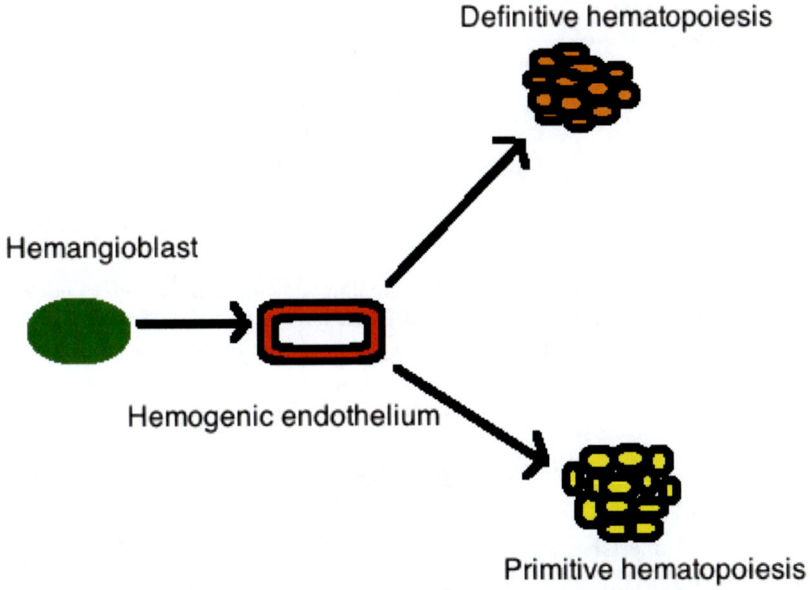

Figure 1. The plasticity for dual primitive and definitive hematopoietic differentiation of hemangioblasts through a hemogenic endothelium stage (*Adapted from* Lancrin C, *et al*, 2009) [20].

HEMANGIOBLASTS, ANGIOTENSIN CONVERTING ENZYME AND ANGIOTENSIN II

Significant further progress in the field occurred following the identification of ACE (also known as CD143) as a cellular marker for primitive hematopoietic stem cells during human hematopoietic ontogeny [22]. Further work revealed ACE as a novel marker for hemangioblasts and the vital role of the RAS through ATII, in regulating the proliferation and differentiation of hemangioblasts [23]. Although the effect of ATII in promoting proliferation of hematopoietic progenitors had been known since the turn of the 21st century [24], it was not until the discovery by Zambidis *et al*, that the extent of both ACE in generating ATII and the differential effects of ATII on its two receptors was better appreciated [23]. They showed that ATII cause preferential effect on endothelial or hematopoietic differentiation in hemangioblasts via activation of ATIIR1 or ATIIR2 respectively (Figure 2) [23].

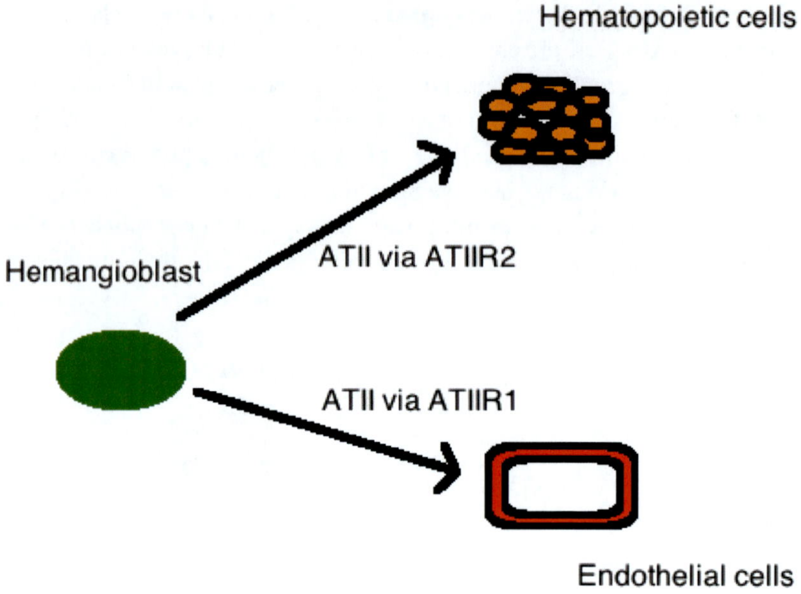

Figure 2. The differential effects of angiotensin II signaling on hemangioblast differentiation, with preferential differentiation towards hematopoietic cells via angiotensin II receptor 2 activation and towards an endothelial lineage via angiotensin II receptor 1 activation (*Adapted from* Zambidis ET, *et al*, 2008) [23].

Infantile Hemangioma

Infantile hemangioma (IH) is the most common tumor of infancy affecting up to 10% of the population, with a predilection for Caucasian, female and premature infants [25,26]. It is typified by excessive vasculogenesis during infancy (proliferative phase), followed by spontaneous slow involution in which the cellular elements are gradually replaced by fibro-fatty tissues over the next 1-5 years (involuting phase), with continued improvement up to 10 years, often leaving behind a fibro-fatty residuum (involuted phase) (Figure 3) [27].

During the proliferative phase the excessive vasculogenesis leads to accumulation of immature endothelial cells organized into capillaries composed of an inner luminal layer characterized by the expression of endothelial markers such as CD31, CD34, and von Willebrands factor [28]. This endothelial layer is surrounded by an outer concentric pericyte layer, expressing smooth muscle actin (Figure 4) [28,29].

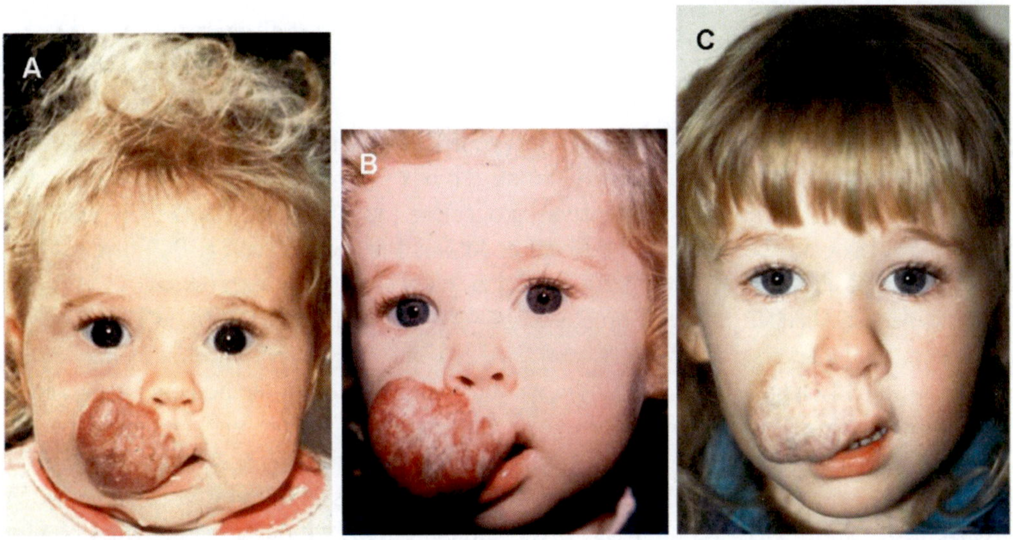

Figure 3. Serial photographs showing a typical infantile hemangioma progression; at 8 months of age (proliferative phase) (A); at 3 years of age (involuting phase) (B); and at 8 years of age (involuted phase) (C).

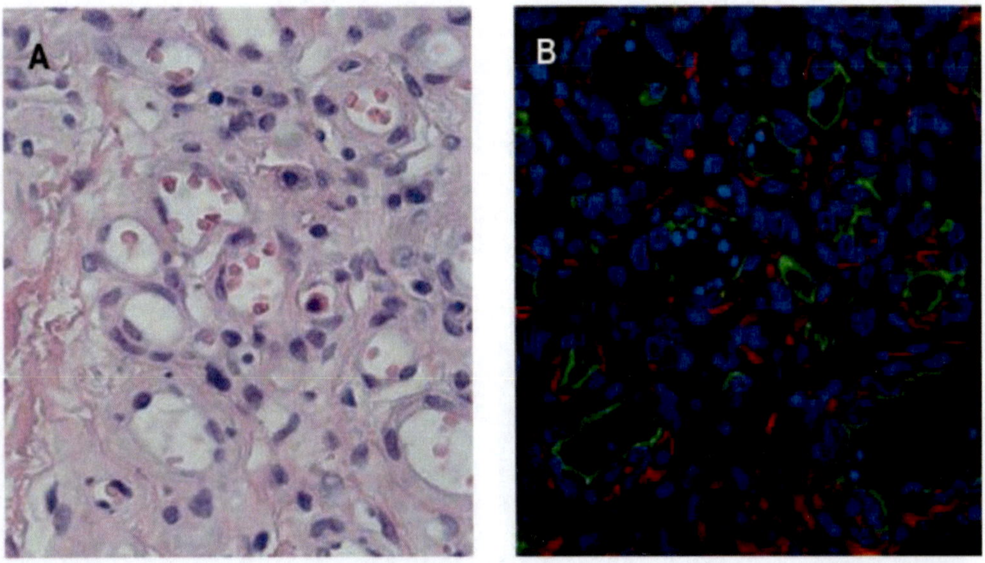

Figure 4. Hematoxylin & eosin staining of a proliferating infantile hemangioma showing an abundance of micro-vessels (A) consisting of an inner endothelial layer expressing CD34 (green) with an outer concentric pericyte layer expressing smooth muscle actin (red) (B). Original magnification: 100X.

Infantile Hemangioma and Hemogenic Endothelium

The endothelial layer of proliferating IH has been shown to possess a primitive phenotype typically associated with an embryonic-like expression pattern [30]. The exact origin of the micro-vessels within proliferating IH, has previously been suggested as arising *de novo* through a primitive process of vasculogenesis [31], with later studies hypothesizing 'a more downstream' bone marrow derived endothelial progenitor cell (EPC) origin [32]. It was not until 2010, that we first revealed the unique co-expression of primitive hematopoietic-associated markers (brachyury, GATA-2, Tal-1 and CD133), as well the neural crest stem cell markers (p75, Sox 9, and Sox-10) on the phenotypic endothelial layer of proliferating IH [33,34]. This novel finding and the appreciation of the hemogenic endothelial nature of the micro-vessels of proliferating IH led to the better understanding of these enigmatic tumors. We also provided evidence of the first trimester placental chorionic villous mesenchymal core origin of IH [35], supporting the findings of Bree *et al*, [36] on the null involvement of placental trophoblasts in IH. This chorionic villous mesenchymal core cell origin of IH concept supports previous theories of placental embolization as a cause for IH [37], based on the unique co-expression of certain proteins in the endothelium of IH and placenta [29,37].

Infantile Hemangioma, Angiotensin Converting Enzyme and Angiotensin II

We have also demonstrated the expression of ACE on the same phenotypic hemogenic endothelium of IH and that cells derived from IH form blast colonies *in vitro* [38,39]. This coupled with the expression of the ATIIR2 isoform (Figure 5), and the proliferative effect of exogenous ATII on the IH derived blast colonies *in vitro*, point to the crucial involvement of the RAS in the regulation of these tumors [38].

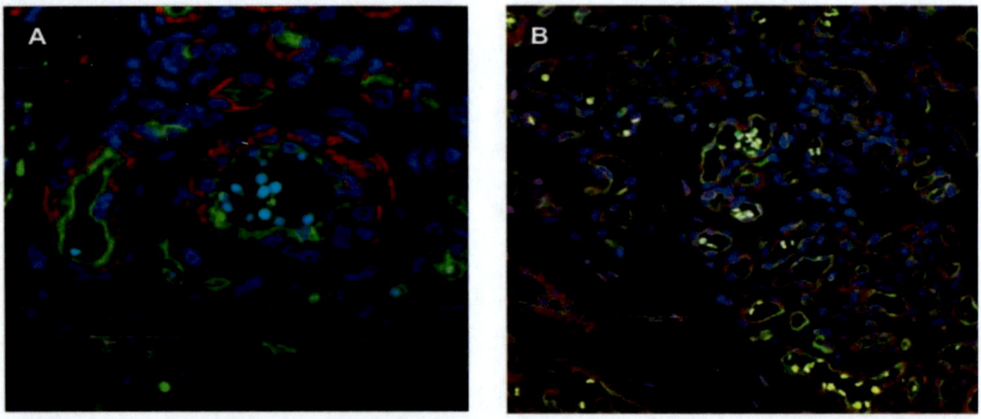

Figure 5. Immunohistochmical staining of proliferating infantile hemangioma showing expression of ACE (green) on the inner endothelial layer with the outer pericyte layer expressing smooth muscle actin (red) (A); and the expression of ATIIR2 (red) also localizing to the hemogenic endothelial layer highlighted by ACE expression (green) (B). Original magnifications: (A) 100X, (B) 40X.

INFANTILE HEMANGIOMA AND ANGIOTENSIN CONVERTING ENZYME INHIBITORS

Our discovery of the involvement of the RAS in IH underscores the basis of the treatment of this condition with β-blockers [38] and led to a prospective observational clinical trial demonstrating the clinical effect of captopril on IH [40] (Figure 6). Accelerated involution of IH was observed in seven out of the eight subjects, with a more gradual response in the remaining patient [40]. Although the clinical response was not as dramatic for one-third of the patients treated with captopril compared to those treated with propranolol [41,42], it is worth noting that the upper limit of the dosage of captopril of 1.5mg/kg/day used in this study was low compared with the maximal cardiovascular dosage of 2mg/kg thrice daily [43]. For safety reasons a low maximum dosage of captopril was used in that pilot study [40]. A retrospective study by Christou *et al* [44], based on a review of IH patients they had been treated with captopril for steroid-induced cardiomyopathy showed no effect of captopril in inducing involution. However, there were flaws in that study as there was no documentation of the dosage and the duration of captopril treatment [44].

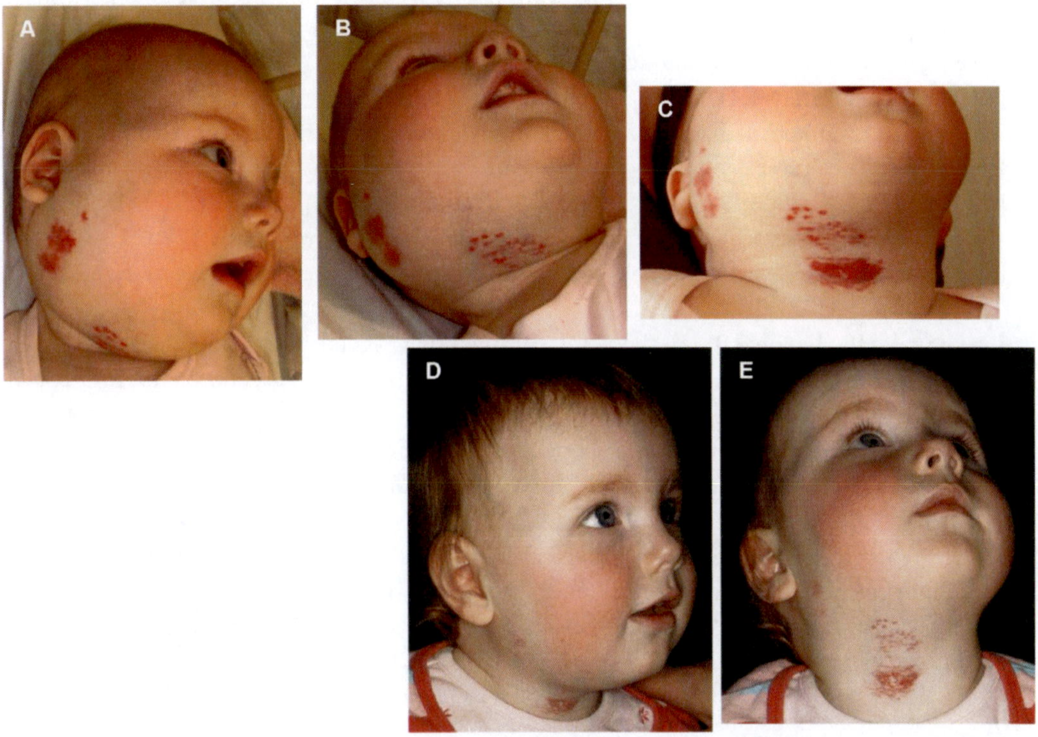

Figure 6. A 22 week-old girl (A,B) with a large right cervico-facial infantile hemangioma 3 weeks (C); and 6 months (D,E) after administration of captopril at a dosage of 1.5mg/kg/day, resulting in accelerated involution (*Reproduced from* Tan ST, *et al*, 2012) [40].

CONCLUSION

Recent studies into the biology of IH reveal the developmental anomalous nature of IH caused by aberrant proliferation and differentiation of a primitive mesoderm-derived hemogenic endothelium with a neural stem phenotype [33]. The involvement of the RAS with expression of ACE [38] on this phenotypic hemogenic endothelium of IH [34] is critical in the modulation of stem cell proliferation in these tumors. These new insights highlight a paradigm shift in the understanding of the biology of IH and underscores the novel treatment of this vascular tumor, through the modulation of RAS using β-blockers [41,45] and ACEi [44]. These recent discoveries have implications in tumor biology in general and the understanding of human development.

REFERENCES

[1] Skeggs LT, Kahn JR, Shumway NP. The preparation and function of the hypertension-converting enzyme. *J Exp Med.* 1956; 103: 295-299.

[2] Skeggs LT. Discovery of the two angiotensin peptides and the angiotensin converting enzyme. *Circ* 1993; 21: 259-260.

[3] Yang HYT, Erdos EG, Levin Y. Characterization of a dipeptide carboxypeptidase that converts angiotensin I and inactivates bradykinin. *Biochem Biophys Acta.* 1970; 214: 374-376.

[4] Yang HYT, Erdos EG, Levin Y. Characterization of a dipeptide hydrolase (kininase II; angiotensin I converting enzyme). *J Pharmacol Exper Therap.* 1971; 177: 291-300.

[5] Gavras H, Brunner HR, Laragh JH, Sealey JE, Gavras I, Vukovich RA. *N Engl J Med.* 1974; 291: 817-821.

[6] Gavras HP, Faxon DP, Berkoben J, Brunner HR, Ryan TJ. Angiotensin converting enzyme inhibition in patients with congestive heart failure. *Circulation* 1978; 58: 770-776.

[7] Smith CG, Van JR. The discovery of captopril. *FASEB J.* 2003; 17: 788-789.

[8] Erdos EG. The ACE and I: how ACE inhibitors came to be. *FASEB J.* 2006; 20: 1034-1038.

[9] van Vark LC, Bertrand M, Akkerhuis KM, Brugts JJ, Fox K, Mourad JJ, Boersma E. Angiotensin-converting enzyme inhibitors reduce mortality in hypertension: a meta-analysis of randomized clinical trials of renin-angiotensin-aldosterone system inhibitors involving 158998 patients. *Eur Heart J.* 2012; 33: 2088-2097.

[10] Sweitzer NK. What is an angiotensin converting enzyme inhibitor. Circ 2003; 108: e16-e18.

[11] Bicket DP. Using ACE inhibitors appropriately. *Am Fam Physician* 2002; 66: 461-468.

[12] Persson PB. Renin: origin, secretion and synthesis. J Physiol. 2003; 552: 667-671.

[13] Neubauer B, Machura K, Schnermann J, Wagner C. Renin expression in large renal vessels during fetal development depends on functional β1/ β2- adrenergic receptors. *Am J Physiol* 2011; 301: F71-77.

[14] Kalupahana NS, Massiera F, Quignard-Boulange A, Ailhaud G, Voy BH, Wasserman DH, Moustaid-Moussa N. Overproduction of angiotensinogen from adipose tissue

induces inflammation, glucose intolerance, and insulin resistance. *Obesity*. 2012; 20: 48-56.

[15] Paul M, Mehr AP, Kreutz R. Physiology of local renin-angiotensin system. *Physiol Rev*. 2006; 86: 747-803.

[16] Huber TL, Kouskoff V, Fehling HJ, Palis J, Keller G. Haemangioblast commitment is initiated in the primitive streak of the mouse embryo. *Nature* 2004; 432: 625-630.

[17] Eichmann A, Corbel C, Nataf V, Vaigot P, Breant C, Le Douarin NM. Ligand-dependent development of the endothelial and hemopoietic lineages from embryonic mesodermal cells expressing vascular endothelial growth factor receptor 2. *Proc Natl Acad Sci USA*. 1997; 94: 5141-5146.

[18] Sugiyama D, Ogawa M, Hirose I, Jaffredo T, Arai K, Tsuji K. Erythropoiesis from acetyl ldl incorporating endothelial cells at the preliver stage. *Blood* 2003; 101: 4733-4738.

[19] Eliken HM, Nishikawa S, Schroeder T. Continuous single-cell imaging of blood generation from haemogenic endothelium. *Nature* 2009; 457: 896-900.

[20] Lancrin C, Sroczynska P, Stephenson C, Allen T, Kouskoff V, Lacaud G. The haemangioblast generates haematopoietic cells through a haemogenic endothelium stage. *Nature* 2009; 457: 892-896.

[21] Gordon-Keylock S, Medvinsky A. Endothelio-hematopoietic relationship: getting closer to the beginnings. *BMC Biology* 2011; 9: 88.

[22] Jokubaitis VJ, Sinka L, Driessen R, Whitty G, Haylock DN, Bertoncello I, Smith I, Peault B, Tavian M, Simmons PJ. Angiotensin-converting enzyme (CD143) marks hematopoietic stem cells in human embryonic, fetal, and adult hematopoietic tissues. *Blood* 2008; 111: 4055-4063.

[23] Zambidis ET, Park TS, Yu W, Tam A, Levine M, Yuan X, Pryzhkova M, Peault B. Expression of angiotensin-converting enzyme (CD143) identifies and regulates primitive hemangiobalsts derived from human pluripotent stem cell. *Blood* 2008; 112: 3601-3614.

[24] Rodgers KE, Xiong S, diZerega GS. Accelerated recovery from irradiation injury by angiotensin peptides. *Cancer Chemother Pharmacol*. 2002; 49: 403-411.

[25] Tan ST. Cellular and molecular basis of haemangioma. (PhD Thesis). *University of Otago*. 2001.

[26] Itinteang T. Haemangioma: a study of the biology. (PhD Thesis). *Victoria University of Wellington*. 2012.

[27] Tan ST, Velickovic, Ruger BM, Davis PF. Cellular and extracellular markers of hemangioma. *Plast Reconstr Surg*. 2000; 106: 529-537.

[28] Tan ST, Wallis RA, He Y, Davis PF. Mast cells in hemangioma. *Plast Reconstr Surg*. 2004; 113: 999-1011.

[29] North PE, Waner M, Mizeracki A, Mihm MC. Glut1: a newly discovered immunohistochemical marker for juvenile hemangiomas. *Hum Pathol*. 2000; 31: 11-22.

[30] Dosanjh A, Chang J, Bresnick S, Zhou L, Reinisch J, Longaker M, Karasek M. *In vitro* characteristics of neonatal hemangioma endothelial cells: similarities and differences between normal neonatal and fetal endothelial cells. *J Cutan Pathol*. 2000; 27: 441-450.

[31] Nguyen VA, Furhapter C, Romani N, Weber F, Sepp N. Infantile hemangioma is a proliferation of B4-negative endothelial cells adjacent to HLA-DR-positive cells with dendritic cell morphology. *Hum Pathol.* 2004; 35: 739-744.

[32] Yu Y, Flint AF, Mulliken JB, Wu JK, Bischoff J. Endothelial progenitor cells in infantile hemangioma. *Blood* 2004; 103: 1373-1375.

[33] Itinteang T, Tan ST, Brasch H, Day DJ. Primitive mesodermal cells with a neural crest stem cell phenotype predominate proliferating infantile hemangioma. *J Clin Pathol.* 2010; 63: 771-776.

[34] Itinteang T, Tan ST, Brasch H, Day DJ. Haemogenic endothelium in infantile haemangioma. *J Clin Pathol.* 2010; 63: 982-986.

[35] Itinteang T, Tan ST, Guthrie S, Tan CES, McIntyre BC, Brasch HD, Day DJ. A placental chorionic villous mesenchymal core cellular origin for infantile haemangioma. *J Clin Pathol.* 2011; 64: 870- 874.

[36] Bree AF, Siegfried E, Sotelo-Avila C, Nahass G. *Arch Dermatol.* 2001; 137: 573-577.

[37] North PE, Waner M, Mizeracki A, Mrak RE, Nicholas R, Kincannon J, Suen JY, Mihm MC. A unique microvascular phenotype shared by juvenile hemangiomas and human placenta. *Arch Dermatol.* 2001; 137: 559-570.

[38] Itinteang T, Brasch HD, Tan ST, Day DJ. Expression of components of the renin-angiotensin system in proliferating infantile haemangioma may account for the propranolol-induced accelerated involution. *J Plast Reconstr Aesthet Surg.* 2011B; 64: 759-765.

[39] Itinteang T, Tan ST, Brasch HD, Vishvanath, A, Day DJ. Primitive erythropoiesis in infantile haemangioma. *Brit J Dermatol.* 2011; 164: 1097-1100.

[40] Tan ST, Itinteang T, Day DJ, O'Donnell C, Mathy JA, Leadbitter P. Treatment of infantile haemangioma with captopril. *Br J Dermatol.* 2012; 167: 619- 624.

[41] Tan ST, Itinteang T, Leadbitter P. Low-dose propranolol for infantile haemangioma. *J Plast Reconstr Aesthet Surg.* 2011; 64: 292-299.

[42] Leaute-Labreze C, de la Roque ED, Hubiche T, Boralevi F. Propranolol for severe hemangiomas of infancy. *N Engl J Med.* 2008; 358: 2649-2651.

[43] Sinaiko AR, Mirkin BL, Hendrick DA, Green TP, O'Dea RF. Antihypertensive effect and elimination kinetics of captopril in hypertensive children with renal disease. *J Pediatr.* 1983; 103: 799-805.

[44] Christou EM, Wargon Q. Effect of captopril on infantile haemangiomas: a retrospective case series. *Australas J Dermatol.* 2012; 53: 216-218.

[45] Itinteang T, Withers AH, Leadbitter P, Day DJ, Tan ST. Pharmacologic therapies for infantile hemangioma: is there a rational basis? *Plast Reconstr Surg.* 2011; 128: 499-507.

SECTION 4. EPILOGUE - ACE INHIBITORS AND ANGIOTENSIN RECEPTOR BLOCKERS AND RENOPROTECTION REVISITED: THE FUTURE OF RENOPROTECTION IN THE 21ST CENTURY

In: ACE Inhibitors. Volume 2
Editor: Macaulay Amechi Onuigbo
ISBN: 978-1-62948-422-8

Chapter 21

EPILOGUE - BOLD PREDICTIONS ON THE FUTURE OF RENOPROTECTION: THE WAY FORWARD WITH MULTIPLE PATHWAY BLOCKERS – MAKING A CASE FOR NOVEL NON-ANGIOTENSIN INHIBITING RENOPROTECTIVE AGENTS LIKE CORTICOTROPIN AND PENTOXIFYLLINE

Macaulay Amechi Onuigbo, MD MSc FWACP FASN MBA*
Mayo Clinic College of Medicine, Rochester, MN, US
Department of Nephrology, Mayo Clinic Health System, Eau Claire, WI, US

EPILOGUE

Just in the last week of April, 2013, our paper titled "Renoprotection and the Bardoxolone Methyl Story – Is This the Right Way Forward? A Novel View of Renoprotection in CKD Trials: A New Classification Scheme for Renoprotective Agents" was published in the journal, *Nephron Extra* [1]. This paper represented a major culmination of this author's clinical research interests, research efforts and perspectives on the very important concept of renoprotection in clinical medicine. The recent failure of the agent, Bardoxolone Methyl, in phase IIIb clinical trial to show safe renoprotection formed the backdrop for this critique of renoproetction as we know it today [1,2]. Despite initial phase II trial results that suggested impressive renoprotection in advanced type 2 diabetic nephropathy, as an add-on to angiotensin inhibition, unfortunately, subsequent phase IIIb trials failed to show that Bardoxolone Methyl was a safe alternative renoprotective agent [1,2]. In October 2012, the BEACON (Bardoxolone Methyl Evaluation in Patients with Chronic Kidney Disease and Type 2 Diabetes: The Occurrence of Renal Events) trial was terminated following observed safety concerns regarding bardoxolone methyl [1].

* Corresponding author: Macaulay Onuigbo MD MSc FWACP FASN MBA; Email: onuigbo.macaulay@mayo.edu.

Whereas current renoprotection archetype is based completely on angiotensin inhibition using ACE inhibitors (ACEIs) and angiotensin receptor blockers (ARBs), however, these agents have repeatedly proved to be imperfect renoprotective agents [3-12]. Despite their widespread use over the last two decades, a dispassionate assessment would describe their performance to be only fair at best [13-24]. Both here and around the world, there is yet to be demonstrated any veritable evidence of true reduction in incident ESRD rates following the common use of the ACEI and the ARB for renoprotection. To the contrary, if anything, all evidence points to an increasing worldwide ESRD pandemic from every region of the world [25-37]. In this 2013 Spring review in the journal, *Nephron Extra*, we had again decisively examined the mechanistic limitations and drawbacks of the several previously published randomized controlled trials (RCTs) on CKD renoprotection, including the high drop-out rates, the failure to study older CKD patients with later stage CKD, the overreliance on the use of renal surrogates and combination renal endpoints, and the paucity of veritable, elaborate and systematic assessment methods for the documentation and reporting of individual patient-level, drug-related adverse events, with particular reference to iatrogenic renal failure or nephrotoxicity [13-24,38,39].

We also had analyzed the evidence-base for the presence of putative, multiple independent and unrelated pathogenetic mechanisms that potentially initiate and further (diabetic and non-diabetic) CKD progression in our patients [1]. What's more, we investigated the validity, or lack thereof, of the overestimated concept that the blockade of a single molecule (angiotensin II), with an ACEI and/or an ARB, and therefore the antagonism of only the angiotensin cascade, could effectively, time after time, and lastingly, produce sufficient and qualitative renoprotection results in (diabetic and non-diabetic) CKD patients [1]. We evidently argued that given the plurality of so many diverse and varied pathogenetic processes, with likely significant interations between them, that both initiate and drive CKD to ESRD progression, it is almost laughable to believe that the blockage of just one moiety (angiotensin II) would result in major renoprotection treatment breakthroughs [1]. We definitely think differently [1]. There are so many potential triggering and propagating factors that drive and modulate CKD-ESRD progression, some of which undoubtedly remain unknown to date. The list, albeit not exhaustive, include the following factors - several predisposing genetic abnormalities including variations of the non-muscle myosin heavy chain 9 gene (MYH9) on chromosome 22 and variants at chromosome 6q24–27 among African-Americans, the role of APOL-1 variants among hypertensive CKD patients of African descent, oxidative stress combined with a paradoxical hypoxic renal environment conditioned by an underlying genetic predisposition, the production of advanced glycosylation end products and the interaction of these end products on the multi-ligand receptor of the immunoglobulin superfamily receptor for advanced glycation end products, intrarenal angiotensin II and/or renin production, inflammation, lipid toxicity, podocyte injury and apoptosis, cytokine/chemokine/growth factor release causing renal injury, asymmetric dimethylarginine and uric acid [1,23,40-65].

We have therefore opined that given the above scenario and realities, that again irrevocably, there is this overarching impetus to infer that multiple, disparately diverse and independent pathways, including any veritable combination of the mechanisms that we have enumerated above, and many more others yet to be identified, do concurrently and asymmetrically contribute to CKD initiation and propagation to ESRD in our CKD patients [1,23,40-65]. Furthermore, we had arrived at the irrevocable conclusion that current knowledge of CKD initiation and progression to ESRD, current knowledge of the natural history of CKD, and current knowledge of the impacts of AKI on this continuum remain in their infancy and call for more research [1,66-69].

Along these lines of thought, we had gone on to suggest a new classification scheme for renoprotective agents as follows [1]:

1. The single-pathway blockers (SPBs) which represent those agents that block a single putative pathogenetic pathway involved in CKD progression, as typified classically by the ACEI and/or the ARB [1].
2. The multiple-pathway blockers (MPBs) that are able to block or antagonize the effects of multiple putative pathogenetic pathways through their ability to simultaneously block, downstream, the effects of several pathways or mechanisms of CKD to ESRD progression and could therefore concurrently interfere with several unrelated upstream pathways or mechanisms [1].

We had proposed that the ideal and truly renoprotective agent must clearly be a MPB and it is our current hypothesis that such an agent may already be available on the horizon, albeit not yet fully evaluated and identified as such. This calls for more research efforts. Very importantly, we submit that it is very vital that such novel renoprotective agent(s) should not in any way exhibit a potential for nephrotoxictity, a factor that, in our strong opinion, has greatly further limited the potential of angiotensin inhibition to produce superior and sustained renoprotection, especially in the older CKD patients [1,13-24].

Our recent elaborate review of related published reports in the renoprotection literature, coming from the above perspectives, has unearthed two potential new pharmaceutical candidates that may blaze the trail for newly 'discovered' renoprotective agents [70-83]. We note, that arguably, these two pharmaceutical agents are both kidney-friendly, both have a proven safety track record over the years for use for several other medical indications, and both agents are MPBs [1,70-83]. The two pharmaceutical agents in question are corticotrophin or ACTH, and pentoxifylline [70-83]. Pentoxifylline is a non-specific phosphor-diesterase inhibitor which suppresses the production of several factors of inflammatory response [71-73]. Corticotrophin or ACTH, on the other hand is a long used pituitary neuroimmunoendocrine polypeptide, which is known to have a multiplicity of actions including controlling steroidogenesis, anti-inflammatory actions via an agonist effect on the melanocortin system, the inhibition of proinflammatory NF-κB activation followed by reduced expression of NF-κB-dependent proinflammatory molecules, including interleukins, chemokines and adhesion molecules, suppression of inflammatory cell proliferation, possibly through inhibition of NF-κB signaling, correction of dyslipidemia, direct effects on kidney cells, and the inhibition of antibodies directed against the M-type phospholipase A2 receptor 1 (PLA2R1), a new focus on the pathogenesis of membranous nephropathy [79-83]. We look forward to more research efforts in the near future along these lines of argument, even as we continue to search for the golden fleece of renoprotection [1,13-24]. We believe that targeted studies directed at certain pre-specified kidney disease states would yield better results [1,84]. Finally, we would argue that hard renal endpoints such ESRD or renal death, only, be used in these renoprotection trials [1]. The abuse of renal surrogates and combination endpoints of these renal surrogates in the last 20 years of nephrology RCTs has not served neither patient nor physicians any better [1,39].

REFERENCES

[1] Onuigbo MAC. Renoprotection and the Bardoxolone Methyl Story - Is this the Right Way Forward? A Novel View of Renoprotection in CKD Trials: A new classification scheme for renoprotective agents. *Nephron Extra* 2013;3:36-49 (DOI: 10.1159/000351044).

[2] Pergola PE, Raskin P, Toto RD, Meyer CJ, Huff JW, et al: Bardoxolone methyl and kidney function in CKD with type 2 diabetes. *N. Eng. J. Med.* 2011; 365: 327–336.

[3] Lewis EJ, Hunsicker LG, Bain RP, Rohde RD. The effect of angiotensin-converting-enzyme inhibition on diabetic nephropathy. The Collaborative Study Group. *N. Engl. J. Med.* 1993; 329(20):1456-1462. Erratum in: *N. Engl. J. Med.* 1993; 330(2):152.

[4] Kasiske BL, Kalil RS, Ma JZ et al. Effect of antihypertensive therapy on the kidney in patients with diabetes: a meta-regression analysis. *Ann. Intern. Med.* 1993; 118: 129–138.

[5] Ruggenenti P, Perna A, Gherardi G, et al. Renoprotective properties of ACE-inhibition in non-diabetic nephropathies with non-nephrotic proteinuria. *Lancet* 1999;354(9176): 359-364.

[6] Effects of ramipril on cardiovascular and microvascular outcomes in people with diabetes mellitus: results of the HOPE study and MICRO-HOPE substudy. Heart Outcomes Prevention Evaluation Study Investigators. *Lancet* 2000;355(9200):253-9. Erratum in: *Lancet* 2000;356(9232):860.

[7] Mogensen CE, Neldam S, Tikkanen I, et al. Randomised controlled trial of dual blockade of renin-angiotensin system in patients with hypertension, microalbuminuria, and non-insulin dependent diabetes: the candesartan and lisinopril microalbuminuria (CALM) study. *BMJ* 2000; 321(7274):1440-1444.

[8] Brenner BM, Cooper ME, de Zeeuw D, et al. Effects of losartan on renal and cardiovascular outcomes in patients with type 2 diabetes and nephropathy. *N. Eng. J. Med.* 2001; 345:861-869.

[9] Parving HH, Lehnert H, Brochner-Mortensen J, Gomis R, Andersen S, Arner P: The effect of irbesartan on the development of diabetic nephropathy in patients with type 2 diabetes. *N. Engl. J. Med.* 2001;345: 870–878.

[10] Lewis EJ, Hunsicker LG, Clarke WR et al. Renoprotective effect of the angiotensin-receptor antagonist irbesartan in patients with nephropathy due to type 2 diabetes. *N. Engl. J. Med.* 2001; 345: 851–860.

[11] Barnett AH, Bain SC, Bouter P, Karlberg B, Madsbad S, Jervell J, Mustonen J; Diabetics Exposed to Telmisartan and Enalapril Study Group. Angiotensin-receptor blockade versus converting-enzyme inhibition in type 2 diabetes and nephropathy. *N. Engl. J. Med.* 2004;351(19):1952-61. Epub 2004 Oct 31. Erratum in *N. Engl. J. Med.* 2005;352(16):1731.

[12] Kunz R, Friedrich C, Wolbers M, Mann JF. Meta-analysis: effect of monotherapy and combination therapy with inhibitors of the renin angiotensin system on proteinuria in renal disease. *Ann. Intern. Med.* 2008;148(1):30-48. Epub 2007 Nov 5.

[13] Onuigbo MA, Onuigbo NT. Late onset renal failure from angiotensin blockade (LORFFAB): a prospective thirty-month Mayo Health System clinic experience. *Med. Sci. Monit.* 2005;11(10):CR462-9. Epub 2005 Sep 26.

[14] Onuigbo MA, Onuigbo NT. Use of ultrahigh RAAS blockade: implications for exacerbation of renal failure. *Kidney Int.* 2006 Jan;69(1):194-5.
[15] Onuigbo MA, Onuigbo NT. Late-onset renal failure from RAAS blockade. *Kidney Int.* 2006 Oct; 70(7):1378-9. PMID:16988746. DOI:10.1038/sj.ki.5001648. (Letter)
[16] Onuigbo MA, Onuigbo NT. Late-onset renal failure from angiotensin blockade (LORFFAB) in 100 CKD patients. *Int. Urol. Nephrol.* 2008;40(1):233-9. Epub 2008 Jan 15.
[17] Onuigbo MA, Onuigbo NT. Late onset azotemia from RAAS blockade in CKD patients with normal renal arteries and no precipitating risk factors. *Ren. Fail.* 2008;30(1):73-80.
[18] Onuigbo MA. The impact of stopping inhibitors of the renin-angiotensin system in patients with advanced chronic kidney disease. *Nephrol Dial Transplant* 2010 Apr; 25(4):1344-5. Epub 2009 Dec 27. PMID:20037177. DOI:10.1093/ndt/gfp678. (Letter)
[19] Onuigbo MA. Reno-prevention vs. reno-protection: a critical re-appraisal of the evidence-base from the large RAAS blockade trials after ONTARGET--a call for more circumspection. *QJM* 2009 Mar;102(3):155-67. Epub 2008 Dec 19.
[20] Onuigbo MA. An analytical review of the evidence-base for reno-protection from the large RAAS blockade trials after ONTARGET. Re-visitation of the potential for iatrogenic renal failure with RAAS blockade ? A call for caution. *Nephron Clin. Pract.* 2009;113(2):c63-9, Epub 2009 Jul 14.
[21] Onuigbo MA. Is renoprotection with RAAS blockade a failed paradigm? Have we learnt any lessons so far? *Int. J. Clin. Pract.* 2010 Sep;64(10):1341-1346.
[22] Onuigbo MA. Can ACE inhibitors and angiotensin receptor blockers be detrimental in CKD patients? *Nephron Clin. Pract.* 2011;118(4):c407-419. doi: 10.1159/000324164. Epub 2011 Mar 7.
[23] Onuigbo MA, Onuigbo N. In: Chronic Kidney Disease and RAAS Blockade: A New View of Renoprotection. London, England: Lambert Academic Publishing GmbH 11 & Co. KG; 2011.
[24] Ahmed AK, Kamath NS, El Kossi M et al. The impact of stopping inhibitors of the renin-angiotensin system in patients with advanced chronic kidney disease. *Nephrol Dial Transplant.* 2009 doi:10.1093/ ndt/gfp511 [Epub ahead of print].
[25] Hsu CY, Vittinghoff E, Lin F, et al. The incidence of endstage renal disease is increasing faster than the prevalence of chronic renal insufficiency. *Ann. Intern. Med.* 2004;141(2):95–101.
[26] Szczech LA, Lazar IL. Projecting the United States ESRD population: Issues regarding treatment of patients with ESRD. *Kidney Int. Suppl.* 2004; 90:S3–S7.
[27] Jones CA, Krolewski AS, Rogus J, Xue JL, Collins A, WarrAm. J.H. Epidemic of end-stage renal disease in people with diabetes in the United States population: do we know the cause? *Kidney Int.* 2005 May;67(5):1684-91.
[28] Chugh KS, Jha V. Differences in the care of ESRD patients worldwide: required resources and future outlook. *Kidney Int. Suppl.* 1995 Aug;50:S7-13.
[29] Ursea N, Mircescu G, Constantinovici N, Verzan C. Nephrology and renal replacement therapy in Romania. *Nephrol Dial Transplant.* 1997 Apr;12(4):684-90.
[30] Jha V. End-stage renal care in developing countries: the India experience. *Ren. Fail.* 2004 May;26(3):201-8.
[31] Perico N, Plata R, Anabaya A, Codreanu I, Schieppati A, Ruggenenti P, Remuzzi G. Strategies for national health care systems in emerging countries: the case of screening

and prevention of renal disease progression in Bolivia. *Kidney Int. Suppl.* 2005 Aug;(97):S87-94.

[32] Badmus TA, Arogundade FA, Sanusi AA, Akinsola WA, Adesunkanmi AR, Agbakwuru AO, Salako AB, Faponle AF, Oyebamiji EO, Adetiloye VA, Famurewa OC, Oladimeji BY, Fatoye FO. Kidney transplantation in a developing economy: challenges and initial report of three cases at Ile Ife. *Cent Afr. J. Med.* 2005 Sep-Oct;51(9-10):102-6.

[33] Liu WJ, Hooi LS. Patients with end stage renal disease: a registry at Sultanah Aminah Hospital, Johor Bahru, Malaysia. *Med. J. Malaysia.* 2007 Aug;62(3):197-200.

[34] Collins AJ, Foley RN, Herzog C, et al. United States Renal Data System 2008 Annual Data Report. *Am. J. Kidney Dis.* 2009 Jan;53(1 Suppl):S1-S374.

[35] Abraham G, Jayaseelan T, Matthew M, Padma P, Saravanan AK, Lesley N, Reddy YN, Saravanan S, Reddy YN. Resource settings have a major influence on the outcome of maintenance hemodialysis patients in South India. *Hemodial Int.* 2010 Apr;14(2):211-217.

[36] Ayodele OE, Alebiosu CO. Burden of chronic kidney disease: an international perspective. *Adv. Chronic Kidney Dis.* 2010 May;17(3):215-24.

[37] Ulasi II, Ijoma CK. The enormity of chronic kidney disease in Nigeria: the situation in a teaching hospital in South-East Nigeria. *J. Trop Med.* 2010;2010:501957. Epub 2010 Jun 2.

[38] U.S. Renal Data System, USRDS 2010 Annual Data Report: Atlas of Chronic Kidney Disease and End-Stage Renal Disease in the United States, National Institutes of Health, National Institute of Diabetes and Digestive and Kidney Diseases, Bethesda, MD, 2010. http://www.usrds.org/2010/ADR_booklet_2010_lowres.pdf, http://www.usrds.org/2009/pdf/V2_02_INC_PREV_09.PDF, accessed December 20, 2010.

[39] Kunz R, Friedrich C, Wolbers M, Mann JF. Meta-analysis: effect of monotherapy and combination therapy with inhibitors of the renin angiotensin system on proteinuria in renal disease. *Ann. Intern. Med.* 2008;148(1):30-48. Epub 2007 Nov 5.

[40] Onuigbo M, Onuigbo N. Aliskiren in Type 2 Diabetes and Cardiorenal End Points. N. Engl. J. Med. 2013 Mar 14;368(11):1064-5. doi: 10.1056/NEJMc1300257#SA1. (http://www.nejm.org/doi/pdf/10.1056/NEJMc1300257).

[41] Freedman BI, Hicks PJ, Bostrom MA, Comeau ME, Divers J, et al. Non-muscle myosin heavy chain 9 gene MYH9 associations in African Americans with clinically diagnosed type 2 diabetes mellitus-associated ESRD. *Nephrol Dial Transplant.* 2009; 24: 3366–3371.

[42] Leak TS, Mychaleckyj JC, Smith SG, Keene KL, Gordon CJ, Hicks PJ, Freedman BI, Bowden DW, Sale MM. Evaluation of a SNP map of 6q24–27 confirms diabetic nephropathy loci and identifies novel associations in type 2 diabetes patients with nephropathy from an African-American population. *Hum. Genet.* 2008; 124: 63–71.

[43] Forbes JM, Coughlan MT, Cooper ME. Oxidative stress as a major culprit in kidney disease in diabetes. *Diabetes* 2008; 57: 1446–1454.

[44] Singh DK, Winocour P, Farrington K. Mechanisms of disease: the hypoxic tubular hypothesis of diabetic nephropathy. *Nat Clin. Pract. Nephrol* 2008; 4: 216–226.

[45] Swaminathan S, Shah SV. Novel approaches targeted toward oxidative stress for the treatment of chronic kidney disease. *Curr. Opin. Nephrol. Hypertens* 2008; 17: 143–148.

[46] Goh SY, Cooper ME. Clinical review: the role of advanced glycation end products in progression and complications of diabetes. *J. Clin. Endocrinol. Metab.* 2008; 93: 1143–1152.

[47] Flyvbjerg A, Denner L, Schrijvers BF, Tilton RG, Mogensen TH, Paludan SR, Rasch R. Long-term renal effects of a neutralizing RAGE antibody in obese type 2 diabetic mice. *Diabetes* 2004; 53: 166–172.

[48] Park S, Bivona BJ, Kobori H, Seth DM, Chappell MC, Lazartigues E, Harrison-Bernard LM. Major role for ACE-independent intrarenal ANG II formation in type II diabetes. *Am. J. Physiol. Renal. Physiol.* 2010; 298:F37–F48.

[49] Matavelli LC, Huang J, Siragy HM. (Pro)renin receptor contributes to diabetic nephropathy by enhancing renal inflammation. *Clin. Exp. Pharmacol. Physiol* 2010; 37: 277–282.

[50] Sasaki H, Kamijo-Ikemori A, Sugaya T, Yamashita K, Yokoyama T, Koike J, et al. Urinary fatty acids and liver-type fatty acid binding protein in diabetic nephropathy. *Nephron Clin. Pract.* 2009;112:c148–c156.

[51] Lennon R, Pons D, Sabin MA, Wei C, Shield JP, Coward RJ, et al. Saturated fatty acids induce insulin resistance in human podocytes: implications for diabetic nephropathy. *Nephrol Dial Transplant.* 2009; 24: 3288–3296.

[52] An WS, Kim HJ, Cho KH, Vaziri ND. Omega-3 fatty acid supplementation attenuates oxidative stress, inflammation, and tubulointerstitial fibrosis in the remnant kidney. *Am. J. Physiol. Renal. Physiol.* 2009; 297:F895–F903.

[53] Yilmaz MI, Saglam M, Qureshi AR, Carrero JJ, Caglar K, Eyileten T, et al. Endothelial dysfunction in type-2 diabetics with early diabetic nephropathy is associated with low circulating adiponectin. *Nephrol Dial Transplant* 2008; 23: 1621–1627.

[54] Yamaguchi Y, Iwano M, Suzuki D, Nakatani K, Kimura K, Harada K, et al. Epithelial-mesenchymal transition as a potential explanation for podocyte depletion in diabetic nephropathy. *Am. J. Kidney Dis.* 2009; 54: 653–664.

[55] Yokoi H, Mukoyama M, Mori K, Kasahara M, Suganami T, Sawai K, et al. Overexpression of connective tissue growth factor in podocytes worsens diabetic nephropathy in mice. *Kidney Int.* 2008; 73: 446–455.

[56] Jaffa AA, Usinger WR, McHenry MB, Jaffa MA, Lipstiz SR, Lackland D, et al. Connective tissue growth factor and susceptibility to renal and vascular disease risk in type 1 diabetes. *J. Clin. Endocrinol. Metab* 2008; 93: 1893–1900.

[57] Fujimi-Hayashida A, Ueda S, Yamagishi S, Kaida Y, Ando R, Nakayama Y, Fukami K, Okuda S. Association of asymmetric dimethylarginine with severity of kidney injury and decline in kidney function in IgA nephropathy. *Am. J. Nephrol* 2011; 33: 1–6.

[58] Chonchol M, Shlipak MG, Katz R, Sarnak MJ, Newman AB, Siscovick DS, et al. Relationship of uric acid with progression of kidney disease. *Am. J. Kidney Dis* 2007; 50: 239–247.

[59] Yen CJ, Chiang CK, Ho LC, Hsu SH, Hung KY, Wu KD, Tsai TJ. Hyperuricemia associated with rapid renal function decline in elderly Taiwanese subjects. *J. Formos Med. Assoc.* 2009; 108: 921–928.

[60] Feig DI. Uric acid: a novel mediator and marker of risk in chronic kidney disease? *Curr. Opin. Nephrol. Hypertens* 2009; 18: 526–530.

[61] Kuo CF, Luo SF, See LC, Ko YS, Chen YM, Hwang JS, et al. Hyperuricaemia and accelerated reduction in renal function. *Scand. J. Rheumatol.* 2011; 40: 116–121.

[62] Bellomo G, Venanzi S, Verdura C, Saronio P, Esposito A, Timio M. Association of uric acid with change in kidney function in healthy normotensive individuals. *Am. J. Kidney Dis* 2010; 56: 264–272.

[63] Tzur S, Rosset S, Shemer R, Yudkovsky G, Selig S, Tarekegn A, et al. Missense mutations in the APOL1 gene are highly associated with end stage kidney disease risk previously attributed to the MYH9 gene. *Hum. Genet.* 2010; 128: 345–350.

[64] Behar DM, Kedem E, Rosset S, Haileselassie Y, Tzur S, Kra-Oz Z, et al. Absence of APOL1 risk variants protects against HIV-associated nephropathy in the Ethiopian population. *Am. J. Nephrol.* 2011; 34: 452–459.

[65] Kopp JB, Nelson GW, Sampath K, Johnson RC, Genovese G, An P, et al. APOL1 genetic variants in focal segmental glomerulosclerosis and HIV-associated nephropathy. *J. Am. Soc. Nephrol.* 2011; 22: 2129–2137.

[66] Papeta N, Kiryluk K, Patel A, Sterken R, Kacak N, Snyder HJ, et al. APOL1 variants increase risk for FSGS and HIVAN but not IgA nephropathy. *J. Am. Soc. Nephrol.* 2011; 22:1991–1996.

[67] Onuigbo MA. The natural history of chronic kidney disease revisited--a 72-month Mayo Health System Hypertension Clinic practice-based research network prospective report on end-stage renal disease and death rates in 100 high-risk chronic kidney disease patients: a call for circumspection. *Adv. Perit. Dial* 2009; 25:85-8. PMID:19886324.

[68] Keith DS, Nichols GA, Gullion CM, Brown JB, Smith DH. Longitudinal follow-up and outcomes among a population with chronic kidney disease in a large managed care organization. *Arch. Intern. Med.* 2004;164:659–663.

[69] Menon V, Wang X, Sarnak MJ, et al. Long-term outcomes in nondiabetic chronic kidney disease. *Kidney Int.* 2008;73:1310–1315.

[70] Onuigbo MA. The CKD Enigma with Misleading Statistics and Myths about CKD, and Conflicting ESRD and Death Rates in the Literature: Results of a 2008 US Population-Based Cross-Sectional CKD Outcomes Analysis. *Ren. Fail.* 2013;35(3):338-43. doi: 10.3109/0886022X.2013.764272. Epub 2013 Feb 8.

[71] Ravera M, Re M, Weiss U, Deferrari L, Deferrari G. Emerging therapeutic strategies in diabetic nephropathy. *J. Nephrol.* 2007 Nov-Dec;20 Suppl 12:S23-32.

[72] Renke M, Tylicki L, Rutkowski P, Knap N, Zietkiewicz M, Neuwelt A, Aleksandrowicz E, Łysiak-Szydłowska W, Woźniak M, Rutkowski B. Effect of pentoxifylline on proteinuria, markers of tubular injury and oxidative stress in non-diabetic patients with chronic kidney disease – placebo controlled, randomized, cross-over study. *Acta Biochim. Pol.* 2010; 57: 119–123.

[73] Navarro-González JF, Muros M, Mora-Fernández C, Herrera H, Meneses B, García J.Pentoxifylline for renoprotection in diabetic nephropathy: the PREDIAN study. Rationale and basal results. *J. Diabetes Complications* 2010, E-pub ahead of print.

[74] Barkhordari K, Karimi A, Shafiee A, Soltaninia H, Khatami MR, Abbasi K, Yousefshahi F, Haghighat B, Brown V. Effect of pentoxifylline on preventing acute kidney injury after cardiac surgery by measuring urinary neutrophil gelatinase – associated lipocalin. *J. Cardiothorac Surg* 2011; 6: 8.

[75] Perkins RM, Aboudara MC, Uy AL, Olson SW, Cushner HM, Yuan CM. Effect of pentoxifylline on GFR decline in CKD: a pilot, double-blind, randomized, placebo-

controlled trial. *Am. J. Kidney Dis.* 2009;53(4):606-16. doi: 10.1053/j.ajkd.2008.11.026. Epub 2009 Feb 12.

[76] Navarro-González JF, Muros M, Mora-Fernández C, Herrera H, Meneses B, García J. Pentoxifylline for renoprotection in diabetic nephropathy: the PREDIAN study. Rationale and basal results. *J. Diabetes Complications.* 2011;25(5):314-9. doi: 10.1016/j.jdiacomp.2010.09.003. Epub 2010 Dec 8.

[77] Badri S, Dashti-Khavidaki S, Lessan-Pezeshki M, Abdollahi M. A review of the potential benefits of pentoxifylline in diabetic and non-diabetic proteinuria. *J. Pharm. Pharm. Sci.* 2011;14(1):128-37.

[78] Badri S, Dashti-Khavidaki S, Ahmadi F, Mahdavi-Mazdeh M, Abbasi MR, Khalili H. Effect of add-on pentoxifylline on proteinuria in membranous glomerulonephritis: a 6-month placebo-controlled trial. *Clin. Drug Investig.* 2013 Mar;33(3):215-22. doi: 10.1007/s40261-013-0057-1.

[79] Fervenza FC, Sethi S, Specks U. Idiopathic membranous nephropathy: diagnosis and treatment. *Clin. J. Am. Soc. Nephrol.* 2008 May;3(3):905-19. doi: 10.2215/CJN.04321007. Epub 2008 Jan 30.

[80] Gong R. The renaissance of corticotropin therapy in proteinuric nephropathies. *Nat. Rev. Nephrol.* 2011 Dec 6;8(2):122-8. doi: 10.1038/nrneph.2011.190. MPB.

[81] Bomback AS, Canetta PA, Beck LH Jr, Ayalon R, Radhakrishnan J, Appel GB. Treatment of resistant glomerular diseases with adrenocorticotropic hormone gel: a prospective trial. *Am. J. Nephrol.* 2012;36(1):58-67. doi: 10.1159/000339287. Epub 2012 Jun 19.

[82] Appel GB, Appel AS. New diagnostic tests and new therapies for glomerular diseases. *Blood Purif.* 2013;35(1-3):81-5. doi: 10.1159/000345185. Epub 2013 Jan 22.

[83] Herrmann SM, Sethi S, Fervenza FC. Membranous nephropathy: the start of a paradigm shift. *Curr. Opin. Nephrol. Hypertens.* 2012 Mar;21(2):203-10. doi: 10.1097/MNH.0b013e32835026ed.

[84] Si J, Ge Y, Zhuang S, Juan Wang L, Chen S, Gong R. Adrenocorticotropic hormone ameliorates acute kidney injury by steroidogenic-dependent and -independent mechanisms. *Kidney Int.* 2013 Apr;83(4):635-46. doi: 10.1038/ki.2012.447. Epub 2013 Jan 16.

[85] Gadegbeku CA, Gipson DS, Holzman LB, Ojo AO, Song PX, et al. Design of the Nephrotic Syndrome Study Network (NEPTUNE) to evaluate primary glomerular nephropathy by a multidisciplinary approach. *Kidney Int.* 2013 Apr;83(4):749-56. doi: 10.1038/ki.2012.428. Epub 2013 Jan 16.

About the Editor

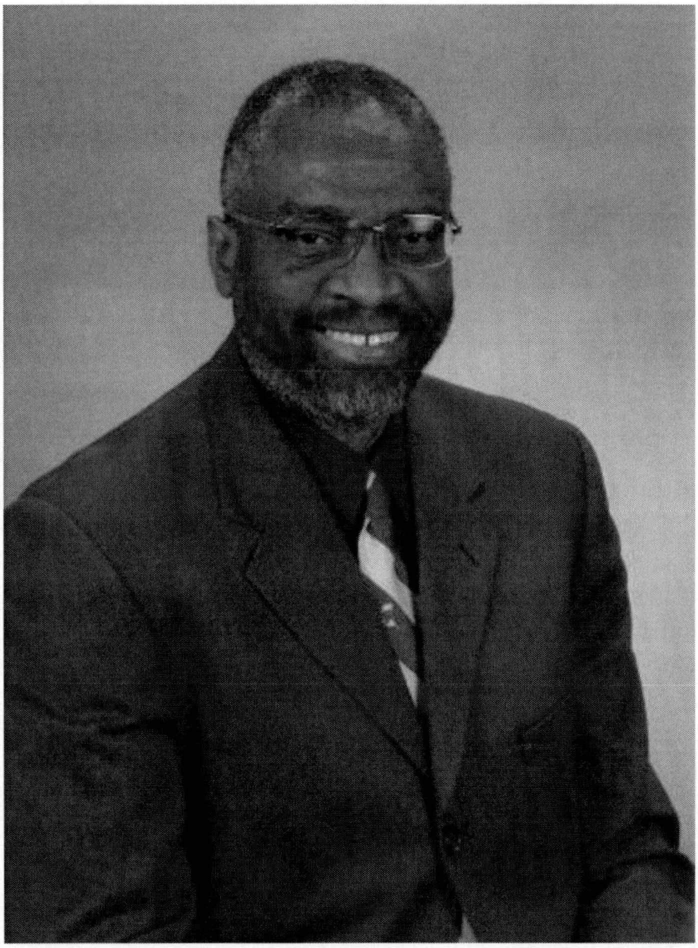

Macaulay Amechi Chukwukadibia Onuigbo MD MSc FWACP FASN MBA, Associate Professor of Medicine, College of Medicine, Mayo Clinic, Rochester, MN; Former Regional Director, North Eastern Region, Mayo Health System Practice-Based Research Network (MHS PBRN); Nephrologist/Hypertension Specialist/Transplant Physician, Department of Nephrology, Mayo Clinic Health System Eau Claire, 1221 Whipple Street, Eau Claire, WI 54702, USA, and MBA Healthcare Executive, Eau Claire, WI, USA.

Dr. Onuigbo received his medical degree from the University of Nigeria in 1981, graduating as the best graduating student in Medicine and Surgery, with distinctions earlier in the medical school in Anatomy, Medical Biochemistry, Physiology, Pharmacology, Pathology and the clinical sciences. He had earlier attended elementary school at St. Barth's Elementary School, Enugu, Nigeria, had his early school life interrupted by the Biafra civil war, 1967-1970, and then completed a blissful secondary school career at the renowned Government College, Umuahia. His post-graduate studies took him to Enugu, Nigeria, Birmingham, United Kingdom, Houston, Texas, and Baltimore, Maryland. He is Double Board Certified in the United States of America in Internal Medicine and Nephrology, with the American Board of Internal Medicine. He had earlier served as an Associate Professor of Medicine/Senior Lecturer, Department of Medicine, College of Medicine, University of Nigeria, Enugu Campus, Nigeria, March 1990 – June 1994. He is a Nephrologist/Transplant Physician/Hypertension Specialist, Mayo Clinic Health System, Eau Claire, WI, USA, September 2002 - 2013. He is an Associate Professor of Medicine, College of Medicine, Mayo Clinic, Rochester, MN, USA, since 2010, and has served as Vice Chairman, Department of Nephrology, Mayo Clinic Health System, Eau Claire, WI, USA. He is a Fellow of the West African College of Physicians (FWACP – Nephrology), a Fellow of the American Society of Nephrology (FASN), and a former Regional Director, North-Eastern Region of the Mayo Health System Practice-Based Research Network. Dr. Onuigbo's recent professional awards include the Mayo Clinic MacMillan Scholar Award (2009-2011) and the Mayo SOAR Research Grant Award in 2011. He has over 100 publications including several book chapters and books. In 2013, he co-edited a major textbook on hemodialysis titled "Hemodialysis, When, How, Why" with Claudio Ronco MD, Biagio Raffaele Di Iorio MD PhD, and August Heidland MD. Dr. Onuigbo described the following previously unreported syndromes - late onset renal failure from angiotensin blockade (LORFFAB) in 2005, the syndrome of rapid onset end stage renal disease (SORO-ESRD) in 2010, and introduced the terms "Ethicomedicinomics" and "Cognitive Drift in the EMR" into current medical literature in 2012. He introduced the concept of "Quadruple Whammy" in the Spring of 2013, in a publication in the British Medical Journal. He has a Master of Science (MSc) degree in Medical Biochemistry from the University of Nigeria (1988). He recently completed an MBA (Healthcare) in May 2012 from the University of Wisconsin Consortium and was named the 2012 University of Wisconsin MBA Consortium Outstanding Graduate. He serves on the editorial boards of several journals including the Quarterly Journal of Medicine, the International Journal of Clinical Practice, and is a member of the Reviewer Panel for the American Society of Nephrology NephSAP publication.

INDEX

B

C

D

E

F

G

H

I

K

L

M

N

O

P

R

S

T

V

W

Z